T0214889

Heinz W. Engl
Alfred K. Louis
William Rundell (eds.)

Inverse Problems
in Medical Imaging and
Nondestructive Testing

Proceedings of the Conference
in Oberwolfach, Federal Republic
of Germany, February 4–10, 1996

SpringerWienNewYork

Prof. Dr. Heinz W. Engl
Institut für Mathematik, Johannes-Kepler-Universität, Linz, Austria

Prof. Dr. Alfred K. Louis
Fachbereich Mathematik, Universität des Saarlandes, Saarbrücken,
Federal Republic of Germany

Prof. Dr. William Rundell
Department of Mathematics, Texas A & M University, College Station,
Texas, U.S.A.

Typesetting: Camera ready by authors
Printing: Druckerei Novographic, A-1238 Wien
Binding: Fa. Papyrus, A-1100 Wien

Graphic design: Ecke Bonk

Printed on acid-free and chlorine-free bleached paper
SPIN: 10631421

With 54 Figures

Die Deutsche Bibliothek – CIP-Einheitsaufnahme

Inverse problems in medical imaging and nondestructive testing /
H. W. Engl ... (ed.). – Wien ; New York : Springer, 1997
ISBN 3-211-83015-4

CIP data applied for

ISBN 3-211-83015-4 Springer-Verlag Wien New York

Preface

The conference on *Inverse Problems in Medical Imaging and Nondestructive Testing* was organized by the editors of these proceedings in the Mathematisches Forschungsinstitut Oberwolfach in the Black Forest in Germany from February 04 to 10, 1996.

Forty participants from thirteen countries presented their research results which can be grouped into the categories:

- overviews on the state of art in medical imaging and nondestructive testing
- x-ray computerized tomography in two and three dimensions
- ultrasound and microwave tomography
- electrical impedance tomography
- electron microscopy
- flow tomography
- inverse scattering
- regularization methods for nonlinear problems
- wavelets and regularization

The common background of the reseach in these fields is inverse problems. It became again evident that much progress in the underlying mathematical research was directly transformed into new algorithms for solving these real world problems in two areas which, at a first glance, seem to be very different. From a mathematical point of view similar principles are applied to measure the data although the realization can be rather different as an example in x–ray computerized tomography shows. In nondestructive testing typically the measured object is rotated and x–ray source and detectors are fixed, which, of course, is impossible in the medical application.

This conference is one of a series of conferences devoted to inverse problems in different fields organized by David Colton, Heinz Engl, Alfred Louis and Bill Rundell. This series is supported by GAMM and SIAM.

The lively scientific atmosphere and the inspiring setting in Oberwolfach stimulated many discussions which certainly will contribute to further progress in the field. Although one is tempted to take this invariably high standard in the Mathematische Forschungsinstitut for granted we thank the staff.

Heinz W. Engl, Alfred K. Louis, William Rundell

Contents

Three-Dimensional Super-Resolving Confocal Scanning Laser Fluorescent Microscopy

Ibrahim Akduman, Jan Grochmalicki and Roy Pike

Physics Department, King's College London, Strand, London WC2R 2LS, UK

1 Introduction

Super-resolution in scanning microscopy has been suggested recently [1]–[3] by using specially designed optical masks and two integrating detectors in place of the single pinhole and detector of a conventional confocal arrangement. The resolving power of such a microscope is significantly improved over the standard confocal one. The method provides an optical implementation of a data inversion algorithm based on singular-system theory.

For incoherent light, the practical realization of the theoretically calculated mask, with a continuously changing profile, proves to be prohibitively difficult. A 'binararised' mask [4] that approximates this changing profile and yet preserves as much of the resolving power of the microscope as possible is then designed and is easy to manufacture.

In previous work with both coherent and incoherent light the above programme has been realised for the two-dimensional low numerical aperture case. In this paper we present an extension to the full three-dimensional high-numerical-aperture case.

2 Theory

The Fredholm equation of the first kind, which describes the imaging system, is solved by finding its singular-value spectrum and its 'object' and 'image' singular functions. These functions provide complete orthonormal basis sets for both object and image. The inversion is then performed by finding the coefficients of the singular function expansion up to a point (the truncation index K) determined by the singular value spectrum and the level of noise in the image.

The relationship between the object f and image g, for a given scanning position, can be written as,

$$g(x) = (Af)(x) = \int S_2(x - y, z) S_1(y, z) f(y, z) \, dy dz, \qquad (1)$$

where S_1 and S_2 represent the point spread functions (PSF) of the illuminating and imaging lenses, respectively. The x and y are the 2-dimensional variables, respectively, in the image and object planes and z is the axial variable. In the incoherent case both f and g are intensity distributions.

We wish to recover $f(y, z)$, or, as scanning is involved, just $f(0, 0)$ — the object value at the scanning point. Complete reconstruction of f is then achieved after solving this problem at each scanning position. Our approach is based on calculating the singular-system of the kernel of the imaging equation. The singular system $\{\alpha_k; u_k, v_k\}$, $k = 1, 2, \ldots$ associated with the operator A of Eq. (1), is defined by

$$Au_k = \alpha_k v_k, \qquad A^* v_k = \alpha_k u_k, \tag{2}$$

with A^* denoting the adjoint operator of A

$$(A^* g)(y, z) = S_1(y, z) \int S_2(x - y, z) g(x) \, dx dz. \tag{3}$$

The singular functions u_k and v_k are basis functions for representing object and image, respectively, while α_k denotes the k-th singular value of the system. In these terms we can express the truncated singular value decomposition (TSVD) approximation of $f(0, 0)$ as

$$\tilde{f}(0, 0) = \sum_{k=1}^{K} \frac{(g, v_k)}{\alpha_k} u_k(0, 0). \tag{4}$$

The truncation index K is controlled by the level of noise affecting the data [5]. If we denote now

$$M(x) = \sum_{k=1}^{K} \frac{1}{\alpha_k} u_k(0, 0) v_k(x), \tag{5}$$

we obtain the previous expression for $\tilde{f}(0, 0)$ in a different form

$$\tilde{f}(0, 0) = \int g(x) M(x) \, dx = (g, M). \tag{6}$$

To invert the image $g(x)$ we multiply it by the known function $M(x)$, and follow by a spatial integration of the product. Both these operations can be implemented optically. This is done by placing the optical mask in the image plane with transmission and reflection profiles given by the positive and negative parts of $M(x)$, respectively, then using two spatially integrating detectors. The difference of the outputs of these detectors recovers directly the axial object point $\tilde{f}(0, 0)$.

3 Calculation of the Kernel

Using the Hankel sampling theorem we can reduce the integral eqution to the discretised linear system

$$b_n = \sum_{m=1}^{\infty} \sum_{l=-\infty}^{\infty} A_{n;m,l} a_{m,l} \tag{7}$$

where

$$A_{n;m,l} = \sqrt{\frac{1 + \cos\alpha}{2}} \frac{W_0(\frac{x_n}{2\pi}, \frac{x_m}{4\pi}; z_l) W(\frac{x_m}{4\pi}, z_l)}{4\pi^2 J_1(x_n) J_1(x_m)}, \tag{8}$$

and where x_n denotes the n-th zero of J_0, and $z_l = \left(\frac{1+\cos\alpha}{2}\right) l$. The singular functions $u_k(\rho, z)$ are then formed from the singular vectors $u_{l,m}^{(k)}$ of the matrix A by

$$u_k(\rho, z) = 4 \sqrt{\frac{2\pi}{1 + \cos\alpha}} \sum_{m=1}^{\infty} \sum_{l=-\infty}^{\infty} u_{m,l}^{(k)} \frac{x_m J_0(4\pi\rho)}{x_m^2 - (4\pi\rho)^2} \operatorname{sinc}\left[\frac{2(z - z_l)}{1 + \cos\alpha}\right]. \tag{9}$$

Singular functions $v_{l,m}^{(k)}(\rho, z)$ are obtained similarly. In the above formulas, the imaging kernel $W(\rho, z)$ is given by

$$W(\rho, z) = |I_0(\rho, z)|^2 + |I_1(\rho, z)|^2 + |I_2(\rho, z)|^2, \tag{10}$$

with

$$I_0(\rho, z) = \int_0^\alpha \sqrt{\cos\theta} \sin\theta \, (1 + \cos\theta) J_0(\frac{\sin\theta}{\sin\alpha}\rho) \exp\left(i\frac{\cos\theta}{\sin^2\alpha} z\right) d\theta, \tag{11}$$

$$I_1(\rho, z) = \int_0^\alpha \sqrt{\cos\theta} \sin^2\theta \, J_1(\frac{\sin\theta}{\sin\alpha}\rho) \exp\left(i\frac{\cos\theta}{\sin^2\alpha} z\right) d\theta, \tag{12}$$

$$I_2(\rho, z) = \int_0^\alpha \sqrt{\cos\theta} \sin\theta \, (1 - \cos\theta) J_2(\frac{\sin\theta}{\sin\alpha}\rho) \exp\left(i\frac{\cos\theta}{\sin^2\alpha} z\right) d\theta. \tag{13}$$

(cf. [6]). In our experiment, for the numerical aperture NA = 1.4 the opening angle of the microscope objective $\alpha = 67.260°$. The projection W_0 of the kernel onto the subspace of circularly symmetrical functions is defined by

$$W_0(\rho, \rho'; z) = \int_0^{2\pi} W(\sqrt{\rho^2 + \rho'^2 - 2\rho\rho' \cos\beta}, z) d\beta. \tag{14}$$

Owing to the complicated nature of the expressions (11)–(13) calculation of the above projection is the most difficult part of the whole computation. The straightforward method, where we evaluate numerically the double integral, is painstakingly slow and its accuracy is rather difficult to control. If we notice, however, that the Fourier transform of $W(\rho, z)$, $\hat{W}(\omega, \eta)$ has support

$$\omega \le 2\pi \qquad |\eta| \le \pi/(1 + \cos\alpha), \tag{15}$$

the computation can be greatly speeded up and also made very easy to manage. If we invoke the Hankel sampling theorem over the band 2π we obtain

$$W(\rho, z) = \frac{1}{\pi} \sum_{k=1}^{\infty} w_k(z) h_k(\rho),$$ (16)

where

$$w_k(z) = \frac{2x_k}{\pi J_1(x_k)} W(\frac{x_k}{2\pi}, z),$$ (17)

$$h_k(z) = \frac{J_0(2\pi\rho)}{x_k^2 - (2\pi\rho)^2}.$$ (18)

To compute W_0 we need now to know

$$\int_0^{2\pi} h_k(\sqrt{\rho^2 + \rho'^2 - 2\rho\rho' \cos\theta}, z) d\theta = \frac{1}{\rho'} h_k(\rho) * \delta(\rho - \rho'),$$ (19)

(see [7]), where $*$ denotes convolution and $\delta(\rho)$ is the radial delta function. This convolution can be easily calculated by means of the Hankel transform techniques. We find

$$h_k(\rho) * \delta(\rho - \rho') = \frac{2\pi\rho'}{x_k J_1(x_k)} I(\rho, \rho', \frac{x_k}{2\pi}),$$ (20)

where

$$I(a, b, c) = \int_0^{2\pi} dx \, x \, J_0(ax) J_0(bx) J_0(cx).$$ (21)

As a result we obtain

$$W_0(\rho, \rho'; z) = \frac{1}{\pi} \sum_{k=1}^{\infty} \frac{W(\frac{x_k}{2\pi}, z)}{(J_1(x_k))^2} I(\rho, \rho', \frac{x_k}{2\pi}).$$ (22)

To get $A_{n;m,l}$ we take $\rho = x_n/2\pi$, $\rho' = x_m/4\pi$, so we need to calculate

$$I(\frac{x_n}{2\pi}, \frac{x_m}{4\pi}, \frac{x_k}{2\pi}).$$ (23)

Such integrals were considered by Fettis in [8]. He has shown that in our case

$$I = 4\pi^2 \frac{x_k J_1(x_k)}{x_n x_m} \sum_{p=0}^{\infty} \epsilon_p J_p(x_n) J_p(x_m/2) \frac{e^{-p\theta}}{\sinh(\theta)},$$ (24)

where $\epsilon_0 = 1$ and $\epsilon_p = 2$ for $p > 0$, and $\cosh\theta = (x_n^2 + x_m^2/4 - x_k^2)/(x_m x_n)$ if only $x_n^2 + x_m^2/4 < x_k^2$ and $\left|\frac{x_n^2 + x_m^2/4 - x_k^2}{x_m x_n}\right| > 1$. Similar expressions are also given for the other three regions of x_n, x_m and x_k.

Crucial for our calculation of the discretised operator matrix $A_{n;m,l}$ is the fact, that we can use pre-calculated tables of $J_p(x_n)$ and $J_p(x_m/2)$ as well as of $W(\frac{x_k}{2\pi}, z_l)/(J_1(x_k))^2$. For each pair (m, n) a series of coefficients (23) is calculated, which is then used unchanged for all values of l. Convergence of the final series is dynamically controlled, further reducing unnecessary computation. The simplicity of the resulting algorithm makes it very easy to implement and also susceptible to compiler optimisations.

Having calculated the kernel in this manner, its SVD was computed using a standard package and the mask form is obtained using Eq. (5). A binary form of this mask has been inserted in a forward calculation of the microscope performance and shows the expected increase in resolution in both axial and transverse directions of the order of a factor of two.

4 Applications in Theoretical Physics

First-kind Fredholm equations appear in a number of analytic- continuation problems in theoretical physics and can be solved satisfactorily by TSVD methods. We have implemented this technique successfully to invert data from Monte Carlo simulations of high temperture superconductors [9] and have also made preliminary studies of the problem of inversion of lattice Quantum Chromodynamic point to point correlation functions of hadronic currents. The spectral weight of the excitatons present in each of the channels (determined by the structure of the currents-eg. vector: $\bar{\psi}\gamma_m u\psi$) can be obtained by solving Fredholm equations of the type $R(x) = 1/x \int ds f(s)\sqrt{(s)}K_n(\sqrt{(s)}x)$ where $R(x)$ is the point to point correlator, $f(s)$ is the spectral density function and $\sqrt{(s)}K_n(\sqrt{(s)}x)$ is the kernel of the equation. K_n is the modified Bessel function (the order n depends upom the channel. By solving for $f(s)$ one can obtain the spectrum of discrete excitations and the point where the continuum starts.

Two other areas are the calculation of transport coefficients in quark-gluon plasmas and rates of baryon-number non-conservation.

5 Acknowledgements

This work was partially funded by the SERC Grant GR/K19150.Some of the material was presented at the ICIAM conference in Hamburg, July 5th -7th 1995. We are grateful to Bio-Rad Ltd and to the US Army (Grant No. DAAH04-95-1-0280) for support.

References

[1]   Walker, J.G., Pike, E.R, Davies, R.E., Young, M.R., Brakenhoff, G.J., Bertero, M.: Superresolving Scanning Optical Microscopy using Holographic Optical Processing. J. Opt. Soc. Am. 10 (1993), 59–64

[2]   Bertero, M., Boccacci, P., Davies, R.E., Malfanti, F., Pike, E.R., Walker, J.G.: Superresolution in confocal scanning microscopy: IV. Theory of Data Inversion by the use of Optical Masks. Inverse Probl. 8 (1992), 1–23

[3]   Young, M.R., Jiang, S.H., Davies, R.E., Walker, J.G, Pike, E.R., Bertero, M.: Experimental confirmation of super-resolution in coherent confocal scanning microscopy using optical masks. J. Microsc. 165 (1992), 131–138

6

[4]   Grochmalicki, J., Pike, R.E., Walker, J.G, Bertero, M., Boccacci, P., Davies, R.E.: Superresolving masks for incoherent scanning microscopy. J. Opt. Soc. Am. **10** (1993), 1074–1077

[5]   Bertero, M., Boccacci, P., Defrise, M., De Mol, C., Pike, E.R.: Superresolution in confocal scanning microscopy: II. The incoherent case. Inverse Probl. **5** (1989), 441–461

[6]   Richards, B.and Wolf, E.,: Electromagnetic diffraction in optical systems: II. Structure of the image field in aplanatic system. Proc. Roy. Soc. (London) **A253** (1959), 358–379

[7]   Papoulis, A.,: Systems and transforms with applications in Optics. McGraw-Hill (1968). Chapter 5: Hankel Transforms

[8]   Fettis, H.E.: Lommel-type integrals involving three Bessel functions. J. Math. and Phys. **36** (1957), 88–95

[9]   Creffield, C. E., Klepfish, E. G., Pike, E. R. and S Sarkar Spectral weight function for the half-filled Hubbard model: a singular value decomposition approach. Physical Review Letters, **75** (1995), 517–520

Wavelets and Waves in Optical Signal Preprocessing

Th. Beth, A. Klappenecker, M. Schmid and D. Zerfowski

Institut für Algorithmen and Kognitive Systeme,
Universität Karlsruhe, 76128 Karlsruhe, Germany

1 Introduction

Wavelets are versatile tools in signal analysis and representation, complementing existing tools from harmonic analysis. In recent years, an upsurge of interest in wavelet methods influenced the area of image processing. Wavelet techniques combine traditional methods from imaging and harmonic analysis, thus yealding powerful and efficient algorithms for various applications.

Using wavelet transforms it is possible to build highly reliable compression schemes for pictures, providing bandwidth economic preview and browsing schemes. Taking the underlying semantics of the signal into account, a comprehensive description of the signal can also be obtained by an adapted coding of the occurring elementary features or objects. Using this semantics leads to a high level description of the signal. For this reason an image preprocessing step, a feature extraction has to be involved, which can again be achieved by using wavelet methods, e.g. for edge detection and segmentation. In this paper we discuss wavelet based feature extraction methods and we describe an optical implementation using diffractive elements.

2 Wavelets

We briefly recall some basic notions from wavelet analysis. The elementary building blocks of wavelet analysis are obtained by translations and unitary dilations from a single square integrable function ψ – the wavelet. A square integrable signal $s \in L^2(\mathbf{R})$ can then be analysed by the scalar products

$$s \longmapsto \left\langle \frac{1}{\sqrt{a}} \psi \left(\frac{\cdot - b}{a} \right) \Big| s \right\rangle, \qquad a, b \in \mathbf{R},\ a > 0. \tag{1}$$

The wavelet ψ is usually assumed to be a function that is sufficiently localized in time as well as in frequency and has some vanishing moments.

A typical example for a wavelet is given by the *mexican hat function* $\psi(x) = (x^2 - 1)e^{-x^2/2}$.

The continuous wavelet transform (1) can be generalized to higher dimensions where we have in addition to the dilation and translation operations a rotation operation. Clearly, the rotation is superfluous, if rotation symmetric wavelets are use. For example, a rotation symmetric 2D mexican hat function is given by $(\|x\|_{R^2}^2 - 2) \cdot \exp(-\|x\|_{R^2}^2/2)$ We will use this wavelet later in an optical implementation for edge detection.

The continuous wavelet transform (1) is rarely used in applications because it leads in general to a highly redundant representation of the signal that is rather expensive from a computational point of view. Typically, only a part of the wavelet coefficients is necessary for feature detection. For example, in edge detection applications only a few scales have to be considered.

Compression applications lead to a natural interest in non-redundant representations of a signal. The most compact way is to express the signal with respect to a basis of the Hilbert space L^2. A particularly nice class of wavelets leads to *biorthogonal wavelet bases* of the Hilbert space $L^2(\mathbf{R})$. A biorthogonal wavelet basis is given by a Riesz basis of the form $\psi_{j,k}(x) = 2^{-j/2}\psi(2^{-j}x - k)$, with $j, k \in \mathbf{Z}$, that has a dual basis[1] $\tilde{\psi}_{j,k}$ of the same form. A pair of biorthogonal wavelet bases allows the representation of a signal as follows:

$$s = \sum_{j,k \in \mathbf{Z}} \langle \tilde{\psi}_{j,k} \mid s \rangle \psi_{j,k} = \sum_{j,k \in \mathbf{Z}} \langle \psi_{j,k} \mid s \rangle \tilde{\psi}_{j,k}.$$

3 Compression

Radiologic image data in the order of at least several peta bytes comes up every year. Clearly, there is a natural demand for effective compression methods, since archiving of radiologic images over several years is legally obliged. Wavelets can be used successfully in radiologic image compression applications. We sketch the main ideas of a wavelet based compression method in this section.

The basic principle of a wavelet based compression scheme can be subdivided into three major steps: the input signal is transformed in order to decorrelate adjacent signal samples, then the entropy of the resulting coefficients is reduced by quantization. In a final step the redundancy is removed by passing the quantized coefficients through an entropy coder.

---

[1] A Riesz basis of a Hilbert space H is a family of linear independent vectors v_i, $i \in I$, that constitute a frame. The dual basis is defined as usual by $\langle \psi_{j,k} \mid \tilde{\psi}_{l,m} \rangle = \delta_{j,l}\,\delta_{k,m}$.

An implementation of this scheme should be as fast as possible. If we use scalar quantization, i.e. a quantization operation that can be applied independently to each coefficient, then the quantization has linear complexity. The entropy coding can for example be done by arithmetic coding. A method with particular high throughput was developed recently at the authors' institution [9]. It remains to give a fast algorithm for the wavelet transform.

All well-behaved biorthogonal wavelet bases can be constructed with the help of multiresolution analyses. For compactly supported biorthogonal wavelets this construction leads directly to a fast algorithm for the discrete wavelet transform. For the ease of exposition we leave out some details that can be found for example in [8] and mainly focus on the points that are relevant for our application.

A multiresolution analysis of $L^2(\mathbf{R})$ is a sequence of nested closed subspaces $V_j \subset V_{j-1}$ of $L^2(\mathbf{R})$ such that $\bigcap_{j \in \mathbf{Z}} V_j = \{0\}$ and $\bigcup_{j \in \mathbf{Z}} V_j$ is dense in L^2. Moreover, the subspaces are linked by $f(x) \in V_j \Leftrightarrow f(2x) \in V_{j-1}$ and the subspace V_0 is supposed to have a Riesz basis of the form $\varphi(x - k)$, $k \in \mathbf{Z}$. The function φ is called *scaling function*. We use again the convenient abbreviation $\varphi_{j,k}(x)$ to denote the dilated and translated functions $2^{-j/2}\varphi(2^{-j}x - k)$. The scaling function manifests the connection between two different scales through the following formula: $\varphi(x/2) = \sum_{n \in \mathbf{Z}} h_n \sqrt{2}\varphi(x - n)$, which can be written in Fourier space as $\hat{\varphi}(2\omega) = m_0(\omega)\hat{\varphi}(\omega)$, with $m_0(\omega) = 2^{-1/2} \sum h_n e^{-in\omega}$. We call $m_0(\omega)$ the scaling filter associated with φ.

A pair of multiresolution analyses V_j and $\widetilde{V}_j$ of $L^2(\mathbf{R})$ is called biorthogonal with compactly supported dual scaling functions iff the scaling functions φ, $\widetilde{\varphi}$ are dual in the sense that $\langle \varphi(x) | \widetilde{\varphi}(x - k) \rangle = \delta_{k,0}$ holds and φ and $\widetilde{\varphi}$ are compactly supported functions. Such a pair of multiresolution analyses allows us to define the functions

$$\hat{\psi}(2\omega) = e^{-i\omega}\overline{m_0(\omega + \pi)}\hat{\varphi}(\omega), \qquad \hat{\widetilde{\psi}}(2\omega) = e^{-i\omega}\overline{\widetilde{m}_0(\omega + \pi)}\hat{\widetilde{\varphi}}(\omega),$$

where we used $\hat{f}$ to denote the Fourier transform of a function f; m_0, $\widetilde{m}_0$ denote the scaling filters associated to φ, $\widetilde{\varphi}$. It turns out that $\psi_{j,k}$, $j, k \in \mathbf{Z}$, is a Riesz basis of $L^2(\mathbf{R})$ with dual $\widetilde{\psi}_{j,k}$, see [6] for a proof. Thus, we can construct biorthogonal wavelet bases from multiresolution analyses.

The structure of the multiresolution analysis allows in a natural way to define certain approximations to the signal. For all $s \in L^2(\mathbf{R})$ a projection on V_j in the direction of $\widetilde{V}_j^{\perp}$ is given by

$$P_j s = \sum_{k \in \mathbf{Z}} \langle \widetilde{\varphi}_{j,k} | s \rangle \varphi_{j,k}.$$

The details missing in a coarse approximation can be described by wavelets; this is the key idea of Mallat's fast wavelet transform algorithm. Given a fine approximation of a signal s, say in terms of the coefficients $s_{j-1,k} = \langle \tilde{\varphi}_{j-1,k} | s \rangle$, $k \in \mathbf{Z}$, then it is possible to calculate efficiently the coefficients $s_{j,k} = \langle \tilde{\varphi}_{j,k} | s \rangle$ and $d_{j,k} = \langle \tilde{\psi}_{j,k} | s \rangle$. In fact, the corresponding operations can be realized by a 2-channel perfect reconstruction filter bank. Similarly, we can again calculate efficiently the coefficients $s_{j+1,k}$ and $d_{j+1,k}$ from the coefficients $s_{j,k}$. The dataflow of Mallat's algorithm is shown in Figure 1.

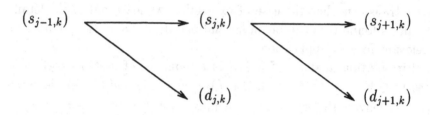

Figure 1. Dataflow of Mallat's fast wavelet transform algorithm.

This algorithm can be extended without any difficulty to higher dimensions using tensor products. It is very convenient from a practical point of view that smooth signals give wavelet coefficients $d_{j,k}$ near zero, provided the wavelet is smooth enough. Hence, after the quantization a large part of the wavelet coefficients is zero, so that for a proper choice of the wavelet we obtain a compact description of the signal. The results of such a compression scheme are exemplified in Figure 2 for a medical image. For the same compression ratio, the JPEG compression standard leads to significantly higher degradation of the image. Wavelet compression is in terms of peak-signal-to-noise-ratio 2dB better.

4 Optical Signal Preprocessing

In recent image processing applications large amount of data has to be manipulated under hard time constraints, especially in real time or medical applications. Fast digital algorithms for signal preprocessing have been developed and proposed but for high resolution applications the needed performance has not been reached yet. For this reason alternative highly parallel methods like optical signal processing seems to be a promising new way. Nowadays optical preprocessing becomes in range of

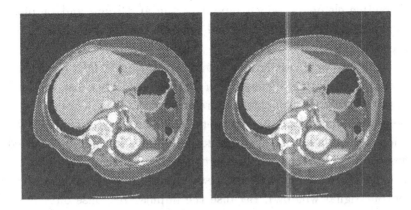

Figure 2. Computer tomographic image of a human body. Left: original image. Right: wavelet compressed image with rate 17.8:1.

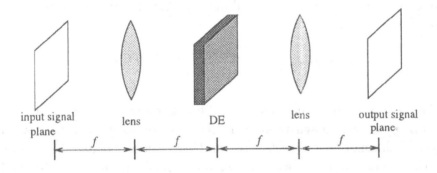

| input signal plane | lens | DE | lens | output signal plane |

Figure 3. $4f$-setup

current technology due to fast and high resolution spatial light modulators (SLM), which are already commercially available.

In principle every linear transform in $L^2(\mathbf{R}^2)$ can be implemented by an optical setup [1]. The input, a complex two dimensional signal, is represented as a wave front on which the optical system operates at highest possible parallelism. Convolutional operators are of special interest in signal preprocessing. These operators can be build in an optical system by the well-known $4f$-setup, which is based on the convolutional theorem of the Fourier transform. A schematic view of a $4f$-setup is given in Figure 3. A monochromatic, coherent, two dimensional input signal from the left is propagated through a lens with focus f, performing the Fourier transform. In the Fourier plane at the distance $2f$ a pre-calculated diffractive element (DE) performs the pointwise multiplication in the frequency space and can be viewed as an adaptable filter. There are several types of diffractive elements, which modulate the amplitude and/or phase of an incoming wavefront. The second lens on the right realizes a second Fourier transform.

Due to the practical restrictions of manufacturing of DEs only phase or amplitude modulating elements can be produced. Because of the light efficiency phase-only elements are preferred.

In general the kernel of the intendend convolution is a complex valued function with non-constant amplitude and thus can not be realized by a phase-only DE. A method to overcome this problem is to search for a phase-only DE with the same impulse response in a given detection area (or output signal window). Because the impulse response outside of the signal window can freely be chosen, we gain some parameters of freedom for the design of the DE.

Given an impulse response $h_0(x, y)$ in the domain S (the signal window) we search for a bandlimited signal $h(x, y)$ which is equal to h_0 in S and satisfies the conditions

$$\left(\mathcal{F}^{-1}h\right)(u, v) = \begin{cases} e^{i\varphi(u,v)} & \text{if } (u, v) \in D \\ 0 & \text{else,} \end{cases} \tag{2}$$

where D describes the domain of the diffractive element. The calculation of $h(x, y)$ is an ill-posed problem in the sense of Hadamard, because in general all conditions for well-posed problems can be violated [3]. In spite of the freedom outside the signal window normally no solution exists and therefore we are interested in a good approximation. Furthermore, for a given impulse response inside the signal window there might exist several diffractive elements, where the impulse responses differ only outside the signal window.

After this preparation we are ready to give an iterative algorithm based on generalized projections for calculating phase-only DEs for the desired filter transfer function. One special method is the so-called IFTA algorithm [10] (Iterative Fourier Transform Algorithm) which is a slight modification of the Gerchberg-Saxton Algorithm [4] for DEs. The main idea of these algorithms is the following: We consider one arbitrary initial point f_0 and two convex sets $M_1, M_2, M_c := M_1 \cap M_2 \neq \emptyset$ in a Hilbert space, with two projections $\mathcal{P}_1, \mathcal{P}_2$ onto the two sets. Applying one projection on the initial point, it is mapped into the corresponding set. In the sequel the alternating use of both projection converges to some point in the intersection M_c. Thus $f_{n+1} = \mathcal{P}_1 f_n$ and $f_{n+2} = \mathcal{P}_2 f_{n+1}$ imply

$$\lim_{n \to \infty} \|\mathcal{P}_c f_n - f_n\| = 0 \tag{3}$$

for the unknown projection $\mathcal{P}_c$ on M_c [5].

In our special application the set of all desired impulse responses with the fixed signal window and the set of the Fourier transformed phase-only elements represent the two sets M_1, M_2. The projection operators $\mathcal{P}_1$ and $\mathcal{P}_2$ are given by

$$(\mathcal{P}_1 g)(x, y) := \begin{cases} h_0(x, y) & \text{if } (x, y) \in S \\ g(x, y) & \text{else,} \end{cases} \tag{4}$$

$$\mathcal{P}_2 := \mathcal{F} \mathcal{P}'_2 \mathcal{F}^{-1} \quad \text{with} \tag{5}$$

$$\left(\mathcal{P}'_2 \hat{h}\right)(u, v) := \begin{cases} \frac{\hat{h}(u,v)}{|\hat{h}(u,v)|} & \text{if } \hat{h}(u, v) \neq 0 \\ 1 & \text{else.} \end{cases} \tag{6}$$

At this point we have to mention that in this special case the set M_1 is not convex and we even can not guarantee that the intersection M_c is not empty. For this reason we have to consider a generalized version to non convex sets [7], for which the convergence can not be guaranteed, too. This lack of convergence is partially compensated by the use of the square distance error, which can be minimized in the iteration process. For the projections

$$h_n = \mathcal{P}_1 g_n \quad \text{and} \quad g_{n+1} = \mathcal{P}_2 h_n \tag{7}$$

we use the squared distance errors $SDE_{M_i}(f) := ||f - \mathcal{P}_i f||$, $i = 1, 2$ related to M_1 and M_2 and it holds

$$SDE_{M_1}(g_{n+1}) \leq SDE_{M_1}(g_n) \text{ and } SDE_{M_2}(h_{n+1}) \leq SDE_{M_2}(h_n). \tag{8}$$

At this point of our discussion we posses an iterative tool to calculate a phase-only DE for a desired convolutional filter.

We now consider implementations of filter functions, which promise great advantages, e.g., in the area of medical imaging: the optical wavelet transforms. One main advantage of using wavelet transforms in image preprocessing is their signal analysing properties at different scales and orientations. For example, different kinds of vertices, sharp or smooth ones, can be detected in different scales. With the knowledge of this kind of information succeeding image processing steps like feature extraction can be made more efficient.

In the previously described design process of the DEs was restricted to one filter function, but for a multiresolution analysis a family of wavelets has to be used. In the optical implementation we overcome this problem by tiling the signal output of the different wavelets spatially in the signal window. Because a translation in the spatial domain results in a linear phase shift in the frequency domain of the DEs we only have to add linear phases to the corresponding wavelet filter functions and superpose them. Taking a two dimensional version of the continuous wavelet transform (1) results in an impulse response

$$W(\mathbf{x}) = \sum_{j=1}^{n} \psi_j(\mathbf{x}) * \delta(\mathbf{x} - \mathbf{t_j}), \tag{9}$$

which leads to a filter function

$$\widehat{W}(\mathbf{u}) = \sum_{j=1}^{n} \hat{\psi}_j(\mathbf{u}) e^{2\pi i \mathbf{u} \mathbf{t_j}}, \tag{10}$$

in the plane of the DE, where $\mathbf{t_j}$ stands for the translation vector of the different tiles in the signal window.

In the following example we use the mexican hat wavelet, defined in section 2, with four different scales $a = 8, 4, 2, \sqrt{2}$, which can immediately be seen in the rightmost image from the upper left to the bottom right. Also in the amplitude image of the complex filter the superposition of the four scaled mexican hats are visible as rings with different diameters. This filter function or rather its Fourier transform serves as the initial point h_0 for the calculation of the phase-only DE shown in the middle of figure 4. Remark that edges contained in the input signal transforms to nullstellen in the output signal.

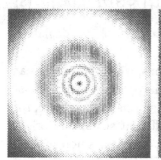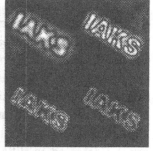

Figure 4. Left: Amplitude of complex filter. Center: Calculated phase-only DE. Right: Output signal window.

The calculated DE is producable using standard techniques, e.g. with lithographic methods. Using spatial light modulators (SLM) is another, more flexible way to realize the DE, because of the dynamical optical or electronical addressing possibilities of SLMs.

5 Conclusion

Wavelets are a flexible language to describe signals. We sketched how they can be used for an efficient signal representation in compression applications. So wavelet bases can be interpreted as "universal dictionary" for signal and image description. If we restrict our interest to special features of the images it may be adequate to use a more expressive "specialized dictionary".

We described an optical implementation of the wavelet transform that allows an extremely fast image preprocessing. This implementation is suitable for pattern recognition applications such as texture analysis or feature extraction. Intelligent medical imaging systems require more elaborated non-linear image processing transforms. This can be achieved with a combination of optical and traditional computation technologies. Some promising experiments with such an hybrid opto-electronical setup have been performed at the authors' institution [2].

References

1. H. Aagedal, Th. Beth, J. Müller-Quade, and M. Schmid. Algorithmic design of diffractive optical systems for information processing. Submitted to: PhysComp96, Boston, November 1996.
2. H. Aagedal, Th. Beth, H. Schwarzer, and S. Teiwes. Modern concepts for computer-aided design in diffractive optics. In G. W. Forbes, editor, *OSA Proceedings of the International Optical Design Conference*, volume 22, pages 257–260. Optical Society of America, Washington DC), 1994.
3. R. Barakat and G. Newsam. Algorithms for reconstruction of partially known, bandlimited fourier-transform pairs from noisy data. *Journal of the Optical Society of America*, 2:2027–2039, 1985.
4. R. W. Gerchberg and W. O. Saxton. A practical algorithm for the determination of phase from image and diffraction plane pictures. *Optik*, 35:237–246, 1972.
5. L. G. Gubin, B. T. Poljak, and E. V. Raik. The method of projections for finding the common point of convex sets. *USSR Computational Mathematics and Mathematical Physics*, 3(6):1–24, 1967.
6. J. P. Kahane and P.-G. Lemarié-Rieusset. *Fourier Series and Wavelets*, volume 3 of *Studies in the Development of Modern Mathematics*. Gordon and Breach Publishers, 1995.
7. A. Levi and H. Stark. Image restoration by the method of generalized projections with application to restoration from magnitude. *Journal of the Optical Society of America*, 1:932–943, 1984.
8. A. K. Louis, P. Maaß, and A. Rieder. *Wavelets*. Teubner, 1994.

9. F. May, A. Klappenecker, V. Baumgarte, A. Nückel, and T. Beth. A high through-put multiplication free approximation to arithmetic coding. To appear in: Proceedings 1996 International Symposium on Information Theory and Its Applications, 1996.

10. F. Wyrowski and O. Bryngdahl. Digital holography as part of diffractive optics. *Reports on Progress in Physics*, 54:1481–1571, 1991.

Regularization Methods for Nonlinear Ill–Posed Problems with Applications to Phase Reconstruction

Barbara Blaschke-Kaltenbacher and Heinz W. Engl

Institut für Mathematik, Johannes Kepler Universität, A-4040 Linz, Austria [*]

1 Introduction

This conference has shown again that many inverse problems arise in medical imaging and nondestructive testing. Mathematically, such problems involve e.g. parameter identification from boundary measurements (see e.g. [36]), inverse scattering (see e.g. [12], [13], [14]), or phase reconstruction (see e.g. [40]). The mathematical formulation of inverse problems usually gives rise to ill–posed problems in Hadamard's sense, where especially the lack of stability causes numerical difficulties. We take this as a motivation to survey some results about convergence and convergence rates for regularization methods for nonlinear ill–posed problems, which have to be used to deal with the instability issue. Again motivated by some talks at this conference, we illustrate our results by some phase reconstruction problems.

As a model for nonlinear inverse problems we consider the abstract operator equation

$$F(x) = y \tag{1}$$

where $F : \mathcal{D}(F)(\subseteq X) \to Y$ is a nonlinear operator between Hilbert spaces X and Y. We are interested in the situation that a solution $x^\dagger$ does not depend continuously on the data. Since in practice only approximate data y^δ with

$$\|y - y^\delta\| \leq \delta \tag{2}$$

are available, problem (1) has to be regularized (see e.g. [20], [27], [28], [48], [51], [52], [64]). Even for linear problems, the speed of convergence to an exact solution of (1) of the approximations produced by any regularization method can be arbitrarily slow (see [62]). Like in the linear case, also for nonlinear ill–posed probems, rates of convergence of regularized solutions can only be obtained under so-called "source conditions" on the difference between an a–priori guess x_* and

[*] Supported by Christian Doppler Forschungsgesellschaft and by Jubiläumsfonds d. österr. Nationalbank, grant no. 5391

an unknown solution $x^\dagger$, which in the nonlinear situation have the form

$$x_* - x^\dagger = \left(F'(x^\dagger)^* F'(x^\dagger)\right)^\nu w$$
$$\text{for some } w \in \mathcal{N}(F'(x^\dagger))^\perp \text{ with } \|w\| \text{ sufficiently small,}$$

(3)

where $\nu \geq 0$ and $\mathcal{N}$ denotes the nullspace of an operator. In applications, they can often be interpreted as smoothness and smallness conditions on $x_* - x^\dagger$, and are the stronger, the larger the exponent ν is.

Like in the well–posed situation, solution methods for nonlinear problems cannot be expected to converge globally unless some additional globalization strategy is applied. Therefore we concentrate on the local convergence properties of the regularization methods under consideration, i.e., we assume that a solution $x^\dagger$ of (1) exists and that we have an initial guess x_* that is sufficiently close to $x^\dagger$:

$$x^\dagger \in B_\rho(x_*)$$

(4)

for some (small) $\rho > 0$, where $B_\rho(x_*) := \{x \in X \,/\, \|x - x_*\| \leq \rho\}$.

In this paper we will first of all (Section 1) give a survey on some of the regularization methods for the general equation (1) that have been studied in the last few years and quote some results about their convergence behaviour. At the end of Section 1 we put an example of a parameter identification problem in order to illustrate the theoretically required conditions like (3) for convergence and convergence rates and show that they can be expected to be fulfilled in practically relevant applications. Section 2 is concerned with the problem of phase reconstruction in two different settings. The methods presented in the first section are applied and, on the basis of the results in Section 1, shown to converge with appropriate rates under certain conditions.

2 Regularization Methods for Nonlinear Ill–Posed Problems

2.1 Tikhonov Regularization

The theory of regularization methods for linear ill–posed problems

$$Ax = y$$

(5)

is already well–established (for a recent account, cf. [20]). Certainly the most widely used regularization technique for linear ill–posed problems is Tikhonov regularization. Here, a solution of (5) is approximated by a solution of the problem

$$\|Ax - y^\delta\|^2 + \alpha\|x\|^2 = \min!$$

(6)

or, equivalently, of the regularized normal equations

$$(A^*A + \alpha I)x = A^*y^\delta$$

(7)

where α is a (small) regularization parameter.

It is near at hand to carry over the principle of Tikhonov regularization in the variational form (6) to the nonlinear situation and use a minimizer x_α^δ of

$$\|F(x) - y^\delta\|^2 + \alpha\|x - x_*\|^2 = \min!\,,\tag{8}$$

where x_* is some a priori guess, as an approximation for a solution $x^\dagger$ of (1).

As already mentioned (and like in [21],) we here consider only the case that the exact data y are attainable, i.e., that there exists a solution of (1). For the more general case that only a least–squares solution of (1) exists, see [6]. The solution that is actually approximated by (8) turns out to be an "x_*–minimum–norm solution" (i.e., a solution of (1) which is closest to x_* among all solutions).

Some basic analysis of Tikhonov regularization for nonlinear problems was done in [63], [21], [53], and [11]. The most important conditions that are needed there in order to establish well–definedness (by (8)) of x_α^δ, and its continuous dependence on the data y^δ for fixed $\alpha > 0$, are continuity and weak sequential closedness of F (cf. [21], [63]).

Under these general assumptions and if the regularization parameter is chosen appropriately in dependence of the noise level δ in (2), one can also prove (see [63]) convergence of the approximations x_α^δ to a solution $x^\dagger$ in the following sense: If

$$\alpha(\delta) \to 0 \quad \text{and} \quad \frac{\delta}{\sqrt{\alpha(\delta)}} \to 0 \qquad \text{as } \delta \to 0\,,\tag{9}$$

then every sequence $(x_{\alpha_k}^{\delta_k})$ where $\|y^{\delta_k} - y\| \le \delta_k$, $\delta_k \to 0$, $\alpha_k := \alpha(\delta_k)$ and $x_{\alpha_k}^{\delta_k}$ is a minimizer of (8) (with y^δ replaced by y^{δ_k}), has a convergent subsequence and the limit of every convergent subsequence is an x_*–minimum–norm solution of (1). If, in addition, the x_*–minimum–norm solution $x^\dagger$ of (1) is unique, then

$$\lim_{\delta \to 0} x_{\alpha(\delta)}^\delta = x^\dagger\,.\tag{10}$$

For the linear case (5), it is a classical result (cf. [27]) that convergence rates can be obtained under source conditions that have the form

$$x^\dagger = (A^*A)^\nu w$$

for some $w \in X$, $\nu > 0$; a natural generalization to the nonlinear situation is (3). As it was proven in [21] under the assumptions that $D(F)$ is convex, that F is Fréchet differentiable with Lipschitz continuous Fréchet derivative, and that

$$x_* - x^\dagger = F'(x^\dagger)^* w$$

for some sufficiently small w (i.e., (3) with $\nu = \frac{1}{2}$), one gets the rates

$$\|x_\alpha - x^\dagger\| = O(\sqrt{\alpha})$$

if $\delta = 0$ in (2) and, if $\delta \neq 0$ and α is chosen according to

$$\alpha \sim \delta\,,\tag{11}$$

then

$$\|x_\alpha^\delta - x^\dagger\| = O(\sqrt{\delta}).\tag{12}$$

Respective rates

$$\|x_\alpha - x^\dagger\| = O(\alpha^\nu), \qquad (\delta = 0),$$
$$\|x_\alpha^\delta - x^\dagger\| = O(\delta^{\frac{2\nu}{2\nu+1}})\tag{13}$$

for arbitrary $\nu \in (0,1]$ in (3) were shown in [53] for $\nu \geq \frac{1}{2}$ and in [34] for $0 < \nu \leq \frac{1}{2}$ with the choice

$$\alpha^{\nu+\frac{1}{2}} c_{\alpha,\nu} \sim \delta,\tag{14}$$

$c_{\alpha,\nu} = 1$ for $0 < \nu \leq \frac{1}{2}$, $c_{\alpha,\nu}^2 := \int_0^\infty \frac{\alpha^{2(1-\nu)}\lambda^{2\nu}}{(\alpha+\lambda)^2} dE_\lambda \|w\|^2$ for $\frac{1}{2} < \nu \leq 1$, where $\{E_\lambda\}$ is the spectral family of $F'(x^\dagger)^* F'(x^\dagger)$. The conditions on F' that are needed to obtain these rates are, as above, local Lipschitz continuity, if $\nu \geq \frac{1}{2}$ and, as long as $\nu < \frac{1}{2}$,

$$\|F(\bar{x}) - F(x) - F'(x)(\bar{x}-x)\| \leq K \|F(\bar{x}) - F(x)\|^\beta \|\bar{x} - x\|^\gamma \qquad \bar{x}, x \in B_{2\rho}(x_*),\tag{15}$$

for some $K > 0$, $\rho > 0$ (cf. (4)), where

$$\beta \geq 1 + 2\nu(1 - \beta - \gamma) > 0,\tag{16}$$

the latter being basically a restriction on the nonlinearity of F.

In actual computation, the exponent ν in the source condition is usually not available, so that one cannot calculate the regularization parameter α *a priori* according to (9), (11), or (14). Instead, one has to choose α depending on quantities that appear in the computations like the residual (*a posteriori* parameter choice). Probably the most widely used a posteriori parameter choice strategy is the discrepancy principle ([50]), where α is defined by the one–dimensional nonlinear equation

$$\|F(x_\alpha^\delta) - y^\delta\| = c\,\delta\tag{17}$$

for some constant $c > 0$. Under certain conditions (see [42]) it can be shown that (17) has a solution for all sufficiently small δ and that this parameter choice rule yields convergence (10) (if $x^\dagger$ is unique). In [21] it was proven that also the convergence rate (12) can be obtained. However, (17) never yields a better rate than (12), even if $\nu > \frac{1}{2}$ in (3). Therefore, first of all in the linear ([18], [26]) and later on in the nonlinear situation ([61]), alternative a posteriori parameter choice strategies have been developed that yield the optimal rate (13) for all $\nu \in (0,1]$.

An alternative choice for the regularizing term (i.e., $\alpha\|x - x_*\|^2$) in (8), namely $\alpha\|D(x) - D(x_*)\|^2$ with a closed linear operator D (in applications often a differential operator; "seminorm regularization"), was proposed in [44], where also convergence results analogous to those in [21] were proven.

Examples of practical inverse problems where this theory of Tikhonov regularization can be applied are given e.g. in [8], [23], [24], [25], [59], [60].

We mention in passing that based on this theory one can do a convergence analysis for the maximum entropy method (see [22], [45]); the method of proof used there seems to be applicable to show convergence rates for total–variation–based regularization, a method which has also been discussed at this conference (see e.g. [1]).

2.2 Iterative Methods

For reasons of computational effort it is, especially in large scale problems, of interest to avoid solving the linear system (7) or the global minimization problem (8). Therefore an attractive alternative to Tikhonov regularization are *iterative* methods (see e.g. [10], [16], [17], [29], [30], [46], [47], [65], [66] for the linear case and [5], [9], [32], [56], [57], [58] for the nonlinear case), where a *stopping index* plays the role of the regularization parameter.

Landweber Iteration

Since it is a fully explicit method and relatively simple to implement, *Landweber iteration* (see, for the linear case, [46], [48], [65]) is of special interest. For nonlinear problems it was studied in [32]:

$$x_{n+1}^\delta = x_n^\delta + F'(x_n^\delta)^*(y^\delta - F(x_n^\delta)). \tag{18}$$

There, under the scaling assumption

$$\|F'(x)\| \leq 1, \qquad x \in \mathcal{B}_{2\rho}(x_0), \tag{19}$$

and the condition

$$\|F(\bar{x}) - F(x) - F'(x)(\bar{x} - x)\| \leq \eta \|F(\bar{x}) - F(x)\| \qquad \bar{x}, x \in \mathcal{B}_{2\rho}(x_0) \tag{20}$$

with $\eta < \frac{1}{2}$ and ρ as in (4) (with x_* replaced by x_0), convergence for $n \to \infty$ in the noise–free case and, with the a posteriori stopping rule

$$\|F(x_{N(\delta)}^\delta) - y^\delta\| \leq \bar{\tau}\delta < \|F(x_n^\delta) - y^\delta\|, \qquad 0 \leq n < N(\delta), \tag{21}$$

(being motivated by the discrepancy principle (17)), convergence with $\delta \to 0$ in the case of noisy data, are proven. Note that (20) with $\eta < 1$ implies that if $x_0 - x^\dagger \in \mathcal{N}(F'(x^\dagger))^\perp$ then $x^\dagger$ is the unique x_0-minimum–norm solution in $\mathcal{B}_\rho(x_0)$ (cf. [9]).

A source condition

$$x_0 - x^\dagger = \left(F'(x^\dagger)^* F'(x^\dagger)\right)^\nu w$$
$$\text{for some } w \in \mathcal{N}(F'(x^\dagger))^\perp \text{ with } \|w\| \text{ sufficiently small,} \tag{22}$$

with $0 < \nu \leq \frac{1}{2}$ is shown in [32] to lead to convergence rates

$$\|x_{N(\delta)}^\delta - x^\dagger\| = O(\delta^{\frac{2\nu}{2\nu+1}}) \tag{23}$$

with the stopping criterion (21) and, for $\delta = 0$, to

$$\|x_n - x^\dagger\| = O((n+1)^{-\nu}),$$

if F is Fréchet differentiable and the derivative F' fulfills the assumption

$$F'(\bar{x}) = R(\bar{x}, x)F'(x)$$
$$\|R(\bar{x}, x) - I\| \leq C_R\|\bar{x} - x\| \qquad \bar{x}, x \in \mathcal{B}_{2\rho}(x_0). \tag{24}$$

Note that (20), (24), like (15), (16), can be interpreted as assuming that F should not be "too nonlinear".

In [31], Landweber iteration in the form (18) is applied to an inverse scattering problem; although some of the theoretical conditions on F (especially (24)) could not be verified for this special problem, the numerical results reported in [31] are quite promising.

Newton Type Methods

Because of their superior convergence properties in the well–posed situation, Newton–like methods should also be attractive for solving ill–posed problems, and therefore have already been applied to several inverse problems (cf. e.g. [15], [37], [41], [43], [49], [55],). However, so far only little is known rigorously about convergence of Newton type methods for nonlinear ill–posed problems (cf. [2], [4]).

As usual in deriving a Newton type method we linearize equation (1) at some current iterate x_n and obtain the linearized equation

$$F'(x_n)(x - x_n) = y - F(x_n), \tag{25}$$

whose solution we define to be the next iterate x_{n+1}. However, (25) is in general ill–posed (e.g. if F is completely continuous, so that $F'(x)$ is compact). Therefore we cannot simply invert $F'(x_n)$ (or solve (25) by a conventional method for linear operator equations), but have to use some regularization technique for the linearized problem. If, e.g., linear Tikhonov regularization is applied to (25), one gets the so–called *Levenberg Marquardt method*:

$$x^\delta_{n+1} = x^\delta_n - (F'(x^\delta_n)^* F'(x^\delta_n) + \alpha_n I)^{-1} F'(x^\delta_n)^* (F(x^\delta_n) - y^\delta), \tag{26}$$

with α_n being a sequence of regularization parameters that should obviously go to zero as $n \to \infty$. It is, however, not yet clear how (α_n) should in fact be chosen to make the iteration (26) converge and, to our knowledge, there exists no convergence proof for the Levenberg–Marquardt method for ill–posed problems yet.

A few years ago Bakushinskii ([2]) proposed what he calls the *iteratively regularized Gauß–Newton method*:

$$x^\delta_{n+1} = x^\delta_n - (F'(x^\delta_n)^* F'(x^\delta_n) + \alpha_n I)^{-1} \left(F'(x^\delta_n)^* (F(x^\delta_n) - y^\delta) + \alpha_n (x^\delta_n - x_0) \right), \tag{27}$$

The role of the additional term $(F'(x^\delta_n)^* F'(x^\delta_n) + \alpha_n I)^{-1} \alpha_n (x^\delta_n - x_0)$ in (27) compared to (26) is clarified by the fact that the $(n+1)$st iterate of the Levenberg–Marquardt method solves

$$\|F(x^\delta_n) + F'(x^\delta_n)(x^{LM}_{n+1} - x^\delta_n) - y^\delta\|^2 + \alpha_n \|x^{LM}_{n+1} - x^\delta_n\|^2 = \min!, \tag{28}$$

while the $(n+1)$st iterate of the iteratively regularized Gauß–Newton method is a minimizer of

$$\|F(x^\delta_n) + F'(x^\delta_n)(x^{GN}_{n+1} - x^\delta_n) - y^\delta\|^2 + \alpha_n \|x^{GN}_{n+1} - x_0\|^2 = \min!. \tag{29}$$

Both (28) and (29) can be regarded as Tikhonov regularization in the variational form (6) or (8) with F linearized around x_n^δ. In (28), the "a priori guess" x_* in the regularizing term $\alpha_n \|x - x_*\|$ is the last iterate and therefore changes in each Newton step, while in (29), x_* is fixed to x_0, whence it is intuitively clear, that there the regularizing term keeps all the iterates near to x_0, which should have a stabilizing effect. This explains why the analysis of (26) might be more complicated than that of (27).

Linear Tikhonov regularization is only one example of a linear regularization method based on so-called "filter functions", i.e., methods where the generalized inverse $A^\dagger$ of a linear operator A is approximated by $g(A^*A, \alpha)A^*$, with a real-valued function $g : (\mathbb{R}^+)^2 \to \mathbb{R}$ with $g(\lambda, \alpha) \to \frac{1}{\lambda}$ as $\alpha \to 0$, where $|\lambda \cdot g(\lambda, \alpha)|$ is bounded by a constant C independent of α and λ (cf. [20], [48]). By applying those linear methods to the linearized problem (25) and taking Bakushinskii's additional term into account, one obtains a class of iterative methods for the solution of the nonlinear problem (1) of the form

$$x_{n+1}^\delta = x_0 - g(F'(x_n^\delta)^* F'(x_n^\delta), \alpha_n) F'(x_n^\delta)^* (F(x_n^\delta) - y - F'(x_n^\delta)(x_n^\delta - x_0)). \quad (30)$$

This idea was already proposed by Bakushinskii in [3] where he also gives some first convergence results, assuming that F' is Lipschitz continuous and that the source condition (22) with $\nu = 1$ is fulfilled, the latter being a quite strong assumption. There, and later also in [9] and [7], (α_n) was chosen to be a fixed sequence of parameters satisfying

$$\alpha_n > 0, \quad 1 \le \frac{\alpha_n}{\alpha_{n+1}} \le r, \quad \lim_{n\to\infty} \alpha_n = 0$$

for some $r > 1$.

Here we concentrate on two special choices for g: First, the case that $g(\lambda, \alpha) = g^T(\lambda, \alpha) := \frac{1}{\lambda+\alpha}$ (i.e., linear Tikhonov regularization) which, as already mentioned, leads to the iteratively regularized Gauß–Newton method (27). Secondly, in order to avoid the direct inversion $(F'(x_n^\delta)^* F'(x_n^\delta) + \alpha_n I)^{-1}$ in each Newton step, $F'(x_n^\delta)^\dagger$ is approximated by an iterative procedure, namely linear Landweber iteration: $g(\lambda, \alpha) = g^L(\lambda, \alpha) := \sum_{k=1}^{k_n}(1-\lambda)^k$, where $k_n := [\frac{1}{\alpha_n}]$, (i.e., instead of the the regularization parameter $\alpha_n \in \mathbb{R}_+$ one uses a stopping index $k_n \in \mathbb{N}$), yielding the "Landweber type iteration"

$$\begin{aligned}
x_{n,0}^\delta &= x_0 \\
x_{n,k+1}^\delta &= x_{n,k}^\delta - F'(x_n^\delta)^* (F(x_n^\delta) + F'(x_n^\delta)(x_{n,k}^\delta - x_n^\delta) - y^\delta), \quad 1 \le k < k_n \\
x_{n+1} &= x_{n,k_n}^\delta ;
\end{aligned}$$

$$(31)$$

(note that like in the linear case and in (18) (cf. (19)), problem (1) has to be properly scaled).

Thus, one has an outer iteration — namely the Newton iteration for the nonlinear problem — and an inner iteration — the linear Landweber iteration for the linearized problem — which, if one would not have to "restart" the inner iteration at $x_{n,0}^\delta = x_0$ in each Newton step, would just be (18) with performing k_n (instead of only one) Landweber iterations per evaluation of F and F'. Although it seems to be more natural to start the inner iteration at x_n^δ instead of x_0, it is not yet clear how to prove convergence rates for the resulting method; note that the restart at x_0 corresponds to Bakushinskii's additional term, cf. (26), (27), and might thus have some additional stabilizing effect.

As it was shown in [9], Bakushinskii's convergence proof for the *iteratively regularized Gauß–Newton method* from [3] can, without any additional assumptions on F', be extended to the situation that $\nu \geq \frac{1}{2}$ in (22), so that one obtains

$$\|x_n - x^\dagger\| = O(\alpha_n^\nu), \tag{32}$$

if $\delta = 0$ in (2), and, for non–vanishing noise, (23) if the stopping index $N(\delta)$ is chosen a priori according to

$$\alpha_{N(\delta)}^{\nu+\frac{1}{2}} \sim \delta. \tag{33}$$

However, in the case that $0 \leq \nu < \frac{1}{2}$, it turns out that a convergence proof for the iteratively regularized Gauß–Newton method seems not to be possible analogously to the one of [3]. Especially, the conditions on F' have to be strengthened: for the convergence analysis in [9], [7] it is assumed that

$$F'(\bar{x}) = R(\bar{x}, x)F'(x) + Q(\bar{x}, x)$$
$$\|I - R(\bar{x}, x)\| \leq C_R \qquad\qquad \bar{x}, x \in \mathcal{B}_{2\rho}(x_0) \tag{34}$$
$$\|Q(\bar{x}, x)\| \leq C_Q \|F'(x^\dagger)(\bar{x} - x)\|^\beta \|\bar{x} - x\|^\gamma,$$

holds with

$$\beta(\tfrac{1}{2} + \nu) + \gamma\nu \geq \tfrac{1}{2}, \tag{35}$$

and ρ, C_R and C_Q sufficiently small. These assumptions are again conditions on the degree of nonlinearity of F and similar to the ones that were made for proving convergence (without source condition, i.e., $\nu = 0$ in (22)) and convergence rates for the nonlinear Landweber iteration (18) (cf. (20), (24)) and also to those needed in [34] for proving convergence rates for Tikhonov regularization in the case $0 < \nu \leq \frac{1}{2}$ (cf. (15)). Although no such condition is required for proving convergence (without rates) for Tikhonov regularization, there is still a need for a similar assumption when it comes to the numerical implementation, i.e., the determination of the actual global minimizer of the Tikhonov functional (see [11]). The condition (34) (with $Q \equiv 0$) was verified in [32] for two parameter estimation problems (from interior measurements) and for a Hammerstein integral equation and in [5] for a special class of operator equations that can be represented as the combination of a well–posed nonlinear and an ill–posed linear problem.

With (34), one obtains convergence in the noise–free case and, with the a priori stopping rule

$$N(\delta) \to \infty \quad \text{and} \quad \frac{\delta}{\sqrt{\alpha_{N(\delta)}}} \to 0 \qquad \text{as } \delta \to 0, \tag{36}$$

(which is analogous to (9)), convergence as $\delta \to 0$, and the rates (32) and (23), respectively, for $0 < \nu \leq \frac{1}{2}$. (cf. [9]). Note that due to the saturation phenomenon for (linear) Tikhonov regularization (see e.g. [20], Section 4.2), no better rates can be expected for $\nu > 1$ than for $\nu = 1$.

The same convergence results for $0 \leq \nu \leq \frac{1}{2}$ can also be obtained by using the a posteriori stopping rule (21) ([9]).

For the *Landweber type iteration* (31) the same convergence and convergence rates assertions under the same conditions hold true ([7]), except for two points: instead of (21), a modified posteriori stopping rule is used, and there is no saturation at $\nu = 1$, i.e., for (31), the rate (23) is achieved for all $\nu > 0$, whence by choosing x_0 with $x_0 - x^\dagger$ sufficiently smooth in the sense of (22), one can come arbitrarily close to the "ideal" rate $O(\delta)$.

As can be seen from the proofs in [9] and [7], the convergence and convergence rates results stated there can still obtained if instead of $F'(x_n^\delta)$ an approximation A_n is used, satisfying either

$$A_n = \tilde{R}_n F'(x_n^\delta) + \tilde{Q}_n$$
$$\|I - \tilde{R}_n\| \leq C_{\tilde{R}} \qquad n \in \mathbb{N} \qquad (37)$$
$$\|\tilde{Q}_n\| \leq C_{\tilde{Q}} \sqrt{\alpha_n},$$

with $\tilde{R}_n \in L(Y,Y)$, $\tilde{Q}_n \in L(X,Y)$, $C_{\tilde{Q}} > 0$, and $C_{\tilde{R}} > 0$ a sufficiently small constant, if $0 \leq \nu \leq \frac{1}{2}$ in the source condition (22), or

$$\|A_n - F'(x_n^\delta)\| \leq \tilde{L}\alpha_n^\nu, \quad n \in \mathbb{N} \qquad (38)$$

for some $\tilde{L} > 0$, if $\frac{1}{2} \leq \nu \leq 1$.

Moreover, $\|I - R(x_n^\delta, x^\dagger)\|$ need not decrease as $n \to \infty$, but only uniform boundedness (by a sufficiently small constant C_R) of $\|I - R(x_n^\delta, x)\|$ is needed. As a consequence, if a linear operator A_0 is available such that

$$A_0 = R F'(x^\dagger) \qquad (39)$$

with $\|I - R\|$ sufficiently small, (e.g., if $Q = 0$ in (34), $A_0 := F'(x_0)$ can be used; note that $F'(x^\dagger)$ need not be known explicitly, as it would seem at a first look at (39)) then one can set

$$A_n := A_0, \qquad n \in \mathbb{N}, \qquad (40)$$

in (27) and gets a method that also converges at the rates given above for $0 \leq \nu \leq \frac{1}{2}$. For $A_0 = F'(x_0)$, one obtains

$$x_{n+1}^\delta = x_n^\delta - (F'(x_0)^* F'(x_0) + \alpha_n I)^{-1}\left(F'(x_0)^*(F(x_n^\delta) - y^\delta) + \alpha(x_n^\delta - x_0)\right), \quad (41)$$

and

$$x_{n,0}^\delta = x_0$$
$$x_{n,k+1}^\delta = x_{n,k}^\delta - F'(x_0)^*(F(x_n^\delta) + F'(x_0)(x_{n,k}^\delta - x_n^\delta) - y^\delta), \quad 1 \leq k < k_n$$
$$x_{n+1} = x_{n,k_n}^\delta,$$
$$(42)$$

respectively.

In this way, the iteratively regularized Gauß–Newton method (27) or the Landweber type method (31), respectively, can be generalized to a method of quasi–Newton type and even to a frozen Newton method (i.e., (41)) that only needs one single linear operator all over the iteration and is therefore computationally much cheaper.

Unfortunately, (34) and especially (24) seem to be hard or even impossible to verify for some inverse problems (see e.g. [31], [33]). Especially problems concerned with parameter identification from boundary measurements, as they frequently arise in medical imaging and in nondestructive testing, where one often wants to get information inside some inaccessible part of a body from boundary data, in general do not fulfill

$$F'(\bar{x}) = R(\bar{x}, x)F'(x), \qquad (43)$$

for any bounded and continuously invertible linear operator $R(\bar{x}, x)$; note that by taking the adjoints one sees that (43) would mean that the range of the adjoint $F'(x)^*$ of $F'(x)$ is invariant, which is in general not the case for that type of problems.

However, in some of these examples it can be shown that the range of $F'(x)$ itself does remain unchanged for all $x \in \mathcal{B}_{2\rho}(x_0)$, and even

$$\begin{aligned} F'(x) &= F'(x^\dagger)R(x) \\ \|R(x) - I\| &\leq C_R\|x - x^\dagger\| \end{aligned} \qquad x \in \mathcal{B}_{2\rho}(x_0) \qquad (44)$$

holds, which means that the linearized operator $F'(x)$ (e.g. for a parameter identification problem from boundary measurements, the trace of the linearized parameter–to–solution map) remains in principle the same for all $x \in \mathcal{B}_{2\rho}(x_0)$, up to some modification by $R(x)$ of the input. Thus, (44) seems to be a more natural condition than (43) for this type of problems.

It was shown in [7], that the convergence results quoted above for the iteratively regularized Gauß–Newton method (27) and the Landweber type iteration (31) with the a priori stopping rule (36), (33), can also be proven under the condition (44) instead of (34).

In [7], (44) is also established for a concrete example of parameter identification from boundary measurements, namely the simple model problem of estimating c in

$$\begin{aligned} -\Delta u + cu &= f && \text{in } \Omega \\ u &= g && \text{on } \partial\Omega, \end{aligned} \qquad (45)$$

where Ω is a bounded domain in $\mathbb{R}^2$ or $\mathbb{R}^3$ with smooth boundary $\partial\Omega$, $f \in L^2(\Omega)$, $g \in H^{\frac{3}{2}}(\partial\Omega)$, and c is assumed to lie inside the set

$$\mathcal{D}(F) := \{c \in L^2(\Omega)/\|c - \hat{c}\| \leq \gamma \text{ for some } \hat{c} \geq 0 \text{ a.e. }\}.$$

The additional data is the normal derivative of the solution u at the boundary, so that F is defined by

$$F := T \circ G : \mathcal{D}(F) \rightarrow L^2(\partial\Omega),$$

where T is the trace operator

$$T : H^2(\Omega) \rightarrow L^2(\partial\Omega)$$
$$v \mapsto \frac{\partial v}{\partial n}\big|_{\partial\Omega}$$

and G is the parameter–to–solution map, mapping $c \in \mathcal{D}(F)$ into the corresponding solution of (45). It can be shown that F is well–defined on $\mathcal{D}(F)$, if γ in the definition of $\mathcal{D}(F)$ is small enough, and that the Fréchet derivative of F is given by

$$F'(c)h = -TA(c)^{-1}\Big(h \cdot G(c)\Big),$$

with $A(c) : H^2(\Omega) \cap H_0^1(\Omega) \rightarrow L^2(\Omega)$ defined by $A(c)v := -\triangle v + cv$ (see [21]). If for the exact solution $u = G(c^\dagger)$, $|u(x)| \geq \kappa > 0$ holds for all $x \in \Omega$, then one can show ([7]) that

$$F'(c) = F'(c^\dagger)R(c)$$
$$\|R(c) - I\| \leq C_R\|c - c^\dagger\| \qquad c \in \mathcal{D}(F)$$

holds with

$$R(c) := \frac{1}{G(c^\dagger)}A(c^\dagger)A(c)^{-1}\Big(h \cdot G(c)\Big).$$

Therefore, the iteratively regularized Gauß–Newton method (27) or the Landweber iteration (31) can be applied to this problem and yield convergence and the convergence rates quoted above.

3 Phase Reconstruction

The problem of reconstructing the phase of a function or of its Fourier transform from amplitude measurements in time and/or frequency space arises in diverse fields such as microscopy, analysis of neutron reflective data, astronomy, and optical design. An introduction to the problem, a description of some applications and some solution techniques together with an extensive bibliography are given in the book [35] as well as the survey article [40]. Also at this meeting, the phase reconstruction problem was addressed in several talks.

We will here consider two different versions of the problem of phase reconstruction:

- Given the intensity $r : \mathbb{R} \rightarrow \mathbb{R}^+$ of the Fourier transform of a real–valued function f, reconstruct f, i.e., find $f : \mathbb{R} \rightarrow \mathbb{R}$ such that $|\mathcal{F}f|^2 = r$ (cf. [38], [8]).
- Given the magnitude $f : \mathbb{R}^d \rightarrow \mathbb{R}^+$ ($d \in \mathbb{N}$) of a complex–valued function and the intensity $r : \mathbb{R}^d \rightarrow \mathbb{R}^+$ of its Fourier transform, reconstruct the phase, i.e., find $\phi : \mathbb{R}^d \rightarrow \mathbb{R}$ such that $|\mathcal{F}(f \cdot e^{i\phi})|^2 = r$ (cf. [15]).

Both of these problems are nonlinear and ill–posed: The first one due to non–uniqueness and, if uniqueness is enforced by using partial knowledge of f (see [38]), due to instability, as an example given in [8] shows. For the second problem, instability of the linearized problem was shown in [15]. (See [21] for the connection between ill–posedness of a nonlinear problem and of its linearization.)

Therefore, some regularization technique has to be applied when solving these problems; in the following, we will consider the use of some of the methods surveyed in Section 1.

3.1 Reconstruction of f from $|\mathcal{F}f|^2$

Formulating this problem as a nonlinear operator equation

$$F(f) = r \tag{46}$$

leads to the definition

$$F(f)(s) := |\mathcal{F}f|^2(s), \quad s \in \mathbb{R}. \tag{47}$$

The formal derivative of F is given by

$$F'(f)h = 2\Re(\mathcal{F}f\overline{\mathcal{F}h}),$$

where $\Re$ denotes the real part. Two possible choices of Hilbert spaces on which F as a function mapping into $Y := L^2_{\mathbb{R}}(\mathbb{R})$ is well–defined and Fréchet differentiable are

1. A space of time–limited square integrable functions:

$$X := L^2_{\mathbb{R}}[0, a],$$

   for some fixed $a > 0$.
2. A weighted L^2-space

$$X := L^{1,2}_{\mathbb{R}}(\mathbb{R}),$$

   where $\|f\|^2_{L^{1,2}} := \int_{\mathbb{R}} (1 + t^2) f(t)^2 dt$.

In both cases it can be shown that F is weakly sequentially closed and that F' is Lipschitz continuous (see [8]). As a consequence, when applying Tikhonov regularization (8) to the operator equation (46), one gets stability for fixed $\alpha > 0$ and (subsequential) convergence if (9) as $\delta \to 0$.

To obtain convergence rates for regularized solutions according to the results quoted in Section 2, one has to make sure that (22) is fulfilled for some $\nu > 0$. Sufficient for (22) with $\nu = \frac{1}{2}$ and therefore, with the choice $\alpha \sim \delta$ or $\alpha_{N(\delta)} \sim \delta$, for the rate

$$\|f^\delta_\alpha - f^\dagger\|_X = O(\sqrt{\delta})$$

for Tikhonov regularization (8) or

$$\|f_{N(\delta)} - f^\dagger\|_X = O(\sqrt{\delta})$$

for the iteratively regularized Gauß–Newton method (27) and the Landweber type iteration (31), respectively, are:

1.

$$w := \frac{\mathcal{F}(f^\dagger - f_0)}{\mathcal{F} f_0} \quad \text{real--valued and } \|w\|_{L^2} < \sqrt{\frac{\pi}{2a}}$$

if $X = L^2_{\mathbb{R}}[0, a]$.

2.

$$w := \frac{\mathcal{F}(f^\dagger - f_0) - (\mathcal{F}(f^\dagger - f_0))''}{\mathcal{F} f_0} \quad \text{real--valued and } \|w\|_{L^{1,2}} < 1 \quad (48)$$

if $X = L^{1,2}_{\mathbb{R}}(\mathbb{R})$.

For proofs and an interpretation of these conditions see [8]; the condition (48) in the second case $X = L^{1,2}_{\mathbb{R}}(\mathbb{R})$ can — under some further assumptions — be fulfilled if f is known outside some compact set $[-N, N]$, which is related (though not identical) to a band–limitedness condition, thus somehow complementing the time–limited case $X = L^2_{\mathbb{R}}[0, a]$.

Under such a kind of band-limitedness condition, one can also verify (44) with

$$R(f)h := \mathcal{F}^{-1}\left(\frac{\mathcal{F} f}{\mathcal{F} f^\dagger} \cdot \mathcal{F} h\right) \quad (49)$$

(see Appendix). Therefore, an application of the iteratively regularized Gauß–Newton method (27) or the Landweber type iteration (31) together with the stopping rule (36) yields a stable and (as $\delta \to 0$) convergent approximation scheme for the solution of the phase reconstruction problem considered in this Subsection.

3.2 Reconstruction of ϕ from $|\mathcal{F}(f \cdot e^{i\phi})|^2$

Motivated by diffractive optics, this problem was studied in [15], where Tikhonov regularization (with fixed $\alpha > 0$) was applied to it and the minimizer of the Tikhonov functional (8) was found by Newton's method, which was shown to be locally almost quadratically convergent. The question of $\alpha \to 0$ remained open there, and can now be answered on the basis of the theory presented in the foregoing Section:

Here, the nonlinear operator in

$$F(\phi) = r \quad (50)$$

is defined by

$$F(\phi)(\xi) := |\mathcal{F}(f \cdot e^{i\phi})|^2(\xi), \quad \xi \in \mathbb{R}^d.$$

If $f \in L^1_{\mathbb{R}}(\mathbb{R}^d) \cap L^2_{\mathbb{R}}(\mathbb{R}^d) \cap L^\infty_{\mathbb{R}}(\mathbb{R}^d)$, then F is well–defined, Lipschitz continuous and Fréchet differentiable as a function from $L^2_{\mathbb{R}}(\mathbb{R}^d)$ to $Y := L^2_{\mathbb{R}}(\mathbb{R}^d)$ ([15]) and F', given by

$$F'(\phi)h := 2\Re(\mathcal{F}(f \cdot e^{i\phi})\overline{\mathcal{F}(i\,h\,f \cdot e^{i\phi})},$$

is Lipschitz continuous. Since in applications, f is typically compactly supported (see [15]), it is natural to assume that $supp(\phi) \subseteq K$ for some bounded set

$K \subset \mathbb{R}^d$; defining F on $X := H^s_{\mathbb{R}}(K)$ for some $s > 0$ one can also show weak sequential closedness of F.

Consequently, under these assumptions, Tikhonov regularization, applied to (50), is stable and convergent as $\alpha \to 0$.

Since the adjoint of $F'(\phi)$ is given by

$$F'(\phi)^* z = 2J^s \Re\left(i\, f \cdot e^{i\phi}\, \overline{\mathcal{F}^{-1}\left(\mathcal{F}(f \cdot e^{i\phi}) \cdot z\right)} \right),$$

where J^s is the adjoint of the embedding operator of H^s into L^2, (e.g., $J^1 = B^{-1}$ with $Bv := v - \Delta v$), a sufficient condition for (22) with $\nu = \frac{1}{2}$ is the existence of a $b \in L^2_{\mathbb{R}}(\mathbb{R}^d)$ such that

$$w := \frac{\mathcal{F}\left(\frac{1}{f} \cdot e^{i\phi} \left(b + i J^s(\phi^\dagger - \phi_0) \right) \right)}{2\mathcal{F}(f \cdot e^{i\phi})}$$

is real–valued and $\|w\|_{L^2}$ sufficiently small. If this is the case, then again the results in [21], [9], [7], imply the convergence rates

$$\|\phi_\alpha^\delta - \phi^\dagger\|_{H^s} = O(\sqrt{\delta})$$

with $\alpha \sim \delta$ for (8), or

$$\|\phi_N - \phi^\dagger\|_{H^s} = O(\sqrt{\delta})$$

with $\alpha_N \sim \delta$ for (27), (31), respectively.

Also (44) can probably be obtained if one (formally) sets

$$R(\phi) := \frac{1}{if} e^{-i\phi^\dagger} \mathcal{F}^{-1}\left(\frac{\mathcal{F}(f \cdot e^{i\phi})}{\mathcal{F}(f \cdot e^{i\phi^\dagger})}\, \mathcal{F}(i\,h\,f \cdot e^{i\phi}) \right).$$

Therefore, under some appropriate conditions on f, the theory presented in Section 2 about convergence and convergence rates for the iteratively regularized Gauß–Newton method (27) and the Landweber iteration (31) for the case $\nu < \frac{1}{2}$ in (22) should be applicable to the phase reconstruction problem considered in this Subsection, although it seems to be quite involved to verify (44) rigorously.

Appendix

We prove that under certain conditions (44) is fulfilled for the problem of reconstructing f from $|\mathcal{F}f|^2$ as considered in Subsection 3.1:

The most important assumption we make is that the Fourier transform $\mathcal{F}f^\dagger$ of a solution $f^\dagger$ of (46) is known outside some set $[-N, N]$, where $N > 0$ is fixed. Then, assuming that $\mathcal{F}f^\dagger \in L^4_{\mathbb{C}}(\mathbb{R})$, we can re–define the problem with a slightly different operator:

$$\bar{F}(\tilde{f})(s) := |\mathcal{F}\tilde{f} + \psi|^2(s), \quad s \in \mathbb{R}, \quad \tilde{f} \in X,$$

with

$$X := \mathcal{F}^{-1} E\left(H^1_{\mathbb{C}}[0, N] \right),$$

where

$$(Ev)(s) := \begin{cases} v(s) & s \in [0, N] \\ v(-s) & s \in [-N, 0] \\ 0 & s \in \mathbb{R} \setminus [-N, N] \end{cases},$$

$$\psi := \mathcal{F}f^\dagger \cdot \chi_{\mathbb{R} \setminus [-N, N]},$$

(note that ψ is know according to our assumption,) and X is equipped with the inner product

$$\langle \tilde{f}_1, \tilde{f}_2 \rangle_X := 2\Re \left(\int_0^N (\mathcal{F}\tilde{f}_1)(s)\overline{(\mathcal{F}\tilde{f}_2)(s)} + (\mathcal{F}\tilde{f}_1)(s)'\overline{(\mathcal{F}\tilde{f}_2)'(s)} ds \right)$$

which on X is just the $L^{1,2}$ inner product; as can be easily seen, X is in fact a subset of $L_{\mathbb{R}}^{1,2}(\mathbb{R})$, especially, all functions in X are real–valued due to the symmetry property $v(-s) = \overline{v(s)}$ of the elements v of $E(H_{\mathbb{C}}^1[0, N])$. The Fréchet derivative of $\tilde{F}$ and its adjoint are given by

$$\tilde{F}'(\tilde{f})h = 2\Re \left((\mathcal{F}\tilde{f} + \psi)\overline{\mathcal{F}h} \right),$$
$$\tilde{F}'(\tilde{f})^* z = \mathcal{F}^{-1}B^{-1} \left((\mathcal{F}\tilde{f} + \psi)(z + z(-\cdot)) \right),$$

where

$$B : H_{\mathbb{C}}^1(\mathbb{R}) \to H_{\mathbb{C}}^1(\mathbb{R})^*$$
$$v \mapsto v - v''.$$

Therefore, (22) with $\nu = \frac{1}{2}$ holds if there exists a sufficiently small $w \in L_{\mathbb{R}}^2(\mathbb{R})$ such that

$$w(s) + w(-s) = \begin{cases} \dfrac{(\mathcal{F}(f^\dagger - \tilde{f}_0))(s) - (\mathcal{F}(f^\dagger - \tilde{f}_0))''(s)}{\mathcal{F}f^\dagger(s)} & s \in [-N, N] \\ 0 & s \in \mathbb{R} \setminus [-N, N] \end{cases},$$

which is e.g. the case if there exists a real–valued function $\Phi \in L_{\mathbb{R}}^2(\mathbb{R})$ (sufficiently near to the characteristic function on $[-N, N]$) such that

$$(\mathcal{F}f^\dagger)''(s) = \Phi(s)(\mathcal{F}f^\dagger)(s), \qquad s \in [-N, N],$$

since then one can set $\tilde{f}_0 :\equiv 0$ and

$$w := \frac{1}{2}(\chi_{[0, N]} - \Phi).$$

If $|\mathcal{F}f^\dagger|$ is bounded away from zero on $[-N, N]$, i.e. $|\mathcal{F}f^\dagger|(s) \geq \kappa > 0$, $s \in [-N, N]$, and $(\mathcal{F}f^\dagger)|_{[-N, N]} \in H_{\mathbb{C}}^1([-N, N])$, then one can also prove that

$$\tilde{F}'(\tilde{f}) = \tilde{F}'(\tilde{f}^\dagger)R(\tilde{f}) \qquad \tilde{f} \in X, \tag{51}$$
$$\|R(\tilde{f}) - I\| \leq C_R \|\tilde{f} - \tilde{f}^\dagger\|$$

where $\tilde{f}^\dagger := \mathcal{F}^{-1}(\mathcal{F}f^\dagger \cdot \chi_{[-N, N]})$, holds with

$$R(\tilde{f})h := \mathcal{F}^{-1}\left(\frac{\mathcal{F}\tilde{f}}{\mathcal{F}f^\dagger} \cdot \mathcal{F}h \right) :$$

Due to

$$\frac{(\mathcal{F}\tilde{f})(-s)}{(\mathcal{F}f^{\dagger})(-s)} \cdot (\mathcal{F}h)(-s) = \overline{\frac{(\mathcal{F}\tilde{f})(s)}{(\mathcal{F}f^{\dagger})(s)} \cdot (\mathcal{F}h)(s)},$$

we have that $R(\tilde{f})h \in X$ if $\frac{\mathcal{F}\tilde{f}}{\mathcal{F}f^{\dagger}} \cdot \mathcal{F}h \cdot \chi_{[0,N]} \in H^1_{\mathbb{C}}(\mathbb{R})$, which is the case since

$$\begin{aligned}
\left\| \tfrac{\mathcal{F}\tilde{f}}{\mathcal{F}f^{\dagger}} \cdot \mathcal{F}h \right\|_{L^2} &\leq \tfrac{1}{\kappa} \| \mathcal{F}\tilde{f} \|_{L^\infty} \| \mathcal{F}h \|_{L^2} \\
&\leq \tfrac{C}{\kappa} \| \tilde{f} \|_X \| h \|_{L^2}
\end{aligned} \tag{52}$$

and

$$\begin{aligned}
\left\| \tfrac{d}{ds} \left(\tfrac{\mathcal{F}\tilde{f}}{\mathcal{F}f^{\dagger}} \cdot \mathcal{F}h \right) \right\|_{L^2} &\leq \tfrac{1}{\kappa} \| (\mathcal{F}\tilde{f})' \|_{L^2} \| \mathcal{F}h \|_{L^\infty} \\
&\quad + \tfrac{2}{\kappa^2} \| (\mathcal{F}\tilde{f}) \|_{L^\infty} \| (\mathcal{F}f^{\dagger})' \cdot \chi_{[0,N]} \|_{L^2} \| \mathcal{F}h \|_{L^\infty} \\
&\quad + \tfrac{1}{\kappa} \| \mathcal{F}\tilde{f} \|_{L^\infty} \| (\mathcal{F}h)' \|_{L^2} \\
&\leq \tfrac{C}{\kappa} (1 + \tfrac{1}{\kappa} \| \tilde{f}^{\dagger} \|_X) \| \tilde{f} \|_X \| h \|_X .
\end{aligned} \tag{53}$$

Analogously to (52), (53) one can show that (51) holds for some C_R depending only on $\| \tilde{f}^{\dagger} \|_X$.

From this we can conclude that, due to the results in Section 2, the iteratively regularized Gauß–Newton method (27) as well as the Landweber type iteration (31), applied to the phase reconstruction problem of Subsection 3.1, are convergent regularization methods and, under an additional condition (22), yield the respective convergence rates.

References

1. R. ACAR, C.R. VOGEL, *Analysis of total variation penalty methods*, Inverse Problems 10 (1994), 1217–1229.

2. A.B. BAKUSHINSKII, *The problem of the convergence of the iteratively regularized Gauss–Newton method*, Comput.Math.Math.Phys. 32 (1992), 1353–1359.

3. A.B. BAKUSHINSKII, *Iterative methods for solving non-linear operator equations in the absence of regularity. A new approach.*, Russian Acad.Sci.Dokl.Math. 47 (1993), 451–454.

4. A.B. BAKUSHINSKII AND A.V. GONCHARSKII, *Iterative Methods for the Solution of Incorrect Problems*, Nauka, Moscow, 1989. In Russian.

5. A. BINDER, M. HANKE, O. SCHERZER *On the Landweber iteration for nonlinear ill-posed problems*, to appear in J.Inverse and Ill-Posed Problems.

6. A. BINDER, H.W. ENGL, C.W. GROETSCH, A. NEUBAUER, AND O. SCHERZER, *Weakly closed nonlinear operators and parameter identification in parabolic equations by Tikhonov regularization*, Applicable Analysis 55 (1994), 215–234.

7. B. BLASCHKE, *Some Newton type methods for the solution of nonlinear ill-posed problems*, PhD thesis, Johannes Kepler Universität Linz, 1996.

8. B. BLASCHKE, H.W. ENGL, W. GREVER, M. KLIBANOV, *An application of Tikhonov regularization to phase retrieval*, to appear in Nonlinear World.

9. B. BLASCHKE, A. NEUBAUER, AND O. SCHERZER, *On convergence rates for the iteratively regularized Gauß–Newton method*, to appear in IMA J. Numer. Anal.

10. H. BRAKHAGE, *On ill-posed problems and the method of conjugate gradients*, in [19], 165–175.

11. G. CHAVENT, K. KUNISCH, *On weakly nonlinear ill-posed problems*, to appear in SIAM J. Appl. Math. (1996).

12. K. CHADAN AND P.C. SABATIER, *Inverse Problems in Quantum Scattering Theory*, Springer, New York, 1989.

13. D. COLTON AND R. KRESS, *Integral Equation Methods in Scattering Theory*, Wiley, New York, 1983.

14. D. COLTON AND R. KRESS, *Inverse Acoustic and Electromagnetic Scattering Theory*, Springer, Berlin, 1992.

15. D.C. DOBSON, *Phase reconstruction via nonlinear least-squares*, Inverse Problems 8 (1992), 541-557.

16. B. EICKE, *Iteration methods for convexly constrained ill-posed problems in Hilbert space*, Numer. Funct. Anal. Optim. 13 (1992), 413-429.

17. B. EICKE, A.K. LOUIS, R. PLATO, *The instability of some gradient methods for ill-posed problems*, Numer. Math. 58 (1990), 129-134.

18. H.W. ENGL, H. GFRERER, *A posteriori parameter choice for general regularization methods for solving linear ill-posed problems*, Appl. Numer. Math. 4 (1988), 395-417.

19. H.W. ENGL, C.W. GROETSCH (eds.), *Inverse and Ill-Posed Problems*, Academic Press, Orlando, 1987.

20. H.W. ENGL, M. HANKE, A. NEUBAUER, *Regularization of Inverse Problems*, Kluwer, Dordrecht, 1996.

21. H.W. ENGL, K. KUNISCH, A. NEUBAUER, *Convergence rates for Tikhonov regularization of nonlinear ill-posed problems*, Inverse Problems 5 (1989), 523-540.

22. H.W. ENGL, G. LANDL, *Convergence rates for maximum entropy regularization*, SIAM J. Numer. Anal. 30 (1993), 1509-1536.

23. H.W. ENGL, A. NEUBAUER, *Convergence rates for Tikhonov regularization of implicitly defined nonlinear inverse problems with an application to inverse scattering*, in: S.Kubo, ed., Inverse Problems, Techn. Publ. Atlanta, 1993, 90-98.

24. H.W. ENGL, W. RUNDELL, O. SCHERZER, *A regularization scheme for an inverse problem in age-structured populations*, J. Math. Anal. Appl. 182 (1994), 658-679.

25. H.W. ENGL, O. SCHERZER, M. YAMAMOTO, *Uniqueness and stable determination of forcing terms in linear partial differential equations with overspecified boundary data*, Inverse Problems 10 (1994), 1253-1276.

26. H. GFRERER, *An a posteriori parameter choice for ordinary and iterated Tikhonov regularization of ill-posed problems leading to optimal convergence rates*, Math. of Comp. 49 (1987) 507-522 and S5-S12.

27. C.W. GROETSCH, *The Theory of Tikhonov Regularization for Fredholm Equations of the First Kind*, Pitman, Boston, 1984.

28. C.W. GROETSCH, *Inverse Problems in Mathematical Sciences*, Vieweg, Braunschweig, 1993.

29. M. HANKE, *Accelerated Landweber iterations for the solution of ill-posed equations*, Numer. Math. 60 (1991), 341-373.

30. M. HANKE, H.W. ENGL, *An optimal stopping rule for the ν-methods for solving ill-posed problems using Christoffel functions*, J. Approx. Theory 79 (1994), 89-108.

31. M. HANKE, F. HETTLICH, O. SCHERZER, *The Landweber iteration for an inverse scattering problem*, in: in K.-W. Wang et al., eds., Proceedings of the 1995 Design Engineering Technical Conferences, Vol. 3, Part C, Vibration Control, Analysis, and Identification, The Americal Society of Mechanical Engineers, New York, 1995, 909-915.

32. M. HANKE, A. NEUBAUER, AND O. SCHERZER, *A convergence analysis of the Landweber iteration for nonlinear ill-posed problems*, Numer. Math. 72 (1995), 21–37.

33. F. HETTLICH, J. MORGAN, O. SCHERZER, *On the estimation of interfaces from boundary measurements*, to appear in: Proceedings of the SIAM conference "Symposion on Inverse Problems: Geophysical Applications", Yosemite, USA 1995.

34. B. HOFMANN AND O. SCHERZER, *Influence factors of ill-posedness for nonlinear problems*, Inverse Problems 10 (1994), 1277–1297.

35. N.E. HURT, *Phase Retrieval and Zero Crossings*, Kluwer, Dordrecht, 1989.

36. V. ISAKOV, *Inverse Source Problems*, Math. Surveys and Monographs 34, Amer. Math. Soc., Providence, 1990.

37. M.V. KLIBANOV, J. MALINSKY , *Newton-Kantorovich method for three-dimensional potential inverse scattering problem and stability of the hyperbolic Cauchy problem with time-dependent data*, Inverse Problems 7 (1991), 577–596.

38. M.V. KLIBANOV AND P.E. SACKS, *Phaseless inverse scattering and the phase problem in optics*, J. Math. Phys. 33 (1992), 3913–3821.

39. M.V. KLIBANOV AND P.E. SACKS, *Use of partial knowledge of the potential in the phase problem of inverse scattering*, J. Comput. Phys. 112 (1994), 273–281.

40. M.V. KLIBANOV, P.E. SACKS AND A.V. TIKHONRAVOV, *The phase retrieval problem*, Inverse Problems 11 (1995), 1–28.

41. R. KOHN , A. MCKENNEY, *Numerical implementation of a variational method for electrical impedance tomography*, Inverse Problems 6 (1990), 389-414

42. C. KRAVARIS AND J.H. SEINFELD, *Identification of parameters in distributed parameter systems by regularization*, SIAM J. Contr. and Optimiz. 23 (1985), 217–241.

43. R. KRESS AND W. RUNDELL, *A quasi–Newton method in inverse obstacle scattering*, Inverse Problems 10 (1994), 1145–1158.

44. K. KUNISCH, W. RING, *Regularization of nonlinear illposed problems with closed operators*, Num. Func. Anal. Optim. 14 (1993), 389-404.

45. G. LANDL, R.S. ANDERSSEN, *Non–negative differentially constrained entropy–like regularization*, Inverse Problems 12 (1996), 35–53.

46. L. LANDWEBER, *An iteration formula for Fredholm integral equations of the first kind*, Amer. J. Math. 73 (1951), 615–624.

47. A. K. LOUIS, *Convergence of the conjugate gradient method for compact operators*, in [19], 177–183.

48. A. K. LOUIS, *Inverse und schlecht gestellte Probleme*, Teubner, Stuttgart, 1989.

49. A.K. LOUIS, *Parametric reconstruction in biomagnetic imaging*, in: M. Bertero, E.R. Pike, eds., Inverse Problems in Scattering and Imaging, Hilger, Bristol, 1992, 156-163.

50. V.A. MOROZOV, *On the solution of the functional equations by the method of regularization*, Sov. Math. Dokl. 7 (1966), 414-417.

51. V.A. MOROZOV, *Methods for Solving Incorrectly Posed Problems*, Springer, New York, 1984.

52. V.A. MOROZOV, *Regularization Methods for Ill-Posed Problems*, CRC Press, Boca Raton, 1993.

53. A. NEUBAUER, *Tikhonov regularization for non–linear ill–posed problems: optimal convergence rates and finite–dimensional approximation*, Inverse Problems 5 (1989), 541-557.

54. A. NEUBAUER, *Tikhonov regularization for non–linear ill–posed problems in Hilbert scales*, Applicable Analysis 46 (1992), 59-72.

55. P. SACKS, F. SANTOSA, *A simple computational scheme for determing the sound speed of an acoustic medium from surface impulse response*, SIAM J. Scient. Stat. Comput. 8 (1987), 501-520

56. O. SCHERZER, *A convergence analysis of a method of steepest descent and a two-step algorithm for nonlinear ill-posed problems*, to appear in Num. Func. Anal. Optim.

57. O. SCHERZER, *Convergence criteria of iterative methods based on Landweber iteration for solving nonlinear problems*, J. Math. Anal. Appl. 194 (1995), 911-933.

58. O. SCHERZER, *A modified Landweber iteration for solving parameter estimation problems*, to appear in: Appl. Math. Optim.

59. O. SCHERZER, *The use of Tikhonov regularization in the identification of electrical conductivities from overdetermined boundary data*, Results of Math. 22 (1992), 598-618.

60. O. SCHERZER, H.W. ENGL, R.S. ANDERSSEN, *Parameter identification from boundary measurements in a parabolic equation arising from geophysics*, Nonlinear Anal. 20 (1993), 127-156.

61. O. SCHERZER, H.W. ENGL, K. KUNISCH, *Optimal a-posteriori parameter choice for Tikhonov regularization for solving nonlinear ill-posed problems*, SIAM J. Numer. Anal. 30 (1993), 1796-1838.

62. E. SCHOCK, *Approximate solution of ill-posed equations: arbitrarily slow convergence vs. superconvergence*, in: G. Hämmerlin, K. H. Hoffmann, eds., Constructive Methods for the Practical Treatment of Integral Equations, Birkhäuser, Basel, 1985, 234-243.

63. T. SEIDMAN, C.R. VOGEL, *Well posedness and convergence for some regularisation methods for non-linear ill posed problems*, Inverse Problems 5 (1989), 227-238.

64. A.N. TIKHONOV, V.A. ARSENIN, *Methods for Solving Ill-Posed Problems*, Nauka, Moscow, 1979.

65. G.M. VAINIKKO, A.Y. VETERENNIKOV, *Iteration Procedures in Ill-Posed Problems*, Nauka, Moscow, 1986. In Russian.

66. V.V. VASIN, *Iterative methods for solving ill-posed problems with a priori information in Hilbert spaces*, USSR Comput. Math. Math. Phys. 28 (1988), 6-13.

Qualitative Methods in Inverse Scattering Theory*

David L. Colton

Department of Mathematical Sciences, University of Delaware, Newark, Delaware 19716, U.S.A.

I. Introduction

A major problem in the use of ultrasound or microwaves for purposes of non-destructive testing or medical imaging is the computational complexity of solving the inverse scattering problem that arises in such applications. This is due to the fact that in order to achieve satisfactory resolution and sufficient penetration of the wave into the material it is often necessary to use frequencies in the resonance region. In this case the inverse scattering problem is not only improperly posed but also nonlinear and even in the case of two dimensions the time needed to solve such problems can be prohibitive. To date the time consuming nature of the problem has mainly been dealt with by the introduction of various innovative schemes that avoid the use of volume integral equations and instead rely on finite difference or finite element methods (c.f. [5], [8]). However, for large scale problems (for example those involving imaging of the human body) the problem of computational complexity remains a serious problem for any practitioner. In this paper we would like to propose a different approach to this problem that, although still in its infancy, has the promise of providing rapid solutions to a number of inverse scattering problems of practical significance.

The approach we have in mind is based on the fact that a complete reconstruction of the scattering object is often far more than is needed. For example, in the case of the detection and location of tumors in the body by microwaves, all that is needed is to determine if there are in fact tumors present and if so what is the support of the tumors. The actual value of the index of refraction in the tumor is, by comparison, of little interest. Similarly, if there are flaws in a material (e.g. a crack) the fact that such flaws exist and determining an estimate of their size is the most important consideration rather than a complete reconstruction of the sound speed or refractive index inside the flaw. Hence, having simple methods to determine the qualitative properties of a penetrable scatterer such as bounds on the index of refraction or the support of the scatterer would be highly desirable. The purpose of this paper is to suggest methods for doing

* This research was supported in part by a grant from the Air Force Office of Scientific Research.

this. Motivated by problems in the use of microwaves in medical imaging ([5]), we will restrict our attention to time harmonic waves with fixed frequency in the resonance region.

For the sake of simplicity and to fix our ideas, we consider the two dimensional scalar problem of determining u from the equations

$$\Delta_2 u + k^2 n(x) u = 0 \text{ in } R^2 \tag{1}$$

$$u(x) = e^{ikx \cdot d} + u^s(x) \tag{2}$$

$$\lim_{r \to \infty} \sqrt{r} \left(\frac{\partial u^s}{\partial r} - iku^s \right) = 0 \tag{3}$$

where $x \in R^2$, $r = |x|$, $k > 0$ is the wave number and d is a vector on the unit circle Ω in R^2. The index of refraction n is assumed to be piecewise continuously differentiable such that

$$m : 1 - n \tag{4}$$

has compact support and the *Sommerfeld radiation condition* (3) is assumed to hold uniformly with respect to $\hat{x} = x/|x|$. It is relatively easy to show that there exists a unique solution to (1)-(3) (c.f. [3]) for the case of smooth $n(x)$, $x \in R^3$) and that the scattered field u^s has the asymptotic behavior

$$u^s(x) = \frac{e^{ikr}}{\sqrt{r}} u_\infty(\hat{x}; d) + O(r^{-3/2}) \tag{5}$$

as $r = |x| \to \infty$ where u_∞ is known as the *far field pattern* of the scattered field.

In this paper we will address three problems associated with the inverse scattering problem of determining $n(x)$ from $u_\infty(\hat{x}; d)$. The first question is how much information can, in principle, be determined from $u_\infty(\hat{x}; d)$? Although striking progress for the case of the impedance tomography problem in R^2 has recently been made by Nachman ([7]), uniqueness of a solution to the inverse scattering problem in R^2 at fixed frequency is unknown. The second problem we will address is that of determining an estimate of the magnitude of the index of refraction from a knowledge of u_∞ or, more specifically, from a knowledge of the eigenvalues of the *far field operator* $F : L^2(\Omega) \to L^2(\Omega)$ defined by

$$(Fg)(\hat{x}) := \int_\Omega u_\infty(\hat{x}; d) g(d) ds(d). \tag{6}$$

Finally, we will show how the support of $m = 1 - n$ can be determined by solving the set of linear integral equations of the first kind

$$(Fg)(\hat{x}) = e^{-ik\hat{x} \cdot y_0} \tag{7}$$

where y_0 is on a rectangular grid known a priori to contain the support of m in its interior. In our view, these last two problems represent promising first steps towards the goal of extracting qualitative information about the index of refraction from a knowledge of fixed frequency scattering data and we hope such progress will encourage others to contribute to this new area of inverse scattering theory.

II. Uniqueness Theorems

Suppose $u_\infty(\hat{x}; d)$ is known exactly for a fixed wave number k and all $\hat{x}, d$ on the unit circle Ω. Does this knowledge uniquely determine any specific property of the index of refraction n? Note that, in contrast to the three dimensional case, the problem is not over-determined, i.e. $n(x)$ and $u_\infty(\hat{x}; d)$ are both functions of two independent variables and, as stated in the Introduction, it is not known if u_∞ uniquely determines n. However, Sun and Uhlmann ([11]) have shown that the *discontinuities* of n are uniquely determined by u_∞:

Theorem:(Sun-Uhlmann): Let n_1, n_2 be in $L^\infty(R^2)$ and suppose $m_1 = 1 - n_1$ and $m_2 = 1 - n_2$ have compact support. Then if u_∞^j is the far field pattern corresponding to n_j and $u_\infty^1(\hat{x}; d) = u_\infty^2(\hat{x}; d)$ for all $\hat{x}, d \in \Omega$, then $n_1 - n_2 \in C^\alpha(R^2)$ for every α, $0 \leq \alpha < 1$.

Although uniqueness of the inverse scattering problem is not known for fixed k, if $u_\infty^1(\hat{x}; d) = u_\infty^2(\hat{x}; d)$ for $\hat{x}, d \in \Omega$ and an *interval* of k values then it is relatively easy to show that $n_1 = n_2$. Since the proof of this fact does not appear to be in the literature, we include it here, noting that the proof closely follows that of Karp's theorem given in [1].

Theorem: The index of refraction n is uniquely determined by a knowledge of the far field pattern $u_\infty(\hat{x}; d)$ for $\hat{x}, d \in \Omega$ and an interval of values of k.

Proof: If u_∞ is the far field pattern corresponding to u', then from Green's formula we can deduce that ([1])

$$u_\infty(\hat{x}; d) = -e^{i\pi/4}\sqrt{\frac{k^3}{8\pi}} \int\int_B e^{-ik\hat{x}\cdot y} m(y) u(y; d) dy \tag{8}$$

where B is a ball centered at the origin of radius a containing the support of $m = 1 - n$. Hence, if $u_\infty^1 = u_\infty^2$ for an interval of k values, then by the analyticity of u as a function of k for $k > 0$ and the Jacobi-Anger expansion of $e^{-ik\hat{x}\cdot y}$ we see from (8) that

$$\int\int_B J_p(k\rho)e^{ip\varphi}[m_1(y)u_1(y; d) - m_2(y)u_2(y; d)]dy = 0 \tag{9}$$

for all $k > 0$, $p = 0, \pm 1, \pm 2, \cdots$, where $y = (\rho\cos\varphi, \rho\sin\varphi)$, J_p is a Bessel function of order p and B contains the support of m_1 and m_2.

We now note that

$$\lim_{k\to 0} k^{-p} J_p(kr) = r^p/2^p p! , \qquad p \geq 0 \tag{10}$$

$$J_{-p}(kr) = (-1)^p J_p(kr)$$

and, using the integral equation formulation of the scattering problem (1)–(3), we can deduce that ([1])

$$\frac{1}{2\pi}\int_{-\pi}^\pi u(x; d)e^{iq\alpha}d\alpha = i^q J_q(kr)e^{iq\theta}[1 + O(k^2 \log k)] \tag{11}$$

where $d = (\cos \alpha, \sin \alpha)$ and $x = (r \cos \theta, r \sin \theta)$. Hence, multiplying (9) by $e^{iq\alpha}$, integrating from $-\pi$ to π, dividing by $k^{|p|+|q|}$ and then letting k tend to zero now shows that

$$\iint_B [m_1(y) - m_2(y)]\rho^{|p|+|q|} e^{i(p+q)\varphi} dy = 0 \tag{12}$$

for $p, q = 0, \pm 1, \pm 2, \cdots$.

To complete the proof, we expand $m_1 - m_2$ in a Fourier series

$$m_1(\rho, \varphi) - m_2(\rho, \varphi) = \sum_{l=-\infty}^{\infty} a_l(\rho) e^{il\varphi} \tag{13}$$

and choose p and q such that $p + q = -l$ for some fixed integer l. Then from (12) and (13) we have that

$$\int_0^a \rho^{|p|+|l+p|+1} a_l(\rho) d\rho = 0 \tag{14}$$

for all integers p. By Muntz's theorem ([6]) we can now conclude that $a_l = 0$ for all integers l and hence from (13) that $m_1 = m_2$. Thus $n_1 = n_2$ and the proof is complete.

III. Estimating the Index of Refraction

We will now attempt to obtain information about the magnitude of the index of refraction from a knowledge of the eigenvalues of the far field operator F under the assumption that $Im\, n(x) > 0$ for x in the support of $m = 1 - n$, i.e. the scattering object is a conductor. Since the eigenvalues of F are readily computable using the measured far field data, they are appropriate numbers to use as "target signatures". Unfortunately, since $Im\, n$ is not zero, the far field operator is no longer a normal operator as it is in the case when $Im\, n = 0$ and hence we cannot immediately claim that eigenvalues of F exist. However, due to the smoothness of u_∞ (c.f. (8)), we can conclude that the far field operator F is a trace class operator and in this case we have the following theorem due to Lidskii ([9]):

Theorem (Lidskii): Let $T : L^2(\Omega) \to L^2(\Omega)$ be a trace class operator such that T has finite dimensional null space and $Im\,(Tg, g) \geq 0$ for every $g \in L^2(\Omega)$ where $(\cdot, \cdot)$ denotes the inner product on $L^2(\Omega)$. Then T has an infinite number of nonzero eigenvalues (which, since T is compact, have the origin as their only point of accumulation).

In order to use Lidskii's theorem, we will need the following lemma due to Colton and Kress ([4]) where a *Herglotz wave function* with kernel g is a solution of the Helmholtz equation $\Delta_2 v + k^2 v = 0$ of the form

$$v(x) := \int_\Omega e^{ikx \cdot d} g(d) ds(d). \tag{15}$$

Lemma (Colton and Kress): Let v_g be the solution of (1)–(3) with $e^{ik\boldsymbol{x}\cdot\boldsymbol{d}}$ replaced by a Herglotz wave function with kernel g. Then

$$k^2 \iint\limits_D Im\, n |v_g|^2 d\boldsymbol{x} = \sqrt{8\pi k} Im(e^{-i\pi/4} Fg, g) - k\|Fg\|^2 \qquad (16)$$

where D is the support of $m = 1 - n$.

We want to use this lemma and Lidskii's theorem to deduce that the far field operator has an infinite number of nonzero eigenvalues. First suppose that $Fg = 0$. Then from the lemma and the fact that $Im\, n(\boldsymbol{x}) > 0$ for $\boldsymbol{x} \in D$ we have that $v_g(\boldsymbol{x}) = 0$ for $\boldsymbol{x} \in D$. Hence, the incident field given by (15) must vanish and from this we can deduce that $g = 0$. Thus F has a trivial null space. Since the lemma implies that $Im\,(e^{-i\,\pi/4} Fg, g) \geq 0$, we can now deduce from Lidskii's theorem that F has an infinite number of nonzero eigenvalues.

What information about $n(\boldsymbol{x})$ can be obtained from a knowledge of the eigenvalues of F? To answer this question, we first note that the lemma says that all the eigenvalues lie in the interior of the disk $\sqrt{8\pi k} Im(e^{-i\pi/4}\lambda) - k|\lambda|^2 = 0$. Furthermore, from (8), we can deduce that if $Fg = \lambda g$ then ([4])

$$k^2 \iint\limits_D Im\, n\, |v_g|^2 d\boldsymbol{x} \geq 4|\lambda|^2 \|g\|^2 \left(k \iint\limits_D \frac{|m|^2}{Im\, n} d\boldsymbol{x} \right)^{-1}. \qquad (17)$$

Now let r be the radius of the smallest circle with center on $Im\,\lambda = -Re\,\lambda$, $Im\,\lambda \geq 0$, and passing through the origin which contains all the eigenvalues of F. Then from (17) and the lemma we see that a knowledge of r provides a lower bound for the quantity

$$k \iint\limits_B \frac{|m|^2}{Im\, n} d\boldsymbol{x}. \qquad (18)$$

How useful this bound is of course depends on the particular problem that is being investigated. Improvements on the rather crude inequality (17) can in principle be made by taking into account the oscillatory nature of the kernel of the integral appearing in (8). It would be desirable to have an upper bound for the integral (18). Unfortunately, at the moment, it is not known how to do this.

IV. Determination of the Support of m

We conclude this paper by briefly indicating how the support D of $m = 1 - n$ can be determined from the far field pattern u_∞ by solving the set of linear integral equations

$$(Fg)(\hat{\boldsymbol{x}}) = e^{-ik\hat{\boldsymbol{x}}\cdot\boldsymbol{y}_o} \qquad (19)$$

where y_o is on a rectangular grid known a priori to contain the support of m in its interior. We again assume that $Im\, n(\boldsymbol{x}) > 0$ for $\boldsymbol{x} \in D$ and furthermore that ∂D is smooth. Further technical assumptions, proofs and numerical examples can be found in [2].

The basic idea of the method is to try and find a superposition of plane waves such that the scattered field corresponding to this superposition is a constant multiple of a point source $\Phi(\cdot; y_0)$ located at a point $y_0 \in D$. Since the scattered field is uniquely determined by its far field pattern ([3]), it suffices to have the far field pattern corresponding to this superposition agree with a constant multiple of the far field pattern of $\Phi(\cdot; y_0)$. In particular, if

$$\Phi(x; y_0) = H_0^{(1)}(k|x - y_0|), \quad x \neq y_0 \tag{20}$$

where $H_0^{(1)}$ is a Hankel function of the first kind of order zero then, since $\Phi(\cdot; y_0)$ has a far field pattern given by $\gamma e^{-ik\hat{x}\cdot y_0}$ where

$$\gamma = \sqrt{\frac{2}{\pi k}}\, e^{-i\pi/4}, \tag{21}$$

we want to find a function $g(\cdot; y_0) \in L^2(\Omega)$ such that (19) is satisfied. This can be done if and only if there exists a function w and Herglotz wave function v with kernel $g = g(\cdot; y_0)$ such that w and v satisfy the *interior transmission problem* ([3], [10])

$$\triangle_2 w + k^2 n(x)w = 0 \qquad\qquad \text{in } D \tag{22}$$

$$\triangle_2 v + k^2 v = 0$$

$$w - v = \gamma^{-1} H_0^{(1)}(k|x - y_0|) \qquad \text{on } \partial D \tag{23}$$

$$\frac{\partial}{\partial\nu}(w - v) = \gamma^{-1}\frac{\partial}{\partial\nu}H_0^{(1)}(k|x - y_0|)$$

where ν is the unit outward normal to ∂D. We would like to conclude that, on ∂D, v becomes unbounded as y_0 tends to ∂D (and hence so does $\|g\|_{L^2(\Omega)}$).

Unfortunately, the solution v of (22), (23) is not in general a Herglotz wave function. Even if it is, it is not clear that v (and hence $\|g\|_{L^2(\Omega)}$) becomes unbounded as y_0 tends to ∂D. However, under certain technical assumptions, it was shown in [2] that for every $\epsilon > 0$ and $y_0 \in D\backslash\partial D$ there exists a function $g(\cdot; y_0) \in L^2(\Omega)$ such that

$$\|(Fg)(\hat{x}) - e^{-ik\hat{x}\cdot y_0}\|_{L^2(\Omega)} < \epsilon \tag{24}$$

and

$$\lim_{y_0 \to \partial D} \|g(\cdot; y_0)\|_{L^2(\Omega)} = \infty. \tag{25}$$

From this it can be deduced that if the integral equation (19) is solved (using an appropriate regularization method) then an approximation to ∂D can be found by determining those values of y_0 for which $\|g(\cdot; y_0)\|_{L^2(\Omega)}$ becomes large. Note that this method is a *linear* method and makes no statement about the *values* of the index of refraction in D. The only quantity which is determined is ∂D.

An intriguing and somewhat delicate feature of this approach for determining ∂D is that it makes a very explicit use of the improperly posed nature of the inverse scattering problem by looking for a solution of the improperly posed integral equation of the first kind (19) that becomes unbounded as y_o tends to ∂D. In particular, the regularization method used to solve (19) must allow for the fact that the solution is in fact unbounded as y_o tends to ∂D, e.g. the penalty term in the Tikhonov regularization method should involve the derivative of g rather than g itself.

References

1. D. Colton and A. Kirsch, Karp's theorem in acoustic scattering theory, *Proc. Amer. Math. Soc.* 103 (1988), 783–788.
2. D. Colton and A. Kirsch, A simple method for solving inverse scattering problems in the resonance region, submitted for publication.
3. D. Colton and R. Kress, *Inverse Acoustic and Electromagnetic Scattering Theory*, Springer-Verlag, Berlin, 1992.
4. D. Colton and R. Kress, Eigenvalues of the far field operator for the Helmholtz equation in an absorbing medium, *SIAM J. Appl. Math* 55 (1995), 1724–1735.
5. D. Colton and P. Monk, A new approach to detecting leukemia: using computational electromagnetics, *Computational Sciences and Engineering* 2 (1995), 46–52.
6. P.J. Davis, *Interpolation and Approximation*, Dover, New York, 1975.
7. A. Nachman, Global uniqueness for a two dimensional inverse boundary value problem, *Annals of Mathematics* 143 (1996), 71–96.
8. F. Natterer and F. Wübbeling, A propagation-backpropagation method for ultrasound tomography, *Inverse Problems* 11 (1995), 1225–1232.
9. J. Ringrose, *Compact Non-Self Adjoint Operators*, Van Nostrand Reinhold, London, 1971.
10. B.P. Rynne and B.D. Sleeman, The interior transmission problem and inverse scattering from inhomogeneous media, *SIAM J. Math. Anal.* 22 (1991), 1755–1762.
11. Z. Sun and G. Uhlmann, Recovery of singularities for formally determined inverse problems, *Comm. Math. Physics* 153 (1993), 431–445.

Recovery of Blocky Images in Electrical Impedance Tomography

David C. Dobson

Department of Mathematics, Texas A&M University, College Station, TX 77843-3368
USA

1 Introduction

The techniques of electrical impedance tomography (EIT) have been widely
studied over the past several years, for applications in both medical imaging
and nondestructive evaluation. The goal is to find the electrical conductivity of
a spatially inhomogeneous medium inside a given domain, using electrostatic
measurements collected at the boundary.

One of the primary difficulties with EIT is the instability of the reconstruction problem. This instability has been characterized in various ways by studying
linearized problems [1, 11, 15]. In essence, the difficulty is that the measured data
are very insensitive to certain features in the conductivity profile. For instance,
two profiles that differ primarily in the high-frequency Fourier components may
yield boundary data that are nearly indistinguishable in the presence of measurement noise. This is a manifestation of the information content of the data.
Any reconstruction procedure will be unstable to data errors unless the problem
is properly regularized. Unfortunately, most common regularization techniques
yield reconstructed conductivity images that are often smeared, blurred, or otherwise distorted.

In an effort to reduce the blurring effect, an "image enhancement" technique
was applied to the linearized EIT problem in [13]. The technique is essentially a
nonlinear regularization by total variation, following ideas introduced by Rudin,
Osher, and Fatemi [23] for image denoising. Measuring the total variation has
long been recognized as an effective way to quantify the "simplicity" of a given
signal or function. It measures the oscillations of a given function, but still admits
discontinuities. Ideas incorporating total variation based methods in reconstruction problems have been used successfully in applications such as image reconstruction [5, 6, 7, 8, 17, 22, 23, 24, 27], inverse problems [25, 26], and optimal
design [11].

The motivation for [13] was to try to incorporate *a priori* information about
the unknown conductivity into the problem formulation. The *a priori* information is roughly the knowledge that the unknown conductivity is "blocky". By
"blocky" we mean that the conductivity is a piecewise constant function for

which the set of discontinuities has relatively small measure in codimension 1. Such conductivity functions have small total variation, provided the discontinuities are not large. The problem is formulated as that of finding the conductivity of minimal total variation which fits the data. The conductivity reconstructions obtained in [13] were very good for blocky images. However as with other known techniques, reconstructions of fine details and highly oscillatory features were difficult or impossible to achieve.

One of the key questions arising from the work in [13] is: how does one characterize the set of images which can be recovered reasonably well by minimization of total variation? This question was explored in a general context of linear image processing problems in [14]. As will be outlined in the present paper, the results have some relevance to EIT and give some insight into the kinds of results one can expect.

In this paper we describe some aspects of the application of total variation minimization techniques to the linearized EIT problem. In Section 2, we formulate a reconstruction problem, describing one approach to total variation regularization by constrained minimization. In Section 3, a stabilization strategy for the constraints is described. Section 4 discusses some results on characterizing conductivity images which can be completely recovered, under the assumption that the instability in the problem is restricted to a limited range of frequency components in the image. Section 5 motivates other conditions which are favorable for recovering images when the instabilities are not bandlimited. In Section 6 we describe a very simple minimization scheme for the constrained regularized problem. Finally, some representative numerical results are presented in Section 7.

2 EIT and Minimal Total Variation Regularization

Given some domain $\Omega \subset \mathbb{R}^d$, $d = 2$ or 3, the idealized model problem is to find the conductivity distribution in the interior of Ω from electrostatic measurements on the boundary $\partial\Omega$. In all of the following, we assume $d = 2$. A spatially distributed current flux density pattern f which satisfies $\int_{\partial\Omega} f = 0$ is applied to $\partial\Omega$. The voltage potential u inside Ω then satisfies

$$\nabla \cdot (\sigma \nabla u) = 0 \quad \text{in } \Omega, \tag{1a}$$

where σ is the conductivity of the medium, with the Neumann boundary condition

$$\sigma \frac{\partial u}{\partial \nu} = f \quad \text{on } \partial\Omega. \tag{1b}$$

With the additional normalization constraint $\int_{\partial\Omega} u = 0$, and the assumption that $\sigma \in L^\infty(\Omega)$ is uniformly bounded away from zero, equations (1) uniquely determine the voltage potential u.

For every "current pattern" f, we measure the corresponding voltage potential u on the boundary $\partial\Omega$. Hence, the data in the ideal problem can be viewed as the so-called Neumann-to-Dirichlet map $\Lambda(\sigma; f)$ which takes current patterns to voltage measurements, defined by $\Lambda(\sigma; f) = u|_{\partial\Omega}$, where u satisfies (1). The operator Λ is linear in f but nonlinear in σ.

It is infeasible in practice to measure all of $u|_{\partial\Omega}$. Instead, one generally obtains a finite number of "samples" of u on $\partial\Omega$. For a given current pattern f, let us assume that rather than measuring all of $u|_{\partial\Omega}$, we have access to the finite set of measurements

$$g_i = \int_{\partial\Omega} uq_i \quad i = 1, \ldots, m, \tag{2}$$

where u satisfies (1). Each distribution $q_i \in H^{-1/2}(\partial\Omega)$ can be chosen to represent a measurement process. For example, the q_i's could be concentrated at m distinct points on $\partial\Omega$ to approximate a set of point measurements, or concentrated on a set of characteristic functions to approximate spatially averaged measurements. Naturally, one would wish to choose the q_i's to be orthogonal, or at least linearly independent.

The forward map, which we denote $F(\sigma; f)$, can then be viewed as taking a current pattern f and a conductivity distribution σ to an $I\!\!R^m$ vector of measurements. In practice, one is limited to performing only a finite set of experiments, generally carried out with very specific f, such as those generated by a given number of electrodes in fixed positions. If we make n experiments, that is, we apply n different current patterns

$$f^{(1)}, f^{(2)}, \ldots, f^{(n)},$$

and make m measurements for each pattern

$$g^{(1)}, g^{(2)}, \ldots, g^{(n)},$$

(where $g^{(j)} = (g_1^{(j)}, \ldots, g_m^{(j)})$ according to (2)), then the inverse problem is to determine σ such that

$$F(\sigma; f^{(j)}) = g^{(j)}, \quad j = 1, \ldots, n.$$

A common technique to simplify the analysis of the problem is to linearize F with respect to σ about about a constant background. Thus, we let

$$\sigma = 1 + \delta\sigma$$

where $\|\delta\sigma\|_{L^\infty(\Omega)}$ is "small", and assume that the voltage potential is

$$u = U + \delta u.$$

By considering terms of the same order in (1a), we see that the background potential U satisfies

$$\Delta U = 0 \quad \text{in } \Omega, \tag{3a}$$

$$\frac{\partial U}{\partial\nu} = f \quad \text{on } \partial\Omega. \tag{3b}$$

The linear part δu of the perturbational voltage potential satisfies

$$\Delta \delta u = -\nabla \cdot \delta \sigma \nabla U \quad \text{in } \Omega, \tag{4a}$$

$$\frac{\partial \delta u}{\partial \nu} = 0 \quad \text{on } \partial \Omega, \tag{4b}$$

where we again enforce the normalization $\int_{\partial \Omega} \delta u = 0$. Since U depends linearly on the current pattern f, we see that δu is also linearly dependent on f.

For a given current pattern f, the linearized forward map DF takes a conductivity perturbation $\delta \sigma$ to perturbational measurements on the boundary. The i-th component of this map is

$$(DF(f)\delta \sigma)_i := \int_{\partial \Omega} \delta u \, q_i. \tag{5}$$

Assuming that $\delta \sigma$ is supported in $\Omega' \subset\subset \Omega$, we can view the map as

$$DF(f) : L^2(\Omega') \to I\!R^m. \tag{6}$$

In the linearized inverse problem, the goal is to find $\delta \sigma$ from knowledge of the *differences* between the measured voltages and the background voltages $\int_{\partial \Omega} U \, q_i$ for a set of current patterns $f^{(j)}$, $j = 1, \ldots, n$. Let us denote the background voltage due to current pattern $f^{(j)}$ by $U^{(j)}$. The linearized inverse problem is to determine $\delta \sigma$ in the equation

$$DF(f^{(j)})\delta \sigma = g^{(j)} - TU^{(j)} =: \delta g^{(j)}, \quad \text{for} \quad j = 1, \ldots, n, \tag{7}$$

where $TU^{(j)}$ is the $I\!R^m$-vector whose components are $\int_{\partial \Omega} U^{(j)} \, q_i$. To simplify notation, let us assume that the current patterns $f^{(1)}, \ldots, f^{(n)}$ have been chosen and are henceforth *fixed*. Forming the $I\!R^{n \cdot m}$ data vector

$$\delta g = (\delta g^{(1)T}, \ldots, \delta g^{(n)T})^T$$

and the corresponding operator

$$DF = (DF(f^{(1)})^T, \ldots, DF(f^{(n)})^T)^T,$$

the linearized inverse problem can be written

$$DF \, \delta \sigma = \delta g. \tag{8}$$

Of course, $\delta \sigma \in L^2(\Omega')$ is not determined due to the finite amount of data. Furthermore, even if $\delta \sigma$ is discretized in a straightforward way to a finite number (say $n \cdot m$) of unknowns, the conductivity perturbation $\delta \sigma$ is generally not well-determined by the data due to instability [1, 11, 15]. In particular, information corresponding to high frequency components of $\delta \sigma$ is easily corrupted by noise.

To motivate the use of total variation regularization, assume for a moment that the unknown $\delta \sigma$ can be described as a sum of characteristic functions:

$$\delta \sigma(x) = \sum_{k=1}^{N} a_k \chi(\Omega_k)(x). \tag{9}$$

Here N is unknown but finite, the coefficients a_k are unknown, the subdomains $\Omega_k \subset\subset \Omega$ are unknown, and $\chi(\Omega_k)$ denotes the characteristic function on Ω_k. For convenience, assume that each Ω_k has a C^2 boundary $\partial\Omega_k$. Equation (9) approximates a very wide variety of conductivity profiles which could be encountered in medical imaging and non-destructive testing.

Let $\nabla\delta\sigma$ denote the gradient of $\delta\sigma$ in the sense of distributions; $\nabla\delta\sigma$ is a vector valued Radon measure and

$$TV(\delta\sigma) := \int_\Omega |\nabla\delta\sigma| \tag{10}$$

is the total variation of $\delta\sigma$. We denote by $BV(\Omega)$ the space of functions of bounded variation in Ω, equipped with the norm

$$\|\delta\sigma\|_{BV(\Omega)} = \|\delta\sigma\|_{L^1(\Omega)} + \int_\Omega |\nabla\delta\sigma|$$

(see for example [18]). We observe that $\delta\sigma$ defined by (9) is in $BV(\Omega)$.

Now suppose that we are trying to reconstruct $\delta\sigma$ by solving $DF\,\delta\sigma = \delta g$. Recall that the data is finite-dimensional. Because of the ill-posedness of the problem, we are only able to obtain an approximation $\tilde{\delta\sigma} = \delta\sigma + \eta$, where η is some unknown "error" from the nullspace of DF. Notice that $\nabla\delta\sigma$ is zero except on $\cup_{k=1}^N \partial\Omega_k$. Thus if η happens to have bounded derivatives in the parts of Ω where $\nabla\delta\sigma$ is singular, then necessarily

$$\int_\Omega |\nabla(\delta\sigma + \eta)| \geq \int_\Omega |\nabla\delta\sigma|.$$

This suggests that one might find a better approximation to $\delta\sigma$ by choosing from all possible solutions $\tilde{\delta\sigma} = \delta\sigma + \eta$, one with smallest total variation. Intuitively, at the very least, this strategy rules out a large class of error components η which have oscillations in the parts of Ω where $\delta\sigma$ is constant. We will describe in Section 4 specific (and rather stringent) conditions which ensure that $\delta\sigma$ can be recovered exactly.

Thus our starting point is the optimization problem

$$\min_{\delta\sigma \in \mathcal{A}} \int_\Omega |\nabla\delta\sigma|, \tag{11a}$$

$$\text{subject to: } DF\,\delta\sigma = \delta g, \tag{11b}$$

where $\mathcal{A}$ is some admissible class of conductivity perturbations. The constraint ensures that a feasible conductivity perturbation is one that matches the observed data. A natural choice for the admissible set is $\mathcal{A} = \{\delta\sigma \in BV(\Omega) : \delta\sigma|_{\partial\Omega} = 0\}$. Since the cost functional is convex and the constraints are linear, any local minimizer of problem (11) must be a global minimizer. However, the cost functional is not *strictly* convex, so uniqueness of solutions is not guaranteed in general.

For existence of solutions, one can show the following.

Theorem 1. *Given any data vector $\delta g \in I\!\!R^{n \cdot m}$ in the range of DF, the problem (11) admits at least one solution $\delta \sigma \in \mathcal{A}$.*

The proof follows the direct method in the calculus of variations, using compactness properties of BV. Details can be found in [13].

3 Stabilizing the Constraints

There are two main difficulties associated with the constraint $DF \, \delta \sigma = \delta g$. The first is that if a measured data vector δg is not in the range of DF, the constraints cannot be satisfied and so the problem has no solution. Consider the following "near-null" set associated with DF:

$$V_{\text{near-null}} = \{v \; : \; v \in L^2(\Omega), \|DF\,v\| \leq \epsilon\},$$

for some small ϵ. The second difficulty is that even if δg is in the range of DF, it is still possible for δg to have a component in the set $(DF\,v)$ where $v \in V_{\text{near-null}}$. In this case, small changes in the measurements δg could lead to large changes in the subspace defined by the constraints $\{\delta \sigma \; : \; DF\,\delta \sigma = \delta g\}$, and hence cause instability in the minimization problem.

One remedy for both difficulties can be obtained in the following way. Let ϵ be the "noise level" in the data. Consider the singular value decomposition (SVD):

$$DF = \mathbf{U} \Sigma \mathbf{V}^T,$$

where $\mathbf{U}$ is an $nm \times nm$ orthogonal matrix, $\mathbf{V}$ is an orthogonal operator mapping $L^2(\Omega) \to L^2(\Omega)$, and Σ is a "diagonal" operator with diagonal $\{s_1, \ldots, s_{nm}\}$, where $s_1 \geq s_2 \geq \ldots \geq s_{nm}$ are the singular values of DF. Given any discrete approximation to $L^2(\Omega)$, the corresponding SVD can be calculated numerically by standard methods, see [19]. A slightly different approach is needed if we choose not to discretize. Such an approach is outlined in [15]. The SVD has been used previously to analyze instability in the EIT problem [3].

Let s_p be the smallest singular value greater than ϵ. Form the new operators

$$\Sigma' = \text{diag}\{s_1, \ldots s_p\},$$

$$\mathbf{U}' = (\mathbf{u}_1, \ldots, \mathbf{u}_p),$$

and

$$\mathbf{V}' = (\mathbf{v}_1, \ldots, \mathbf{v}_p),$$

where $\mathbf{u}_j$ denotes the jth column of $\mathbf{U}$, and similarly for $\mathbf{v}_j$. Now we can form the "reduced rank" operator

$$M = \Sigma' \mathbf{V}'^T.$$

The range space of M is p-dimensional, and M has a well-defined pseudo-inverse $M^\dagger$ whose norm is less than or equal to $1/\epsilon$. The "stabilized" linear inverse problem can then be posed as

$$M\delta \sigma = \mathbf{U}'^T \delta g := \delta g'.$$

The effect of this manipulation is that δg has been projected onto the subspace spanned by range vectors of DF whose singular values are greater than ϵ, thus eliminating both difficulties described above. The constraint $M\delta\sigma = \delta g'$ defines a subspace of conductivity perturbations which are consistent with the observed data to within the noise level ϵ.

We emphasize that there are alternate ways of handling the instability in the constraints. The penalty method [27, 25, 26], augmented Lagrangian formulations [20], and the method in [24] are such alternatives. These methods are for the most part more computationally efficient for large problems because they do not require calculating the SVD. However, the approach presented here is useful from a conceptual standpoint.

4 The Case of Band-Limited Instability

In this section we describe some conditions under which blocky images $\delta\sigma_0$ can be fully recovered, under the assumption that there is no instability in recovering the low-frequency Fourier components of $\delta\sigma_0$. This assumption is certainly not true in general, but we outline below that it may be a useful approximation.

From (4a) it follows that

$$(DF(f)\delta\sigma)_i := \int_{\partial\Omega} \delta u \, q_i = \int_{\Omega} \delta\sigma \nabla U \cdot \nabla V_i,$$

where $\Delta V_i = 0$, and $\partial V_i/\partial\nu = q_i$. We may assume without loss of generality that Ω is contained within a unit ball centered at the origin. Based on the approach of Calderon [4], consider the harmonic functions

$$U_\xi(x) = e^{(i\xi+\zeta)\cdot x - |\xi|}, \quad V_\xi(x) = e^{(i\xi-\zeta)\cdot x - |\xi|}$$

where $\xi, \zeta \in \mathbb{R}^n$, with $\xi \cdot \zeta = 0$ and $|\xi| = |\zeta|$ in the expression above to obtain

$$\int_{\partial\Omega} \delta u \, q_\xi = e^{-2|\xi|}|\xi|^2 \int_{\Omega} \delta\sigma \, e^{i\xi \cdot x}, \tag{12}$$

where $q_\xi = \partial V_\xi/\partial\nu$. In other words, one can recover the Fourier coefficients of $\delta\sigma$ by choosing the "current patterns" $f_\xi = \partial U_\xi/\partial\nu$, and appropriate measurement weights. In practice, the weights q_ξ could be approximated by taking appropriate linear combinations of point measurements of δu. Notice that the magnitude of f_ξ and q_ξ is bounded with increasing ξ.

Now suppose as in the previous section that we make a finite number n of experiments, each corresponding to a different frequency ξ_j, $j = 1, \ldots, n$. For each current pattern f_{ξ_j}, we make one measurement with weight q_{ξ_j}. For these particular experiments and measurements,

$$(DF \, \delta\sigma)_j = e^{-2|\xi_j|}|\xi_j|^2 \int_{\Omega} \delta\sigma \, e^{i\xi_j \cdot x}. \tag{13}$$

The operator DF is thus diagonalized and the SVD is simply $U = $ identity, $\Sigma = \text{diag}(e^{-2|\xi_j|}|\xi_j|^2)$, and V is the Fourier transform.

Since the magnitude of the measurements is exponentially decreasing with increasing frequency $|\xi_j|$, one would expect that with a fixed amount of background noise, the relative noise level for low frequency measurements would be very low compared to high frequency measurements. Under this assumption, we use the data as equality constraints to define a set of feasible images. Recall the stabilized operator M as defined in Section 3. The feasible set of images is described by

$$V = \{\delta\sigma \; : \; M\delta\sigma = \delta g'\}.$$

Since M is simply a weighted and truncated Fourier transform, the set V contains all images whose spectrum for frequencies $|\xi_j| \leq R$, for some R defined by the noise level, agree with that of the true image.

The problem is then to solve

$$\min_{\delta\sigma} \; TV(\delta\sigma) \quad \text{subject to} \; \delta\sigma \in V. \tag{14}$$

Note that knowledge about the noise is used to determine R, and hence V.

If the low frequency measurements $\delta g'$ corresponding to a given image $\delta\sigma_0$ are not corrupted by noise, then clearly $\delta\sigma_0 \in V$, since then $M\,\delta\sigma_0 = \delta g'$. Also notice that every $\delta\sigma \in V$ can be written $\delta\sigma = \delta\sigma_0 + \alpha$, where α is from the null space of M. In order to establish that the minimization (14) will successfully recover $\delta\sigma_0$, we must show that any other image $\delta\sigma = \delta\sigma_0 + \alpha \in V$, necessarily has larger total variation than $\delta\sigma_0$. In other words we must show that

$$TV(\delta\sigma_0 + \alpha) > TV(\delta\sigma_0)$$

for all α in the null space of M. Due to the form of M this means simply that high frequency perturbations to $\delta\sigma_0$ should increase its total variation.

4.1 Recovery of Discrete Images

Recall that Ω is assumed to be contained in a unit ball centered at the origin. Assume that the true image $\delta\sigma_0$ is piecewise constant on a uniform square grid on $(-1,1)^2$ with $N \times N$ cells and denote the value of $\delta\sigma_0$ on the (n,m)-th cell by $(\delta\sigma_0)_{n,m}$. To calculate the total variation of $\delta\sigma_0$, we define the horizontal and vertical difference operators D_H and D_V by

$$(D_H\delta\sigma_0)_{n,m} = (\delta\sigma_0)_{n+1,m} - (\delta\sigma_0)_{n,m},$$
$$(D_V\delta\sigma_0)_{n,m} = (\delta\sigma_0)_{n,m+1} - (\delta\sigma_0)_{n,m},$$

where, since $\delta\sigma_0$ is supported away from the boundary, $(\delta\sigma_0)_{N+1,m} \equiv (\delta\sigma_0)_{1,m}$ and $(\delta\sigma_0)_{n,N+1} \equiv (\delta\sigma_0)_{n,1}$. Defining $\|v\|_1 = \sum_{n,m=1}^{N} |v_{n,m}|$, we see that

$$\int_\Omega |\nabla\delta\sigma_0| = \frac{2}{N} \left(\|D_H(\delta\sigma_0)\|_1 + \|D_V(\delta\sigma_0)\|_1 \right), \tag{15}$$

gives the total variation of $\delta\sigma_0$. Let us define the set of all edges upon which $\delta\sigma_0$ is not constant:

$$S = \{(n,m) : (D_H\delta\sigma_0)_{n,m} \neq 0 \text{ or } (D_V\delta\sigma_0)_{n,m} \neq 0\}$$

and assume that there are exactly ν elements in S, numbered (n_r, m_r) for $r = 1, \ldots, \nu$. Notice that ν/N^2 indicates the proportion of edges upon which $\delta\sigma_0$ is not constant.

Assume that α is a *band-limited* perturbation, i.e, we can express

$$\alpha_{n,m} = \frac{1}{N^2} \sum_{(k,l)\in\mathcal{K}} \hat{\alpha}_{k,l} \exp\left(\frac{-2\pi i(n-1)(k-1)}{N}\right) \exp\left(\frac{-2\pi i(m-1)(l-1)}{N}\right)$$

$$(16)$$

where $\mathcal{K}$ is some finite set with K elements. By a direct calculation and an application of the triangle inequality, one finds that

$$\sum_{(n,m)\in S} |D_H(\delta\sigma_0 + \alpha)_{n,m}| \geq \sum_{(n,m)\in S} |(D_H\delta\sigma_0)_{n,m}| - \frac{K\nu}{N^2}\|\hat{\alpha}\|_\infty,$$

where $\|\hat{\alpha}\|_\infty = \max_{n,m} |\hat{\alpha}_{n,m}|$. With a similar calculation, one can show that

$$\left(1 - \frac{K\nu}{N^2}\right)\|\hat{\alpha}\|_\infty \leq \sum_{(n,m)\notin S} |(D_H(\delta\sigma_0 + \alpha)_{n,m}|.$$

Applying the previous two inequalities, it follows that

$$\|D_H(\delta\sigma_0 + \alpha)\|_1 \geq \|D_H\delta\sigma_0\|_1 + \left(1 - \frac{2K\nu}{N^2}\right)\|\hat{\alpha}\|_\infty.$$

The same derivation yields an analogous inequality for the the vertical difference operator D_V. Adding the horizontal and vertical contributions, we find that

$$\int |\nabla(\delta\sigma_0 + \alpha)| \geq \int |\nabla\delta\sigma_0| + \frac{4}{N}\left(1 - \frac{2K\nu}{N^2}\right)\|\hat{\alpha}\|_\infty,$$

$$(17)$$

recalling that $\int |\nabla\delta\sigma_0|$ is given by (15).

The bound (17) indicates that as long as

$$\frac{2K\nu}{N^2} < 1$$

$$(18)$$

and $\alpha \neq 0$, the perturbed signal $\delta\sigma_0 + \alpha$ has higher total variation than the original signal $\delta\sigma_0$. This implies that $\delta\sigma_0$ can be recovered by minimizing $\int |\nabla(\delta\sigma_0 + \alpha)|$ over all perturbations of the form (16).

Estimate (18) indicates a tradeoff between the spectral content of the noise (measured by K) and the proportion of edges upon which $\delta\sigma_0$ is not constant (measured by ν/N^2). This is a form of the uncertainty principle as discussed in Donoho [16]. It is interesting that neither the intensity of any of the frequency components of α, nor distribution of the spectrum of α in important in this condition. Only the *number* of frequencies K allowed in the noise matters.

In terms of the minimization problem (14), if the noise level in the problem is such that the subspace V spans K or fewer frequencies, and the number of non-constant edges ν in $\delta\sigma_0$ satisfies (18), then solving the minimization will recover $\delta\sigma_0$. Note that inherent in this statement is the assumption that the problem is discrete; otherwise V is infinite dimensional.

4.2 Sharpness of the Spectral Bounds

The estimate (18) gives a condition which guarantees that a given image can be recovered from a bandlimited perturbation. It is worthwhile to ask how "sharp" is the bound, e.g., what is the fewest number of frequencies K which can be perturbed in order to decrease the total variation of a given image? The inequality (18) states that if $K < N^2/2\nu$, then the total variation cannot be decreased.

In [14] several numerical experiments were carried out to test the bound. Generally speaking, for "blocky" images $\delta\sigma_0$, it was found to be very difficult to lower the total variation with simple filtering operations. Low-pass and high-pass filters were applied to blocky images. It was generally necessary for the filter to alter substantially more than $K = N^2/2\nu$ frequencies before the total variation of the image was lowered. This indicates that for blurring operators like DF applied to blocky images, the band limit suggested by (18) is too conservative. However, this is only supported by numerical evidence.

Images for which the bound is "least conservative" seem to be composed of a few pure frequencies. For example, images $\delta\sigma_0$ consisting of vertical or horizontal "stripes" of uniform width can be perturbed by $\alpha = -\delta\sigma_0$, thus reducing the total variation to zero with $K = N^2/\nu$, thereby violating the bound (18) by only a factor of two. Similarly, other images with concentrated frequency content are easily diminished by changing a few frequency components, thereby decreasing the total variation.

4.3 Recovery of Nearly Piecewise-Constant Images

Estimates analogous to (17) can be established in an infinite-dimensional setting. Such estimates have implications for denoising and image recovery problems when the spectral content of the noise can be controlled. Here we merely state the main result; the reader is referred to [14] for details.

Let Ω be the unit square and assume as before that $\delta\sigma_0$ is supported away from the boundary. Assume for convenience that $\delta\sigma_0 \in C^1(\Omega)$ and define the set upon which $\delta\sigma$ is not constant:

$$B = \{x \in \Omega : \nabla\delta\sigma_0(x) \neq 0\}.$$

Let the signal perturbation α have the Fourier series representation

$$\alpha(x) = \sum_{k \in Z^2} \hat{\alpha}_k e^{2\pi i x \cdot k},$$

where $Z = \{0, \pm 1, \pm 2, \dots\}$ and

$$\hat{\alpha}_k = \int_\Omega \alpha(x) e^{-2\pi i x \cdot k} dx.$$

Theorem 2. *The total variation of $\delta\sigma_0 + \alpha$ is strictly greater than the total variation of $\delta\sigma_0$ provided that*

$$2|B| \, \|k\hat{\alpha}_k\|_{l^1} < \|k\hat{\alpha}_k\|_{l^\infty}. \tag{19}$$

Condition (19) says that if $\|k\hat{\alpha}_k\|_{l^1}$ is finite, then as long as the nonconstant set B is small enough, $\delta\sigma_0$ can be recovered. On the other hand, if $|B|$ is fixed, condition (19) indicates that $\delta\sigma_0$ can be recovered as long as the spectrum of the noise is not too spread out compared to the magnitude of any one of its Fourier components. So for example, a "nearly piecewise constant" image polluted by a few pure frequencies would be relatively easily recoverable. On the other hand, a smoothly varying function polluted by a spatially localized perturbation (implying that the spectrum of the perturbation is "spread out") may be impossible to recover.

Without additional information about the asymptotic behavior of the spectrum of the noise, the estimate (19) does not give particularly useful information about EIT. On the other hand, suppose we knew that the spectrum of α is bounded by some sequence $\hat{h}_k$. If $|\hat{h}_k|$ decreases quickly enough as $|k| \to \infty$, it follows that $\|k\hat{\alpha}_k\|_1/\|k\hat{\alpha}_k\|_\infty$ must decrease as the frequency cutoff $R \to \infty$. Then (19) shows that $\delta\sigma_0$ can be recovered provided $|B|$ is small enough, and furthermore the constraint on $|B|$ becomes less restrictive as R increases.

In case α is bandlimited, i.e. all but K Fourier components $\hat{\alpha}_k$ are zero, condition (19) becomes

$$2K|B| < 1, \tag{20}$$

in analogy with the discrete case (18).

In the limiting case $|B| = 0$, under the assumption that $\delta\sigma_0$ can be described as a sum of characteristic functions (9), It can easily be shown that if $\alpha \in W^{1,1}(\Omega)$, then

$$\int_\Omega |\nabla(\delta\sigma_0 + \alpha)| = \int_\Omega |\nabla\delta\sigma_0| + \int_\Omega |\nabla\alpha|. \tag{21}$$

Thus, provided $\delta\sigma_0$ is piecewise constant, α has integrable derivatives, and the minimization problem has a unique solution, $\delta\sigma_0$ can be recovered by minimizing the total variation of $\delta\sigma_0 + \alpha$.

It would be interesting to see how results such as these might be combined with other regularization techniques designed to limit the spectral content of α, in order to obtain recoverability results under reasonable assumptions on noise and discretization. This is in effect what took place in Section 4.1, where regularization by discretization truncates the spectrum of α.

5 The Case of Non-Bandlimited Instability

The case of recovering $\delta\sigma$ in the presence of general measurement noise is now considered. We consider the unconstrained minimization

$$\min_u TV(\delta\sigma) + \lambda\|DF\,\delta\sigma - \delta g\|^2_{L^2(\Omega)}. \tag{22}$$

The penalty coefficient λ is chosen so that at minimum, the data mismatch $\|DF\,\delta\sigma - \delta g\|$ is within the estimated signal to noise ratio. If the noise is Gaussian with variance η is γ, then we choose λ to be such that

$$\|DF\,\delta\sigma - \delta g\| \le \gamma. \tag{23}$$

As one might expect, without the assumption of band-limited noise in the problem, results on recoverability are mostly negative. Let $\delta\sigma_0$ be the image we wish to recover; for now assume that $\delta\sigma_0$ is any BV function. First notice that there are *always* perturbations α such that $(\delta\sigma_0 + \alpha)$ has lower total variation than $\delta\sigma_0$ while at the same time $(\delta\sigma_0 + \alpha)$ satisfies the data fit requirement

$$\|DF(\delta\sigma_0 + \alpha) - g\|_2 \leq \gamma,$$

for some "noise level" $\gamma > 0$. For convenience, assume that $DF\delta\sigma_0 = \delta g$. Then the set of feasible perturbations is

$$P_\gamma = \{\alpha : \|DF\alpha\|_2 \leq \gamma\}. \tag{24}$$

One then wishes to determine if

$$\min_{\alpha \in P_\gamma} \int_\Omega |\nabla(\delta\sigma_0 + \alpha)| \tag{25}$$

can be less than $\int_\Omega |\nabla\delta\sigma_0|$. Notice that P_γ contains rough (non-bandlimited) perturbations. We can set $a = \min(\gamma/\|DF\delta\sigma_0\|_2, 1)$ so that

$$\|DF(a\delta\sigma_0)\|_2 \leq \gamma,$$

i.e., $a\delta\sigma_0 \in P_\gamma$. Then by taking the perturbation $\alpha = -a\delta\sigma_0$, we see that

$$\min_{\alpha \in P_\gamma} \int_\Omega |\nabla\delta\sigma_0 + \nabla\alpha| \leq (1 - a) \int_\Omega |\nabla\delta\sigma_0| < \int_\Omega |\nabla\delta\sigma_0|. \tag{26}$$

Thus one cannot recover $\delta\sigma_0$ by solving problem (25).

On the other hand, if $(1 - a)\delta\sigma_0$ *were* the solution to (25), we would probably be quite happy since it differs from the true image only by a multiplicative constant. In this sense, we could say that the image $(1 - a)\delta\sigma_0$ is a "qualitatively correct" reconstruction of $\delta\sigma_0$ (provided $(1 - a) \neq 0$).

However, one is generally not guaranteed a qualitatively correct solution either. Using a blurring operator for which explicit calculations could be made, an example was constructed in [14] of a perturbation which lies inside the constraint set and which lowers the total variation, while making the image qualitatively different from the original image. The same construction could be easily repeated for EIT using the currents and measurements measurements f_{ξ_j}, q_{ξ_j} as used in Section 4. A prominent feature of the example from [14] is that the total variation of the true image $\delta\sigma_0$ is very large relative to its "mass" $\int |\delta\sigma_0|$. This condition seems to characterize most of the images we found hard to reconstruct accurately in the numerical experiments.

6 Minimization of the Total Variation Functional

The main computational difficulty associated with problems (14) and (22) is mainly due to the nondifferentiability of the total variation functional. Rudin and Osher overcome this difficulty by using a nonlinear diffusion equation whose steady state is the Euler-Lagrange equation of the minimization problem [23].

Vogel [27, 28] has introduced a fixed point method to solve this type of problem. In this approach, the total variation seminorm is mollified slightly to get around the nondifferentiability. This method has exhibited rapid convergence in numerical experiments.

Ito and Kunisch [20] have introduced an active set strategy based on the augmented Lagrangian formulation for similar problems in image restoration.

A new class of methods to solve optimization problems with nondifferentiable functional, such as (14), has been proposed by Coleman and Li [9]. An image enhancement method based on the ideas of Coleman and Li has been developed by Li and Santosa. [21]. The method, which works on the original nondifferentiable functional, is based on an affine scaling strategy and appears to be quite efficient for large problems. The code minimizes the total variation while searching in the feasible set (23). To solve the optimization (22), in [14] a quadratic programming method of Coleman and Liu [10] was employed.

Rather than discussing the different algorithmic approaches to this problem, we will describe here a simple gradient-descent type method used in [13], and based on the original scheme of Rudin, Osher and Fatemi [23].

For arbitrary current patterns and measurements, the minimal total variation reconstruction problem with stabilized linear constraints can be formulated:

$$\min_{\delta\sigma \in X} J(\delta\sigma) = \int_\Omega |\nabla\delta\sigma|, \tag{27a}$$

$$\text{subject to } M\delta\sigma = \delta g', \tag{27b}$$

where $M : L^2(\Omega) \to I\!\!R^p$ is the linear operator constructed in Section 3, and $X = \{\delta\sigma \in BV(\Omega) : \delta\sigma|_{\partial\Omega} = 0\}$. In the two-dimensional case we consider here, $BV(\Omega)$ imbeds in $L^2(\Omega)$, so $M\delta\sigma$ is well-defined.

The fact that the cost functional is not smooth creates certain complications from both practical and theoretical standpoints. A common approach is to "mollify" the cost functional J with a small smoothing parameter and solve the resulting problem by straightforward methods. In principle the smoothing parameter can be taken arbitrarily small, so that in the limit one should obtain a solution to problem (27). The problem we try to solve can be written

$$\min_{\delta\sigma \in X} J_\epsilon(\delta\sigma) = \int_\Omega h_\epsilon(|\nabla\delta\sigma|), \tag{28a}$$

$$\text{subject to } M\delta\sigma = \delta g', \tag{28b}$$

where

$$h_\epsilon(s) = \begin{cases} s & \text{if } s > \epsilon, \\ \frac{s^2}{2\epsilon} + \frac{\epsilon}{2} & \text{if } s \le \epsilon. \end{cases}$$

Thus h_ϵ is C^1 for $\epsilon > 0$. The effect of h_ϵ is to "round off" the corner in the absolute value function.

The Euler-Lagrange equations for problem (28) are formally given by

$$\nabla \cdot (q_\epsilon(|\nabla\delta\sigma|)\nabla\delta\sigma) - M^T\lambda = 0, \quad \text{in } \Omega, \tag{29a}$$

$$\delta\sigma = 0, \quad \text{on } \partial\Omega, \tag{29b}$$

$$M\delta\sigma = \delta g', \tag{29c}$$

where $\lambda \in I\!\!R^p$, M^T denotes the L^2 adjoint of M, and the function q_ϵ is defined by

$$q_\epsilon(s) = \frac{h'_\epsilon(s)}{s} = \begin{cases} 1/s \text{ if } s > \epsilon, \\ 1/\epsilon \text{ if } s \le \epsilon. \end{cases}$$

In [23] the approach to solving the Euler-Lagrange equations is to use time as an evolution (iteration) parameter. Applying this idea to our problem, we would solve

$$\delta\sigma_t = \nabla \cdot (q_\epsilon(|\nabla\delta\sigma|)\nabla\delta\sigma) - M^T\lambda, \quad \text{in } \Omega \times (0,\infty), \tag{30a}$$

$$\delta\sigma = 0, \quad \text{on } \partial\Omega \times (0,\infty), \tag{30b}$$

$$\delta\sigma(x,0) = \delta\sigma_0(x), \quad x \in \Omega, \tag{30c}$$

where $\delta\sigma_0$ is a solution of $M\delta\sigma_0 = \delta g'$, given, say, by the pseudo-inverse solution $\delta\sigma_0 = M^\dagger \delta g'$.

To solve the initial boundary value problem in (30), one could apply an explicit time-stepping scheme, that is, starting with the initial step $\delta\sigma_0$, apply the iteration

$$\delta\sigma_{i+1} = \delta\sigma_i + \tau \left[\nabla \cdot (q_\epsilon(|\nabla\delta\sigma_i|)\nabla\delta\sigma_i) - M^T\lambda^{(i)} \right], \tag{31}$$

where τ is the "step length". To solve for the Lagrange multiplier approximation $\lambda^{(i)}$, let $b_j \in L^2(\Omega)$ be a solution of

$$Mb_j = e_j, \quad j = 1,\ldots,p,$$

where e_j denotes the standard unit basis vectors for $I\!\!R^p$. Assuming that the SVD has already been calculated as in the last section, we can set $b_j = v_j/s_j$, where v_j is the j-th column of the orthogonal operator V. We see that if (29a) is satisfied then

$$\int_\Omega \nabla \cdot (q_\epsilon(|\nabla\delta\sigma|)\nabla\delta\sigma)b_j - \int_\Omega (M^T\lambda)b_j = 0,$$

and hence

$$\lambda_j = \langle \lambda, Mb_j \rangle = \int_\Omega (M^T\lambda)b_j = \int_\Omega \nabla \cdot (q_\epsilon(|\nabla\delta\sigma|)\nabla\delta\sigma)b_j. \tag{32}$$

Using equation (32), $\lambda^{(i)}$ can be calculated from $\delta\sigma_i$ and the vectors b_j. This procedure can be viewed as projecting the L^2 gradient

$$D_{\delta\sigma}J_\epsilon = -\nabla \cdot (q_\epsilon(|\nabla\delta\sigma|)\nabla\delta\sigma) \tag{33}$$

of the cost functional J_ϵ onto the linear subspace $\{\delta\sigma : M\delta\sigma = 0\}$. Thus the entire iteration scheme (31) can be viewed as a "projected gradient method". Taking this viewpoint, define the negative "projected gradient"

$$G_i = -D_{\delta\sigma}J_\epsilon(\delta\sigma_i) - M^T\lambda^{(i)}.$$

This leads to the following simple minimization procedure.

1. Choose an initial steplength τ_0, a parameter $\epsilon > 0$, and an initial iterate $\delta\sigma_0$ satisfying the constraint (27b).
2. For $i = 1,\ldots$, convergence do
3.   If $J_\epsilon(\delta\sigma_i + \tau_i G_i) < J_\epsilon(\delta\sigma_j)$ then

           $\delta\sigma_{i+1} = \delta\sigma_i + \tau_i G_i$

           $\tau_{i+1} = \tau_i$

       else

           $\tau_i = \tau_i/2$

           If $\tau_i\|G_i\|$ is too small then stop

           otherwise go to step 3

     end do

A more complicated backtracking strategy that allows an increase as well as a decrease in the step size can also be implemented, however experiments in [13] indicated very little improvement in speed of convergence with such a scheme. Faster convergence is generally observed for larger mollification ϵ, but the scheme seems to converge even for very small positive values of ϵ.

In the next section, we discretize the problem by making the simplifying assumption that $\delta\sigma$ is a piecewise constant function over a square array of square pixels. We note that one does *not* obtain convergence in BV with this discretization as the number of pixels is increased. The intuitive reason for the lack of convergence is that the resulting discrete total variation measure is anisotropic. For example, a discretized function with a discontinuity along a straight line oriented parallel to the gridlines would have smaller total variation than one oriented at a 45 degree angle to the gridlines (independent of the level of discretization). The primary advantage of this discretization is its simplicity. The cost functional $J_\epsilon(\delta\sigma)$ can be calculated in closed form. This leads to a very simple exact formula for the gradient of $J_\epsilon(\delta\sigma)$ and avoids the difficulty of choosing an appropriate approximation of the partial derivatives in G_i.

7 Implementation and Numerical Examples

In this section we describe some numerical computations carried out for a particular linearized EIT problem. We take Ω to be unit disk in $\mathbb{R}^2$. In polar coordinates, $\Omega = \{(r,\theta) : r < 1\}$, and $\partial\Omega = \{(r,\theta) : r = 1\}$. Furthermore, we assume that the current patterns f are generated by a finite number n of fixed electrodes. Thus, in (1b) we can write f in the form

$$f(\theta) = \sum_{i=1}^{n} f_i\chi(\theta,\theta_i), \tag{34}$$

where χ is the characteristic function

$$\chi(\theta, \theta_i) = \begin{cases} 1/h \text{ for} & |\theta - \theta_i| \leq h/2, \\ 0 & \text{otherwise,} \end{cases}$$

h is the electrode width, and $\{\theta_i\}_{i=1}^n$ are the electrode centers. For simplicity set $\theta_i = 2\pi i/n$, $i = 1, \cdots, n$. We identify the current pattern function f with the n-vector $(f_i)_{i=1}^n$. Finally, the measurements are taken as voltage drops between adjacent electrodes. That is, let u_i be the voltage potential at electrode i, then the data, corresponding to a current pattern f, is the $\mathbb{R}^n$ vector

$$g = (g_1, g_2, \cdots, g_n)^T,$$

where $g_i = u_{i+1} - u_i$ (electrode $n + 1$ is identified with electrode 1), and it is understood that u solves (1) with (34). We make n experiments, that is, we apply n different current patterns

$$f^{(1)}, f^{(2)}, \ldots, f^{(n)},$$

and measure the corresponding voltage drops

$$g^{(1)}, g^{(2)}, \ldots, g^{(n)}.$$

The problem is then linearized to obtain $DF\,\delta\sigma = \delta g$, as described in Section 2. We note that this arrangement of current patterns and measurements is similar to one which has been implemented in medical imaging [2].

Extending the domain to the unit square

$$Q = (-1, 1) \times (-1, 1),$$

we discretize the conductivity perturbation $\delta\sigma$ to lie the space of piecewise constant functions on a uniform square grid with $N \times N$ cells. The linearized map DF acting on a $\delta\sigma$ defined over Q is simply defined to be DF acting on the restriction of $\delta\sigma$ to Ω. In this case $h_\epsilon(|\nabla\delta\sigma|)$ is a measure supported on the lines of the grid. Thus if we denote the value of $\delta\sigma$ on the (i, j)-th cell by $\delta\sigma_{i,j}$ then

$$\int_Q h_\epsilon(|\nabla\delta\sigma|) = \frac{1}{N} \sum_{i,j=1}^{N-1} h_\epsilon(|\delta\sigma_{i+1,j} - \delta\sigma_{i,j}|) + h_\epsilon(|\delta\sigma_{i,j+1} - \delta\sigma_{i,j}|).$$

Also discretizing the domain of DF, the stabilized constraint operator M becomes a $p \times N^2$ matrix. From now on we denote the $\mathbb{R}^{N^2}$ vector $(\delta\sigma_{i,j})_{i,j=1}^N$ by $\delta\sigma$. Problem (28) can then be written

$$\min_{\delta\sigma \in X} J_\epsilon^N(\delta\sigma) = \frac{1}{N} \sum_{i,j=1}^{N-1} h_\epsilon(|\delta\sigma_{i+1,j} - \delta\sigma_{i,j}|) + h_\epsilon(|\delta\sigma_{i,j+1} - \delta\sigma_{i,j}|), \tag{35a}$$

$$\text{subject to } M\delta\sigma = \delta g', \tag{35b}$$

where X is the subset of $\mathbb{R}^{N^2}$ with zero boundary values, that is,

$$X = \{\delta\sigma \in \mathbb{R}^{N^2} : \delta\sigma_{1,k} = \delta\sigma_{N,k} = \delta\sigma_{k,1} = \delta\sigma_{k,N} = 0, \quad k = 1, \ldots, N\}.$$

The gradient of the functional $J(\delta\sigma)$ is easy to calculate. For $1 < k, l < N$,

$$\frac{\partial J_\epsilon^N}{\partial \delta\sigma_{k,l}} = q_\epsilon(|\delta\sigma_{k,l} - \delta\sigma_{k-1,l}|)(\delta\sigma_{k,l} - \delta\sigma_{k-1,l}) \tag{36}$$
$$- q_\epsilon(|\delta\sigma_{k+1,l} - \delta\sigma_{k,l}|)(\delta\sigma_{k+1,l} - \delta\sigma_{k,l})$$
$$+ q_\epsilon(|\delta\sigma_{k,l} - \delta\sigma_{k,l-1}|)(\delta\sigma_{k,l} - \delta\sigma_{k,l-1})$$
$$- q_\epsilon(|\delta\sigma_{k,l+1} - \delta\sigma_{k,l}|)(\delta\sigma_{k,l+1} - \delta\sigma_{k,l}) .$$

With the convention that $\partial J_\epsilon^N / \partial \delta\sigma_{k,l} = 0$ for k or l equal to 1 or N, the gradient of $J_\epsilon^N(\delta\sigma)$ over X may be written

$$\mathrm{grad}_{\delta\sigma} J_\epsilon^N = \left(\frac{\partial J_\epsilon^N}{\partial \delta\sigma_{k,l}} \right)_{k,l=1}^N .$$

With this formula, one can easily compute the projected gradient G_i as described in the previous section. The gradient descent method is then applied to solve (35).

In the following experiments we use a 32×32 grid. The number of electrodes is fixed at 20 and we make 20 measurements, so the data vector δg consists of 400 data points. We remark that the method is feasible for finer discretizations. Most of the computational work in the problem is expended computing DF and its singular value decomposition. The SVD can be avoided by considering other equivalent constraints or by incorporating the constraints as penalty as in (22). The data error tolerance is set at 0.0001, which resulted in $p = 150$ "useable" singular values in the SVD of DF. Thus the constraint operator M is a 150×1024 matrix and the reduced data vector $\delta g'$ has 150 elements. The smoothing parameter $\epsilon = 0.001$ for all experiments.

In the first experiment we attempt to recover the separated block profile pictured in Figure 1. The pseudo-inverse solution $\delta\sigma_0 = M^\dagger \delta g'$ was taken as the starting point in the minimization. Figure 2 compares the initial iterate $\delta\sigma_0$ with the final approximate minimizer. As the figure indicates, a near-exact reconstruction is obtained. The reconstruction not only sharpens the edges of the image, but also recovers nearly exactly the true values of the image on the "blocks". This example confirms our expectations from Sections 4 and 5 that good reconstructions can be obtained for images with a relatively small number of non-constant edges ν, and hence relatively small total variation (compared to "mass").

Unfortunately it is not always possible to recover images as accurately as in the previous example. As described in Sections 4 and 5, one should not expect good reconstructions for images $\delta\sigma_0$ with high total variation (or number of non-constant edges) and low "mass". This is illustrated in the following example. Figure 3 shows the true image consisting of a thin curved line. Figure 4 shows the comparison between the pseudo-inverse solution and the minimal total variation reconstruction. As it turns out, in this example the reconstruction has much

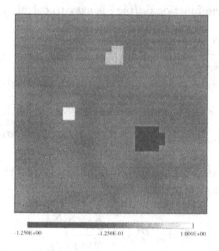

Fig. 1. True profile for the first example.

smaller total variation than the original image: approximately half as much. In fact, even the pseudo-inverse has less total variation than the original image.

The preceding two examples were in some sense extreme cases. For the last example, we try to indicate the behavior of the method in a slightly more realistic situation. A caricature of a cross-section of the human torso is pictured in Figure 5. The large light-colored areas on the right and left indicate the lungs, the slightly darker area between the lungs represents muscle and other tissue, and the two dark areas in the lower center represent heart chambers filled with blood. Many details have been omitted from the image, of course. Since the underlying problem is linearized, one might think of Figure 5 as the difference between the true image and a background conductivity.

As can be seen from Figure 6, the reconstruction recovers some features not visible in the pseudo-inverse, most noticeably the lungs and the tissue between the lungs. In this example as in the previous example, the reconstruction had slightly lower total variation than the original image, however in this case the pseudo-inverse had higher total variation.

In conclusion, we believe that total variation based methods and other edge-preserving regularizations have great potential in electrical impedance tomography, and in numerous other applications involving inverse problems, optimal design, and image processing. Further research is necessary to develop efficient computational techniques, applications to fully nonlinear problems, and to better understand questions of recoverability, such as those touched upon here.

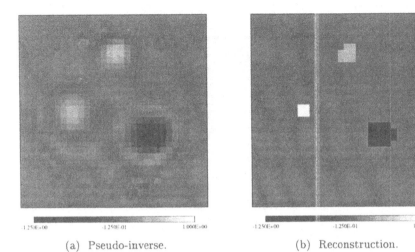

(a) Pseudo-inverse. (b) Reconstruction.

Fig. 2. Comparison of pseudo-inverse solution and minimal total variation reconstruction for the first example.

Acknowledgements

Most of the work reported here was done jointly with Fadil Santosa. The author wishes to express sincere thanks the organizers of the Oberwolfach conference. This work was partially supported by AFOSR Grant number F49620-95-1-0497.

References

1. A. ALLERS AND F. SANTOSA, *Stability and resolution analysis of a linearized problem in electrical impedance tomography*, Inverse Problems, 7 (1991), pp. 515–533.
2. D. BARBER, B. BROWN, AND J. JOSSINET, *Electrical impedance tomography*, Clinical Physics and Physiological Measurements, 9 (1988). Supplement A.
3. W.R. BRECKON AND M.K. PIDCOCK, *Some mathematical aspects of electrical impedance tomography*, in Mathematics and Computer Science in Medical Imaging, M.A. Viergever and Å. Todd-Pokropek, eds., NATO ASI Series, Springer Verlag (1987), pp. 351–362.
4. A.P. CALDERÓN, *On an inverse boundary value problem*, in Seminar on Numerical Analysis and its Applications to Continuum Physics (Soc. Brasiliera de Matematica, Rio de Janerio (1980).
5. F. CATTÉ, P.L. LIONS, J. MOREL, AND T. COLL, *Image selective smoothing and edge detection by nonlinear diffusion*, SIAM J. Numer. Anal., 29 (1992), pp. 182–193.
6. T. F. CHAN, H. M. ZHOU, AND R. H. CHAN, *A Continuation Method for Total Variation Denoising Problems*, UCLA CAM Report 95-18.

62

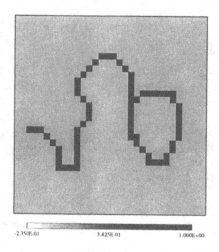

-2.350E-01   3.825E-01   1.000E+00

Fig. 3. True profile for the second example.

7. A. CHAMBOLLE AND P. L. LIONS, *Image recovery via total variation minimization and related problems*, Research Report No. 9509, CEREMADE, Universite de Paris-Dauphine, 1995.

8. P. CHARBONNIER, L. BLANC-FERAUD, G. AUBERT, AND M. BARLAUD, *Deterministic edge-preserving regularization in computed imaging*, Research Report no. 94-01, Univ. of Nice–Sophia Antipolis, 1994.

9. T. COLEMAN AND Y. LI, *A globally and quadratically convergent affine scaling method for linear l_1 problems*, Mathematical Programming, 56 (1992), pp. 189–222.

10. T. COLEMAN AND J. LIU, *An interior Newton method for quadratic programming*, Cornell University Department of Computer Science Preprint TR 93-1388, 1993.

11. D. DOBSON, *Estimates on resolution and stabilization for the linearized inverse conductivity problem*, Inverse Problems, 8 (1992), pp. 71–81.

12. D. DOBSON, *Exploiting ill-posedness in the design of diffractive optical structures*, in "Mathematics in Smart Structures", H. T. Banks, ed., SPIE Proc. **1919** (1993), pp. 248–257.

13. D. DOBSON AND F. SANTOSA, *An image-enhancement technique for electrical impedance tomography*, Inverse Problems 10 (1994) pp. 317–334.

14. D. DOBSON AND F. SANTOSA, *Recovery of blocky images from noisy and blurred data*, SIAM J. Appl. Math., to appear.

15. D. DOBSON AND F. SANTOSA, *Resolution and stability analysis of an inverse problem in electrical impedance tomography—dependence on the input current patterns*. SIAM J. Appl. Math, 54 (1994) pp. 1542-1560.

16. D. DONOHO, *Superresolution via sparsity constraints*, SIAM J. Math. Anal., 23 (1992), pp. 1309–1331.

17. D. GEMAN AND C. YANG, *Nonlinear image recovery with half-quadratic regularization*, IEEE Trans. Image Proc., vol. 4 (1995), pp. 932-945.

18. E. GIUSTI, *Minimal Surfaces and Functions of Bounded Variation*, Birkhauser, Boston, 1984. Monographs in Mathematics, Vol. 80.

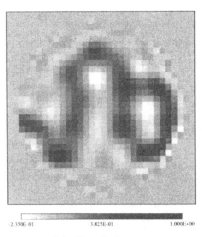

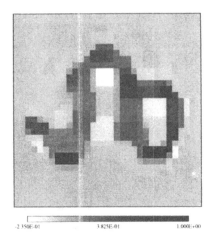

(a) Pseudo-inverse.

(b) Reconstruction.

Fig. 4. Comparison of pseudo-inverse solution and minimal total variation reconstruction for the second example.

19. G. GOLUB AND C. V. LOAN, *Matrix Computations*, Johns Hopkins, 1983.
20. K. ITO AND K. KUNISCH, *An active set strategy based on the augmented Lagrangian formulation for image restoration*, preprint (1995).
21. Y. LI AND F. SANTOSA, *An affine scaling algorithm for minimizing total variation in image enhancement*, Cornell Theory Center Technical Report 12/94, submitted to IEEE Trans. Image Proc.
22. S. OSHER AND L.I. RUDIN, *Feature-oriented image enhancement using shock filters*, SIAM J. Numer. Anal., 27 (1990), pp. 919–940.
23. L.I. RUDIN, S. OSHER, AND E. FATEMI, *Nonlinear total variation based noise removal algorithms*, Physica D., 60 (1992), pp. 259–268.
24. L.I. RUDIN, S. OSHER, AND C. FU, *Total variation based restoration of noisy blurred images*, SIAM J. Num. Anal., to appear.
25. F. SANTOSA AND W. SYMES, *Linear inversion of band-limited reflection seismograms*, SIAM J. Sci. Stat. Comput., 7 (1986), pp. 1307–1330.
26. F. SANTOSA AND W. SYMES, *Reconstruction of blocky impedance profiles from normal-incidence reflection seismograms which are band-limited and miscalibrated*, Wave Motion, 10 (1988), pp. 209–230.
27. C.R. VOGEL AND M. E. OMAN, *Iterative methods for total variation denoising*, SIAM J. Sci. Comput., to appear.
28. C.R. VOGEL AND M. E. OMAN, *Fast numerical methods for total variation minimization in image reconstruction*, in SPIE Proc. Vol. 2563, Advanced Signal Processing Algorithms, July 1995.

This article was processed using the LaTeX macro package with LMAMULT style

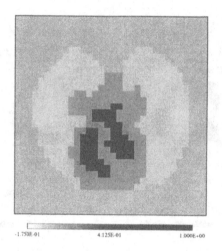

Fig. 5. True profile for the third example.

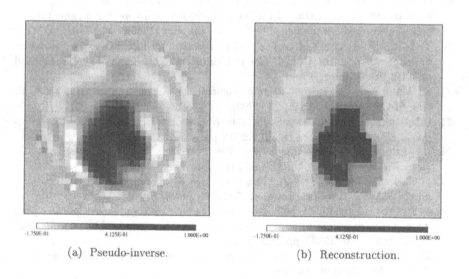

(a) Pseudo-inverse.   (b) Reconstruction.

Fig. 6. Comparison of pseudo-inverse solution and minimal total variation reconstruction for the third example.

Impedance Imaging and Electrode Models

Seppo Järvenpää[1] and Erkki Somersalo[2]

[1] Rolf Nevanlinna Institute, University of Helsinki
[2] Department of Mathematics, Helsinki University of Technology

0 Introduction

In this article, we consider the impedance imaging problem of estimating the unknown resistivity distribution in a body from a finite number of current–voltage measurements on the surface of the body. In practice, the current is injected into the body through electrodes attached on the surface, and usually the same electrodes are used for voltage measurements. The focus of this article is on the effect of the electrodes on the resistivity estimation.

The question of modelling the electrodes has been discussed in the articles [2], [7] and [5]. If the model is furnished with a properly chosen contact impedance between the electrodes and the body, the computed voltages agree with measured voltages with a reasonably high precision, see [2]. To reduce the electrode noise in the inverse solution, one should therefore use algorithms that take the contact impedance into account in one way or another.

In this article, we discuss impedance imaging algorithms that take the electrodes into account. The first algorithm is a Newton type algorithm based on a finite element direct solver using the contact impedance electrode model. The second algorithm is a simple linearized algorithm based on the invariant imbedding equation used in the layer stripping algorithms. In the latter algorithm, we introduce an idea that can be applied to basically any scheme to reduce electrode noise. This idea is called here *quasistatic imaging*.

1 Direct Problem: Electrode Models

In this section, we review the two different electrode models used in this article. For the sake of definiteness, we consider the impedance imaging problem in a unit disc in $\mathbb{R}^2$. We denote by $D \subset \mathbb{R}^2$ the disc, $D = \{x \in \mathbb{R}^2 \mid |x| < 1\}$, and by $\sigma : D \to \mathbb{R}$ the conductivity in D. The electric potential u satisfies the equation

$$\nabla \cdot (\sigma \nabla u) = 0 \tag{1}$$

in D. The electrodes are identified with L non–overlapping intervals e_ℓ on the boundary ∂D. For simplicity, we assume that the electrodes are identical and evenly distributed. By using the polar coordinates (r, θ), we set

$$e_\ell = \{(1, \theta) \in \partial D \mid |\theta - \frac{2\pi}{L}\ell| < \frac{\Delta}{2}\}, \quad 1 \leq \ell \leq L,$$

where $\Delta < 2\pi/L$ is the width of the electrode.

Let I_ℓ be the current injected through the electrode. We call the vector $(I_1, \ldots, I_L)^T \in \mathbb{R}^L$ a *current pattern*. The conservation of charge requires that I must satisfy

$$\sum_{\ell=1}^{L} I_\ell = 0. \tag{2}$$

Similarly, let U_ℓ denote the voltage of the ℓth electrode. The vector $U = (U_1, \ldots, U_L)^T$ is called a *voltage pattern*. The ground voltage is fixed by the condition

$$\sum_{\ell=1}^{L} U_\ell = 0. \tag{3}$$

The electrode models fix the boundary conditions that the potential u must satisfy. We start with a simple model that yields a Neumann boundary condition for the direct problem.

Gap model: In this model, the current flow through each electrode is assumed to be equally distributed along the electrode. We set

$$\sigma \frac{\partial u}{\partial n}\Big|_{e_\ell} = \frac{1}{\Delta} I_\ell, \quad 1 \leq \ell \leq L, \tag{4}$$

and

$$\sigma \frac{\partial u}{\partial n}\Big|_{\partial D \setminus \cup e_\ell} = 0. \tag{5}$$

Hence, with a given current pattern I, the problem (1) with (4) and (5) is a standard Neumann boundary value problem. The voltages U_ℓ are identified here with the values of the potential in the middle of the electrodes,

$$U_\ell = u(1, \frac{2\pi}{L}\ell), \quad 1 \leq \ell \leq L.$$

The uniqueness of the problem is guaranteed by the condition (3).

As it was demonstrated in [2], the gap model fails to agree with measured current–voltage–pairs because the contact impedances between the electrodes and the body are ignored. A better model is the following, called the *complete model*.

Complete model: Let us denote by z_ℓ the contact impedance between the ℓth electrode and the body. For simplicity, we assume here that z_ℓ is real. In the complete model, the voltage U_ℓ on the ℓth electrode is modeled as

$$\left(u + z_\ell \sigma \frac{\partial u}{\partial n}\right)\Big|_{e_\ell} = U_\ell, \quad 1 \leq \ell \leq L. \tag{6}$$

For the uniqueness, we assume the condition (3). The condition (5) is unaltered, while the condition (4) is replaced by a weaker condition,

$$\int_{e_\ell} \sigma \frac{\partial u}{\partial n} dS = I_\ell, \quad 1 \leq \ell \leq L. \tag{7}$$

Note that this seemingly overdetermined problem is well defined beacuse in the mixed type condition (6), the voltages U_ℓ are unknown and part of the boundary value problem.

In [7], a variational formulation corresponding to the complete model was derived. The existence and uniqueness of a weak solution to this problem was proved. More precisely, let us denote

$$H = H^1(D) \oplus \mathbb{R}^L,$$

and by $C_p(\overline{D})$ the space of piecewise continuous functions in $\overline{D}$ that are C^1 in the neighborhood of the boundary ∂D. We equip the space with the sup–norm. We have the following existence and uniqueness result.

Proposition 1. *Assume that $z_\ell > 0$, $1 \leq 1 \leq L$ and $\sigma \in C_p(\overline{D})$ is positive. If $(u, U) \in H$ and u satisfies the equation (1) in the weak sense and the boundary conditions (5), (6) and (7) hold, then (u, U) satisfies the equation*

$$B((u, U), (v, V)) = \sum_{\ell=1}^{L} U_\ell I_\ell \tag{8}$$

for all $(v, V) \in H$, where

$$B((u, U), (v, V)) = \int_D \sigma \nabla u \cdot \nabla v dx + \sum_{\ell=1}^{L} \frac{1}{z_\ell} \int_{e_\ell} (u - U_\ell)(v - V_\ell) dS.$$

Conversely, the equation (8) has a unique solution $(u, U) \in H$ and the solution satisfies the equations (1), (5), (6) and (7) of the complete model.

It has been demonstrated by numerical examples that the current densities in the complete model deviate strongly from the simple condition (4) used in the gap model. Therefore, it is expected that the gap model should lead to erroneous results near the boundary when used in inversion algorithms.

The direct problem corresponding to both the gap model and complete model is solved numerically by finite element method. We have implemented the solver using second order isoparametric triangular elements that are able to approximate well the singular behavior of the fields at the edges of the electrodes. Details are omitted here.

For later reference, we define the *resistance matrix* of the complete model as follows: If $\sigma \in C_p(\overline{D})$, $\sigma > 0$ and $z = (z_1, \ldots, z_L) \in \mathbb{R}^L$, $z_\ell > 0$ are given, the resistance matrix $R(\sigma, z)$ is the $L \times L$–matrix with the property

$$U = R(\sigma, z)I,$$

where I is any current pattern with the property (2).

2 Iterative Solver

In this section we describe an interative inverse solver based on the complete electrode model described in the previous section. Let us denote by V the matrix whose columns are the measured voltage patterns, the corresponding current patterns being collected to the matrix I. The solver is a Newton–Raphson–type algorithm, minimizing the object functional

$$F(\sigma) = \|V - R(\sigma, z)I\|^2.$$

The norm used here is the Frobenius norm. We discretize the disc into pixels of the form $\{(r, \theta) \mid r_1 < r < r_2, \theta_1 < \theta < \theta_2\}$. The pixels are chosen very much like in the "Joshua tree" mesh of the NOSER algorithm, see [3]. In each pixel, the conductivity is assumed to be constant. For the computation of the potential and the voltages, each pixel is divided further to triangular elements.

For the Newton–Raphson algorithm, we need to compute the derivatives with respect to the conductivities and contact impedances. To do this, the following result is needed.

Proposition 2. *The mapping*

$$\mathcal{M} : C_p(\overline{D}) \oplus \mathbb{R}^L \to H, \quad (\sigma, z) \mapsto (u, U),$$

is Frechet differentiable. The derivative $\mathcal{M}'(\sigma, z)$ *satisfies the following equation: Let* $h = (s, \zeta) \in C_p(\overline{D}) \oplus \mathbb{R}^L$, *with* $\sigma + s > 0$ *and* $z_\ell + \zeta_\ell > 0$. *Denoting* $(w, W) = \mathcal{M}'(\sigma, z)h$, *we have*

$$B((w, W), (v, V)) = -\int_D s\nabla u^0 \cdot \nabla v dx + \sum_{\ell=1}^{L} \frac{\zeta_\ell}{z_\ell^2} \int_{e_\ell} \int_{e_\ell} (u^0 - U_\ell^0)(v - V_\ell)dS$$

for all $(v, V) \in H$.

Thus, the derivatives of the functional $F(\sigma, z)$ can be computed by the same FEM solver as the solution (u, U) itself.

To demonstrate the effect of the correct electrode modelling, consider the reconstruction of the conductivity from computed data by a Newton–Raphson based solver using the gap model and on the other hand the complete model.

Figure 1a shows the actual resistivity (i.e. inverse of conductivity) distribution used to generate the data. There is a highly resistive object near the boundary and an conducting object deeper in the body. No artificial noise is added to the data. Figure 1b shows the reconstruction with an algorithm based on the gap model. The algorithm is a linearized Newton–Raphson algorithm, taking one step from the initial constant resistivity distribution. The effect of the missing contact impedance in the model shows as a ringing around the boundary of the body.

Figures 1c and 1d are reconstructions with a Newton–Raphson algorithm based on the complete electrode model. Figure 1c is a linearized reconstruction, one step from the initial constant background. In Figure 1d, three Newton steps

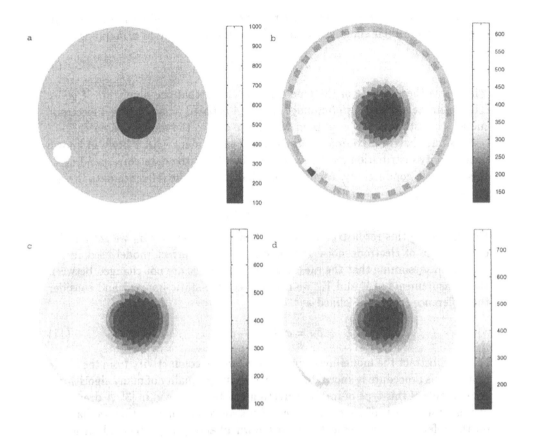

Fig. 1. Original resistivity distribution (a), reconstruction with a one step New-ton–Raphson algorithm based on the gap model (b) and on the complete electrode model (c), and an iterative solution after three steps using the complete model (d).

have been taken. In these reconstructions, the contact impedance was assumed to be known. In pratice, the contact impedances are part of the inverse problem and have to be reconstructed from the data. A more comprehensive study of the full problem will be discussed elsewhere. In this example, the overall image quality seems not to improve by taking more than one iteration step. Only the dynamical range of the image has improved slightly.

3 Linearized Solver and Quasistatic Images

In this section, we discuss a method to reduce electrode noise in reconstruction algorithms that are based on an incorrect electrode model. As an example, this method is applied to a simple linearized inversion algorithm.

Assume that we have an algorithm that maps the given current–voltage mea-surements to an estimate of the conductivity distribution. Hence, if I and V are matrices containing the current patterns and the corresponding measured voltage patterns in their columns, we may define the algorithm as a mapping

$$A : (I, V) \mapsto \tilde{\sigma}, \tag{9}$$

where $\tilde{\sigma}$ is the estimate of the true conductivity σ that the algorithm A gives. This estimate is called a *static image* of σ. If A is based on an incorrect electrode model, the estimate $\tilde{\sigma}$ is corrupted with noise due to the model mismatch.

Assume that we have made a reference measurement with a body of known conductivity distribution σ_0. Let us denote by (I, V_0) the data corresponding to this reference conductivity. Applying the algorithm on the reference data, we get an estimate of σ_0,

$$A : (I, V_0) \mapsto \tilde{\sigma}_0. \tag{10}$$

By comparing this reconstruction to the known conductivity σ_0 we get an idea of the effect of electrode noise that is due to the incorrect model used in the algorithm. Assuming that the measurement conditions are not changed between the measurements of V and V_0, we may correct the static image $\tilde{\sigma}$ and consider the *difference image* $\tilde{\sigma}_d$ defined as

$$\tilde{\sigma}_d = \tilde{\sigma} - (\tilde{\sigma}_0 - \sigma_0), \tag{11}$$

i.e., we substract the modelling error of the reference conductivity from the static image. This procedure is known to improve the image quality of many algorithms. An example of this type of image correction can be found e.g. in [3]. A drawback of this procedure is of course the need of a known reference. Either we have to do the reference measurement with a known phantom (e.g. in nondestructive testing) or we have to settle for considering only temporal changes in the body of interest (e.g. in medical imaging of the thorax). In the former case, there is a risk that the measurement conditions (e.g. electrode contacts) may not remain unaltered when the bodies are swapped, while in the latter case, no estimate of the actual conductivities are obtained. This is the case e.g. in the backprojection algorithm ([1]).

The idea of the *quasistatic images* is to use a computed reference. The image correction is done through the following steps.

1. Compute the static image

$$\tilde{\sigma} = A((I, V)).$$

2. Find an optimal background conductivity σ_0=constant and background contact impedance z_0 from the condition

$$\|V - R(\sigma_0, z_0 \mathbf{1})I\| \longrightarrow \min!,$$

where $\mathbf{1} = (1, 1, \ldots, 1)^T$.

3. Compute the reference image

$$\tilde{\sigma}_0 = A((I, R(\sigma_0, z_0 \mathbf{1})I).$$

4. Define the quasistatic image as

$$\tilde{\sigma}_{qs} = \tilde{\sigma} - (\tilde{\sigma}_0 - \sigma_0).$$

To demonstrate the performance of the correction scheme, we apply it to an algorithm that is based on the gap model. The algorithm is an upgraded version of the one described in [8]. The new feature here is the modelling of the electrodes with the gap model. The algorithm in the cited article ignored the electrodes completely. A brief review of the algorithm is given below.

Denote by $L_0^2([-\pi, \pi])$ the square integrable functions with zero mean over the unit circle and by $P_N : L_0^2([-\pi, \pi]) \to \mathbb{R}^{2N}$ the mapping of the functions to their Fourier coefficients up to order N,

$$P_N : \varphi \mapsto \begin{pmatrix} (\langle \cos n\theta, \varphi \rangle)_{1 \le n \le N} \\ (\langle \sin n\theta, \varphi \rangle)_{1 \le n \le N} \end{pmatrix}.$$

Let j denote the current density corresponding to the current pattern I in the gap model, i.e., u is the solution of the equation (1) with the Neumann boundary condition

$$\sigma \frac{\partial u}{\partial n}\bigg|_{\partial D} = j = \frac{1}{\Delta} \sum_{\ell=1}^{L} \chi_\ell I_\ell.$$

Here, χ_ℓ is the characteristic function of the electrode e_ℓ. We denote

$$J = P_N j = P_N \frac{1}{\Delta} \sum_{\ell=1}^{L} \chi_\ell I_\ell = SI,$$

where S is a $2N \times L$-matrix that is simple to compute. Similarly, denote by U the $2N$-vector

$$U = P_N u\big|_{\partial D},$$

and by T the $L \times 2N$-matrix

$$T : U \mapsto V,$$

where V is a vector whose ℓth component is the value of the truncated Fourier series with the coefficients U at the midpoint of the ℓth electrode e_ℓ.

Let $W = W(\sigma) \in \mathbb{R}^{2N \times 2N}$ be the truncated matrix in the Fourier basis of the Neumann–to–Dirichlet map corresponding to the differential equation (1). Thus, we have

$$W : J \mapsto U.$$

With these notations, we have a Fourier series based approximation for the resistance matrix $R_{\text{gap}}(\sigma)$ in the gap model, mapping the current pattern I to the voltage pattern V,

$$R_{\text{gap}} \approx TW(\sigma)S.$$

The algorithm is based on the minimization of the functional

$$F(\sigma) = \|V - TW(\sigma)SI\|^2$$

with respect to the conductivity σ, where V is the matrix of measured voltage patterns. To this end, we discretize the conductivity as follows. First, the disc D is divided in J rings,

$$A_j = \{x \in D \mid r_{j-1} \leq |x| < r_j\}, \quad 1 \leq j \leq J,$$

where $0 = r_0 < r_1 < \ldots < r_J = 1$. In each ring, the resistivity $\rho = 1/\sigma$ is assumed to be constant in the radial direction,

$$\rho(r, \theta)\big|_{A_j} = \frac{1}{\sigma(r, \theta)}\bigg|_{A_j} = \rho_j(\theta).$$

The resistivities in each ring are approximated with the truncated Fourier series,

$$\rho_j(\theta) \approx \sum_{n=0}^{N} c_{j,n} \cos n\theta + \sum_{n=1}^{N} s_{j,n} \sin n\theta.$$

With this approximation, we write

$$F(\sigma) = f((c, s)),$$

where c and s are matrices containing the coefficients $c_{j,n}$ and $s_{j,n}$, respectively, and minimize f with respect to c and s.

The minimization is based on a Newton–Raphson method. In [8], a method to compute W and the derivatives of W with respect to c and s was given. The key idea is to use the Riccati equation for the Neumann–to–Dirichlet map. More precisely, let $0 < r \leq 1$, and denote by σ_r the restriction of σ to the disc of radius r. If u is a solution of the equation

$$\nabla \cdot \sigma_r \nabla u = 0 \text{ in } D_r = \{x \in \mathbb{R}^2 \mid |x| < r\},$$

we define the operator $\mathcal{R}(r)$ as

$$\mathcal{R}(r) : \sigma_r \frac{\partial u}{\partial n}\bigg|_{\partial D_r} \mapsto u\big|_{\partial D_r},$$

i.e., $\mathcal{R}(r)$ is the Neumann–to–Dirichlet map for the disc D_r. Let us denote $\mathcal{W}(r) = r^{-1}\mathcal{R}(r)$. The operator–valued function $r \mapsto \mathcal{W}(r)$ satisfies the Riccati equation

$$r\frac{d\mathcal{W}}{dr} = \rho + \mathcal{W}\frac{\partial}{\partial\theta}\sigma\frac{\partial}{\partial\theta}\mathcal{W},$$

see e.g. [6] for a derivation. By projecting this equation to the Fourier basis, we find a differential equation for computing the matrix W. What is more, by differentiating the matrix equation with respect to c and s, we get a linear differential equation for computing the derivatives of W. These equations are discussed in more detail in [8].

We restrict ourselves here to a linearized algorithm. Starting with an initial guess ρ=contant, the mapping W and its derivatives can be solved explicitly by this method. Furthermore, it turns out that the updating of the vectors c

and s can be done separately. Moreover, if we denote $c^{(n)} = (c_{1,n}, c_{2,n}, \ldots c_{J,n})$, $0 \leq n \leq N$, and $s^{(n)}$ defined similarly, the coefficient vectors $c^{(n)}$ and $s^{(n)}$ of different order n can be updated separately. The details are omitted here.

The algorithm has been tested with both numerically produced and experimental data, and it seems to give a reasonable reconstruction of the conductivity distributions not too far away from the boundary. For objects close to the center of the body, the ringing due to the use of Fourier basis results in poor resolution in the angular direction.

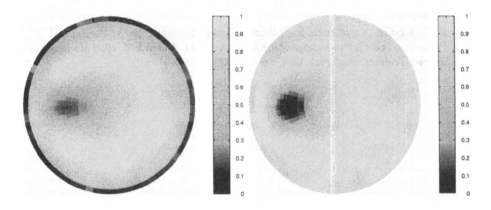

Fig. 2. A static reconstruction of an off-centered target in a saline bath (left) and the corresponding quasistatic reconstruction.

Figure 2 shows a resistivity reconstruction from experimental data. The data is collected with the Rensselaer Polytechnic Institute ACT 2 system (see [4]). The body is a phantom of a saline bath with an off–centered conducting target. The actual dimensions of the target are unknown to us. The image on the left is the static image. Here, the effect of the electrodes is clearly visible as a shading around the rim of the body. The image on the right is the corresponding quasistatic image. The electrode noise is clearly reduced in this image. In these images, the resistivity is scaled to vary from zero to one.

Acknowledgements: The authors wish to thank the RPI impedance imaging group for making the ACT 2 data available to us.

References

1. D. Barber and B. Brown: Applied potential tomography. J. Phys. E: Sci. Instrum 17 (1984) 723–733.
2. K.-S. Cheng, D. Isaacson, J. C. Newell and D. G. Gisser: Electrode models for electric current computed tomography. IEEE Trans. Biomed. Engrg. 3 (1989) 918–914.

3. M. Cheney, D. Isaacson, J. C. Newell, S. Simske and J. Goble: NOSER: An algorithm for solving the inverse conductivity problem. Int. J. Imaging Syst. Tech. 2 (1990) 66–75.

4. J. C. Newell, D. G. Gisser and D. Isaacson: An electric current tomograph. IEEE Trans. Biomed. Eng. 35 (1988) 828–833.

5. K. Paulson, W. Breckon and M. Pidcock: Electrode modelling in electrical impedance tomography. SIAM J. Appl. Math. 52 (1992) 1012–1022.

6. E. Somersalo, M. Cheney, D. Isaacson and E. L. Isaacson: Layer stripping: A direct numerical method for impedance imaging. Inverse Problems 7 (1991) 899–926.

7. E. Somersalo, M. Cheney and D. Isaacson: Existence and uniqueness for electrode models for electric current computed tomography. SIAM J. Appl. Math. 52 (1992) 1023–1040.

8. E. Somersalo: A numerical impedance imaging algorithm. In: A. Fasano and M. Primicerio (Eds.): *Proceedings of the Seventh ECMI, March 2–6, 1993 Montecatini Terme*. Teubner, Stuttgart 1994, pp. 331–338.

Inverse Obstacle Scattering with Modulus of the Far Field Pattern as Data*

Rainer Kress[1] and William Rundell[2]

[1] Institut für Numerische und Angewandte Mathematik,
   Universität Göttingen, 37083 Göttingen, Germany
[2] Department of Mathematics, Texas A&M University,
   College Station, Texas 77843-3368

1 Introduction

For the two-dimensional inverse scattering problem for a sound-soft or perfectly conducting obstacle we may distinguish between uniqueness results on three different levels. Consider the scattering of a plane wave $u^i(x) = e^{ik\,x\cdot d}$ (with wave number $k > 0$ and direction d of propagation) by an obstacle D, that is, a bounded domain $D \subset \mathbb{R}^2$ with a connected boundary ∂D. Then the total wave u is given by the superposition $u = u^i + u^s$ of the incident wave u^i and the scattered wave u^s and obtained through the solution of the Helmholtz equation

$$\Delta u + k^2 u = 0 \quad \text{in } \mathbb{R}^2 \setminus \bar{D} \tag{1}$$

subject to the Dirichlet boundary condition

$$u = 0 \quad \text{on } \partial D \tag{2}$$

and the Sommerfeld radiation condition

$$\lim_{r \to \infty} \sqrt{r}\left(\frac{\partial u^s}{\partial r} - iku^s\right) = 0, \quad r = |x|, \tag{3}$$

uniformly with respect to all directions. The exterior Dirichlet problem (1)–(3) has a unique solution provided the boundary ∂D is of class C^2 (see [1, 2]).

Because of the Sommerfeld radiation condition (3) the scattered wave u^s has the asymptotic behaviour

$$u^s(x) = \frac{e^{ik|x|}}{\sqrt{|x|}}\left\{u_\infty(\hat{x}) + O\left(\frac{1}{|x|}\right)\right\}, \quad |x| \to \infty, \tag{4}$$

where $\hat{x} := x/|x|$ and where the function u_∞, defined on the unit circle Ω in $\mathbb{R}^2$, is called the far field pattern of the scattered wave (see [1, 2]). The fundamental inverse obstacle scattering problem now is, given the far field pattern u_∞ of

---

* This research was supported in part by grants from the Deutsche Forschungsgemeinschaft and the National Science Foundation.

the scattered wave u^s for one incident plane wave $u^i(x) = e^{ik\,x\cdot d}$ with incident direction $d \in \Omega$, to determine the shape of the scatterer D.

For the sake of simplicity we assume that the scatterer is starlike with respect to the origin, i.e.,

$$\partial D = \{x_r = r(\hat{x})\,\hat{x} : \hat{x} \in \Omega\} \tag{5}$$

where $r : \Omega \to \mathbb{R}$ is a positive and twice continuously differentiable function representing the radial distance from the origin. The solution to the direct scattering problem (1)–(3) with a fixed incident wave u^i defines an operator

$$F : C_+^2(\Omega) \to L^2(\Omega)$$

which maps the radial function r into the far field pattern u_∞ of the scattered wave u^s for the obstacle described through (5). Here, by $C_+^2(\Omega)$ we denote the cone of positive functions in $C^2(\Omega)$. Given a (measured) far field pattern u_∞, in terms of the operator F, the inverse problem now is equivalent to solving the equation

$$F(r) = u_\infty \tag{6}$$

for the radial function r representing the boundary curve ∂D.

The modification of Schiffer's classical uniqueness result for the inverse problem with Dirichlet boundary conditions due to Colton and Sleeman [3] (see also [2]) now implies that the operator F is injective on $\{r \in C_+^2(\Omega) : \|r\|_\infty < \zeta_0/k\}$ where $\zeta_0 = 2.40482...$ denotes the smallest positive zero of the Bessel function J_0 of order zero.

Both by using a Hilbert space approach (see [2, 8]) or a boundary integral equation method (see [14]) it has been established that the operator F is Fréchet differentiable. The derivative is given by

$$F'(r)\,q = v_\infty$$

where v_∞ is the far field pattern of the solution v to the Helmholtz equation

$$\Delta v + k^2 v = 0 \quad \text{in } \mathbb{R}^2 \setminus \bar{D} \tag{7}$$

satisfying the Sommerfeld radiation condition and the Dirichlet boundary condition

$$v = -\nu \cdot x_q \, \frac{\partial u}{\partial \nu} \quad \text{on } \partial D. \tag{8}$$

Here, ν denotes the outward unit normal to the boundary ∂D. We note that the ill-posedness of the inverse scattering problem is reflected through the fact that the linear operator $F'(r) : L^2(\Omega) \to L^2(\Omega)$ is compact.

Applying Newton's method to the inverse obstacle scattering problem, given a far field pattern u_∞, the nonlinear equation (6) is replaced by the linearised equation

$$F(r) + F'(r)\,q = u_\infty \tag{9}$$

which has to be solved for q in order to improve an approximate boundary given by the parametrisation r into the new approximation $\tilde{r} = r + q$. Now the second observation on uniqueness for the inverse Dirichlet problem is concerned with the uniqueness for the linearised equation (9). From (8), by a simple application of Holmgren's uniqueness theorem, it follows that for each $r \in C_+^2(\Omega)$ the compact linear operator $F'(r) : C^2(\Omega) \to L^2(\Omega)$ is injective [8, 12].

Of course, for practical computations the equation (9) has to be discretised. One possibility for the discretisation is to take q from a finite dimensional subspace $C^2(\Omega)$ and project (9) orthogonally onto another finite dimensional subspace of $L^2(\Omega)$. Now the third observation on uniqueness is concerned with the obvious choice where both subspaces coincide and are given by the space of trigonometric polynomials T_M of degree less than or equal to M. For the case where r is constant, i.e., for a circle, it has been shown in [12] that for sufficiently small wave numbers k the corresponding finite dimensional operator $F'_M(r) : T_M \to T_M$ is injective. Hence, locally, the first M Fourier coefficients of the far field pattern u_∞ uniquely determine the first M Fourier coefficients of the radial function r representing the boundary of the scatterer.

However, the latter result is unsatisfactory in one respect; the Fourier coefficients of the far field pattern are complex valued whereas for the boundary curve the Fourier coefficients need to be real valued, that is, we have an overdetermined problem with twice as many equations as unknowns. In order to have a problem with the same number of equations and unknowns we posed ourselves the problem whether is is possible to recover the first $2M + 1$ cosine and sine Fourier coefficients of the radial function r from the first $2M + 1$ cosine and sine Fourier coefficients of the modulus of far field pattern u_∞. In this paper we will describe some of the results which we obtained in this attempt to solve the inverse obstacle scattering problem from the modulus of the far field pattern as data. We have to admit that we have only preliminary results. However, we wish to point out, that it seems to be a very difficult problem to obtain analogues both for the Schiffer uniqueness result and for the injectivity of the Fréchet derivative. The proofs of both of these results heavily rely on the fact that, by Rellich's lemma, the far field pattern u_∞ uniquely determines the scattered wave u^s. A corresponding result is not available for the modulus of the far field pattern, even with the translation invariance taken into account.

More recent investigations indicate that regularised Newton methods [9, 10, 11, 13] and Landweber iterations provide efficient [4, 6] tools for the approximate solution for inverse obstacle scattering problems. Therefore, in a first attempt to solving the inverse obstacle problem from the modulus of the far field alone, it seems to be adequate to also try and investigate the applicability of these schemes in the present situation.

The plan of the paper is as follows. In Section 2 we briefly will describe that the modulus of the far field pattern for plane wave incidence is invariant under translations of the scatterer. In Section 3 we will derive an explicit expression for the Fréchet derivative of the operator $G : r \mapsto |F(r)|^2$ for the case of the unit circle $r = 1$. The representation will be in terms of the real cosine and sine coefficients of q and $G'(r)q$, and, in particular, the effect of the translation invariance will be discussed. In the final Section 4 will describe the implementation of frozen regularised Newton and Landweber iterations including some numerical examples which illustrate the feasibility of our approach.

2 Translation Invariance

The problem to recover the shape of an obstacle from the modulus of the far field pattern for one incident plane wave suffers from an inherent ambiguity due to translation invariance of the modulus of the far field pattern. Let $h \in \mathbb{R}^2$ denote a fixed unit vector. For the shifted domain

$$D_\varepsilon := \{x + \varepsilon h : x \in D\}$$

with boundary $\partial D_\varepsilon := \{x + \varepsilon h : x \in \partial D\}$ the scattered field u_ε^s is given by

$$u_\varepsilon^s(x) = e^{ik\varepsilon\,h\cdot d} u^s(x - \varepsilon h), \quad x \in \mathbb{R}^2 \setminus D_\varepsilon, \tag{10}$$

as can be seen by checking the boundary condition $u_\varepsilon^s = -u^i$ on ∂D_ε. The corresponding far field pattern is

$$u_{\infty,\varepsilon}(\hat{x}) = e^{ik\varepsilon\,h\cdot(d-\hat{x})} u_\infty(\hat{x}), \quad \hat{x} \in \Omega, \tag{11}$$

which follows from

$$\frac{e^{ik|x-\varepsilon h|}}{\sqrt{|x - \varepsilon h|}} = e^{-ik\varepsilon\,h\cdot\hat{x}}\, \frac{e^{ik|x|}}{\sqrt{|x|}}\left(1 + O\left(\frac{1}{|x|}\right)\right).$$

This in particular implies that for plane wave incidence the modulus of the far field pattern is invariant under translations of the scatterer D. Therefore, from the modulus of the far field pattern for one incident plane wave we cannot recover the location of the obstacle.

Considering the limit $\varepsilon \to 0$, from Taylor's formula and (10) it follows that

$$v := \lim_{\varepsilon \to 0} \frac{1}{\varepsilon}\,(u_\varepsilon^s - u^s)$$

exists and is given by

$$v = ik\,h\cdot d\,u^s - h\cdot\operatorname{grad} u^s \quad \text{in } \mathbb{R}^2 \setminus \bar{D}. \tag{12}$$

By evaluating the boundary values and the far field pattern of v, with the aid the boundary condition $u^i + u^s = 0$ on ∂D the following result can be established.

Lemma 1. *Let $h \in \mathbb{R}^2$ be a unit vector. Then the function v given by*

$$v = h \cdot (iku^s\,d - \operatorname{grad} u^s) \quad \text{in } \mathbb{R}^2 \setminus \bar{D}$$

satisfies the boundary condition

$$v = -h \cdot \nu\,\frac{\partial}{\partial\nu}\,(u^i + u^s) \quad \text{on } \partial D$$

and has far field pattern

$$v_\infty(\hat{x}) = ik\{h \cdot (d - \hat{x})\}\,u_\infty(\hat{x}), \quad \hat{x} \in \Omega.$$

3 The Fréchet Derivative

Given the (measured) modulus $|u_\infty|$ of the far field pattern, in terms of an operator equation, the inverse scattering problem with the modulus of the far field pattern as data is equivalent to solving the equation

$$G(r) = |u_\infty|^2 \tag{13}$$

for the radial function r describing the boundary ∂D. Here, $G : C_+^2(\Omega) \to L^2(\Omega)$ denotes the operator given by

$$G(r) = |F(r)|^2, \quad r \in C_+^2(\Omega).$$

Clearly, G is Fréchet differentiable, and by the product rule, the derivative is given by

$$G'(r)q = 2 \operatorname{Re} \overline{F(r)} \, F'(r)q. \tag{14}$$

We proceed by deriving an explicit representation of $G'(r)$ for the case where ∂D is the unit circle, i.e., $r = 1$. For $r = 1$ we will write $F(r) = F$, $F'(r)(q) = F'q$ and $G'(r)(q) = G'q$. Without loss of generality, we may assume that $d = (1,0)$. Using polar coordinates (ρ, θ) for $x \in \mathbb{R}^2$, the Jacobi–Anger expansion (see [2]) reads

$$e^{ik\,x\cdot d} = \sum_{n=-\infty}^{\infty} i^n J_n(k\rho)e^{in\theta}, \quad x \in \mathbb{R}^2,$$

where the J_n denote the Bessel functions of order n. From this it can be seen that the total field $u = u^i + u^s$ has the form

$$u(x) = \sum_{n=-\infty}^{\infty} \frac{i^n}{H_n^{(1)}(k)} \{J_n(k\rho)H_n^{(1)}(k) - J_n(k)H_n^{(1)}(k\rho)\}e^{in\theta}, \quad |x| > 1, \tag{15}$$

where the $H_n^{(1)}$ denote the Hankel functions of the first kind of order n. From the asymptotics of the Hankel functions, and by evaluating the far field pattern of $u^s = u - u^i$ from (15), we find that

$$F(\theta) = -e^{-\frac{\pi i}{4}}\sqrt{\frac{2}{\pi k}} \sum_{n=-\infty}^{\infty} \frac{J_n(k)}{H_n^{(1)}(k)} e^{in\theta}, \quad 0 \le \theta \le 2\pi. \tag{16}$$

Using the Wronskian for the Bessel and Hankel functions, from (15) we can deduce that

$$\frac{\partial u}{\partial \nu}(x) = \frac{2}{i\pi} \sum_{n=-\infty}^{\infty} \frac{i^n e^{in\theta}}{H_n^{(1)}(k)}, \quad |x| = 1. \tag{17}$$

We consider perturbations q given by a Fourier expansion

$$q(\theta) = \sum_{m=-\infty}^{\infty} a_m e^{im\theta}, \tag{18}$$

where in order to ensure that q is real valued, the coefficients must satisfy

$$a_{-m} = \overline{a_m}, \quad m = 0, 1, 2, \ldots. \tag{19}$$

Since on the unit circle we have $v \cdot h = q$, the boundary values (8) of the function v determining the Fréchet derivative are obtained by multiplying the series (17) and (18). From this we can conclude that

$$v(x) = \frac{2i}{\pi} \sum_{n=-\infty}^{\infty} c_n \frac{H_n^{(1)}(k\rho)}{H_n^{(1)}(k)} e^{in\theta}, \quad |x| > 1,$$

where we have set

$$c_n := \sum_{m=-\infty}^{\infty} a_m \frac{i^{n-m}}{H_{n-m}^{(1)}(k)}. \tag{20}$$

Evaluating the far field pattern of v we find that

$$(F'q)(\theta) = e^{-\frac{\pi i}{4}} \sqrt{\frac{2}{\pi k}} \frac{2i}{\pi} \sum_{n=-\infty}^{\infty} \frac{c_n}{i^n H_n^{(1)}(k)} e^{in\theta}, \quad 0 \le \theta \le 2\pi. \tag{21}$$

Multiplying the series (21) and the conjugate complex of the series (16) and inserting (20) we arrive at

$$(G'q)(\theta) = -\frac{4}{\pi k} \operatorname{Re} \left\{ \sum_{n=-\infty}^{\infty} \sum_{m=-\infty}^{\infty} M_{nm} a_m e^{in\theta} \right\}, \quad 0 \le \theta \le 2\pi, \tag{22}$$

where

$$M_{nm} = \frac{2}{\pi i^{m-1}} \sum_{j=-\infty}^{\infty} \frac{1}{H_j^{(1)}(k)} \frac{J_{j-n}(k)}{H_{j-n}^{(1)}(k)} \frac{1}{H_{j-m}^{(1)}(k)}. \tag{23}$$

Here we have used the symmetries $J_{-n} = (-1)^n J_n$ and $H_{-n}^{(1)} = (-1)^n H_n^{(1)}$, which also imply that

$$M_{-n,-m} = M_{nm}, \quad m, n = 0, \pm 1, \pm 2, \ldots. \tag{24}$$

However, instead of the complex formulation (22) we need a relation between the real cosine and sine Fourier coefficients of q and $G'(q)$. Therefore, unfortunately, we have to destroy the convolution structure of (22) and (23). We abbreviate

$$g_n := \sum_{m=-\infty}^{\infty} M_{nm} a_m, \quad n = 0, \pm 1, \pm 2, \ldots, \tag{25}$$

and rewrite (22) into the form

$$(G'q)(\theta) = -\frac{4}{\pi k} \left\{ \operatorname{Re} g_0 + \sum_{n=1}^{\infty} [\operatorname{Re}(g_n + g_{-n}) \cos n\theta - \operatorname{Im}(g_n - g_{-n}) \sin n\theta] \right\}.$$

From (19) and (24) it follows that

$$\operatorname{Re}(g_n + g_{-n}) = 2\operatorname{Re} M_{n,0}\operatorname{Re} a_0 + 2\sum_{m=1}^{\infty}\operatorname{Re}(M_{nm} + M_{n,-m})\operatorname{Re} a_m,$$

$$\operatorname{Im}(g_n - g_{-n}) = 2\sum_{m=1}^{\infty}\operatorname{Re}(M_{nm} - M_{n,-m})\operatorname{Im} a_m.$$

Therefore, setting

$$\alpha_0 = \operatorname{Re} a_0, \quad \alpha_m = 2\operatorname{Re} a_m, \quad \beta_m = -2\operatorname{Im} a_m, \quad m = 1, 2, \ldots, \tag{26}$$

we finally can summarise our computations in the following theorem.

Theorem 2. *For*

$$q(\theta) = \sum_{m=0}^{\infty}\alpha_m \cos m\theta + \sum_{m=1}^{\infty}\beta_m \sin m\theta \tag{27}$$

we have that

$$(G'q)(\theta) = \sum_{n=0}^{\infty}\sum_{m=0}^{\infty}T_{nm}^{c}\alpha_m \cos n\theta + \sum_{n=1}^{\infty}\sum_{1=0}^{\infty}T_{nm}^{s}\beta_m \sin n\theta \tag{28}$$

with the coefficients given by

$$T_{0,m}^{c} = -\frac{4}{\pi k}\operatorname{Re} M_{0,m}, \quad m = 0, 1, 2, \ldots,$$

$$T_{n,m}^{c} = -\frac{4}{\pi k}\operatorname{Re}[M_{nm} + M_{n,-m}], \quad n = 1, 2, \ldots, \; m = 0, 1, 2, \ldots$$

$$T_{n,m}^{s} = -\frac{4}{\pi k}\operatorname{Re}[M_{nm} - M_{n,-m}], \quad n, m = 1, 2, \ldots.$$

A remark on the derivation of Theorem 2 seems to be appropriate. Denote by E the operator taking the real cosine and sine coefficients of a Fourier series of the form (27) into the complex coefficients of the series (18). Further denote by R the operator that maps the complex coefficients of a series of the form (18) into the cosine and sine coefficients of the real part of (18). Clearly RE=I, with I the identity operator on the cosine and sine coefficients. Let M and T be the operators described through (22) and (28). Then, of course, the above analysis just reflects the fact that

$$T = -\frac{4}{\pi k}RME. \tag{29}$$

The translation invariance of the far field pattern effects the injectivity of these matrices as we will show through the subsequent analysis.

Lemma 3. *For $q(\theta) = \cos\theta$ we have that*

$$(F'q)(\theta) = ik(1 - \cos\theta)F(\theta). \tag{30}$$

Proof. Setting $a_1 = a_{-1} = 1/2$ and using the recurrence relation

$$H_{n-1}^{(1)}(k) - H_{n+1}^{(1)}(k) = 2H_n^{(1)'}(k),$$

from (20) and (21) we obtain

$$(F'q)(\theta) = -\frac{2}{\pi} e^{-\frac{\pi i}{4}} \sqrt{\frac{2}{\pi k}} \sum_{n=-\infty}^{\infty} \frac{H_n^{(1)'}(k)}{H_{n-1}^{(1)}(k)H_n^{(1)}(k)H_{n+1}^{(1)}(k)} e^{in\theta}. \tag{31}$$

On the other hand, from (16) we derive

$$(1 - \cos\theta)F(\theta) = \frac{1}{2} e^{-\frac{\pi i}{4}} \sqrt{\frac{2}{\pi k}} \sum_{n=-\infty}^{\infty} \frac{A_n(k)}{H_{n-1}^{(1)}(k)H_n^{(1)}(k)H_{n+1}^{(1)}(k)} e^{in\theta}, \tag{32}$$

where we have set

$$A_n(k) = J_{n-1}(k)H_n^{(1)}(k)H_{n+1}^{(1)}(k) + J_{n+1}(k)H_n^{(1)}(k)H_{n-1}^{(1)}(k)$$

$$-2J_n(k)H_{n-1}^{(1)}(k)H_{n+1}^{(1)}(k).$$

Now we use the recurrence relations

$$J_{n+1}(k) = \frac{n}{k} J_n(k) - J_n'(k), \quad J_{n-1}(k) = \frac{n}{k} J_n(k) + J_n'(k) \tag{33}$$

and the corresponding relations for the Hankel functions and the Wronskian to obtain that

$$A_n(k) = 2H_n^{(1)'}(k)\left\{ J_n(k)H_n^{(1)'}(k) - H_n^{(1)}(k)J_n'(k) \right\} = \frac{4i}{\pi k} H_n^{(1)'}(k).$$

Inserting this into (32) and comparing the result with (31) yields (30).

Lemma 4. *For $q(\theta) = \sin\theta$ we have that*

$$(F'q)(\theta) = -ik\sin\theta\, F(\theta). \tag{34}$$

Proof. Setting $a_1 = 1/2i$ and $a_1 = -1/2i$, and using the recurrence relation

$$H_{n-1}^{(1)}(k) + H_{n+1}^{(1)}(k) = 2nH_n^{(1)}(k)/k,$$

from (20) and (21) we obtain

$$(F'q)(\theta) = \frac{2i}{\pi k} e^{-\frac{\pi i}{4}} \sqrt{\frac{2}{\pi k}} \sum_{n=-\infty}^{\infty} \frac{n}{H_{n-1}^{(1)}(k)H_{n+1}^{(1)}(k)} e^{in\theta}. \tag{35}$$

On the other hand, from (16) we derive

$$\sin\theta\, F(\theta) = \frac{i}{2} e^{-\frac{\pi i}{4}} \sqrt{\frac{2}{\pi k}} \sum_{n=-\infty}^{\infty} \frac{B_n(k)}{H_{n-1}^{(1)}(k) H_{n+1}^{(1)}(k)} e^{in\theta} \qquad (36)$$

where we have set

$$B_n(k) = J_{n+1}(k) H_{n-1}^{(1)}(k) - J_{n-1}(k) H_{n+1}^{(1)}(k).$$

Using the recurrence relations (33) and the Wronskian we find

$$B_n = \frac{2n}{k} \left\{ J_n(k) H_n^{(1)\prime}(k) - H_n^{(1)}(k) J_n'(k) \right\} = \frac{4in}{\pi k^2}.$$

Inserting this into (36) and comparing the result with (35) yields (34) $\square$

At this stage we wish to note that the two Lemmata 3 and 4 can also be deduced from Lemma 1 as special cases where $d = (1,0)$ and ∂D is the unit circle. Setting $h = (1,0)$ we have $h \cdot \nu = \cos\theta$ and $h \cdot (d - \hat{x}) = 1 - \cos\theta$. Hence, from Lemma 1 we can conclude that $(F'q)(\theta) = ik(1-\cos\theta)\, F(\theta)$ for $q(\theta) = \cos\theta$. Setting $h = (0,1)$ we have $h \cdot \nu = \sin\theta$ and $h \cdot (d - \hat{x}) = -\sin\theta$. Hence, from Lemma 1 we can conclude that $(F'q)(\theta) = -ik\sin\theta\, F(\theta)$ for $q(\theta) = \sin\theta$. This indicates that the following theorem is indeed a consequence of the translation invariance of the far field pattern.

Theorem 5. *The second column of the matrix T_{mn}^c and the first column of the matrix T_{mn}^s, i.e., the columns corresponding to the coefficients of $\cos\theta$ and $\sin\theta$ in the radial function q vanish.*

Proof. From the Lemmata 3 and 4 it follows that both for $q(\theta) = \cos\theta$ and $q(\theta) = \sin\theta$ the product $\bar{F}\, F'(q)$ is purely imaginary. Therefore, by (14) we have $G'(q) = 0$ in both cases. $\square$

Thus, for plane wave incidence it is impossible to recover the first $2M + 1$ cosine and sine coefficients of q from the first $2M + 1$ cosine and sine coefficients of $|u_\infty|^2$. Hence, we need to modify the problem and try to recover the $2M - 1$ coefficients $\alpha_0, \alpha_2, \alpha_3, \ldots, \alpha_M, \beta_2, \beta_3, \ldots, \beta_M$, that is, reconstruct the shape of the obstacle but not its location. It seems worthwhile noting, that this ambiguity cannot be remedied by using the modulus of the far field pattern for finitely many incident waves with different wave numbers or different incident directions.

For the diagonal elements M_{nn} we can write

$$M_{nn} = \frac{2}{\pi\, i^{n-1}} \sum_{j=-\infty}^{\infty} \frac{1}{H_j^{(1)}(k)} \frac{J_{j-n}(k)}{|H_{j-n}^{(1)}(k)|^2}, \qquad n = 0, 1, 2, \ldots. \qquad (37)$$

From the power series expansion for the Bessel and Hankel functions it follows that

$$M_{nn} = \frac{2}{\pi i^{n-1}} \frac{J_0(k)}{|H_0^{(1)}(k)|^2} \frac{1}{H_n^{(1)}(k)} + O(k^{n+4}), \qquad n = 0, 1, 2, \ldots, \qquad (38)$$

and from this

$$M_{nn} = -\frac{k^n}{i^n 2^{n-1}(n-1)!} \frac{J_0(k)}{|H_0^{(1)}(k)|^2} + O(k^{n+2}), \quad n = 1, 2, \ldots,$$

for small k. For the off-diagonal elements from (23) we obtain that

$$M_{nm} = O(k^{n+|n-m|}) \frac{1}{\ln k}, \quad n, m = 0, 1, 2, \ldots, \quad n \neq m.$$

Since furthermore from (23) it follows that

$$M_{n,-m} = O(k^{2n+m}), \quad n, m = 0, 1, 2, \ldots,$$

the above estimates imply that the matrices $M_{nm} \pm M_{n,-m}$, $n, m = 0, 1, \ldots, N$, are diagonally dominant for sufficiently small wave numbers k.

Since the leading term for the diagonal elements in (38) is purely imaginary for n odd, the diagonal dominance is lost through taking the real part – as we must for the matrices T_{nm}^c and T_{nm}^s. Actually, from (37) it follows that

$$T_{nn}^c = O(k^{3n}), \quad T_{nn}^s = O(k^{3n}), \quad n = 1, 3, 5, \ldots.$$

This has prevented us from proving an invertibility result for the matrices T_{nm}^c, $n = 0, 1, \ldots, N - 1$, $m = 0, 2, 3, \ldots, N$, and T_{nm}^s, $n = 1, 2, \ldots, N - 1$, $m = 2, 3, \ldots, N$. However, the numerical reconstructions obtained through the frozen Newton method (that is, where the direction used is held fixed throughout the iteration process) in the next section are quite sufficient and encourage further research on the reconstruction of obstacles from the modulus of the far field pattern.

In concluding this section, we mention in passing that in the rotationally symmetric case where we choose the radial wave $u^i(x) = J_0(|x|)$ as incident field, the analysis simplifies considerably. Here, corresponding to (16) we have

$$F(\theta) = -e^{-\frac{\pi i}{4}} \sqrt{\frac{2}{\pi k}} \frac{J_0(k)}{H_0^{(1)}(k)}, \quad 0 \leq \theta \leq 2\pi,$$

And for $q(\theta) = \cos n\theta$ the boundary condition (8) reads

$$v(x) = \frac{2i}{\pi} \frac{1}{H_0^{(1)}(k)} \cos n\theta, \quad |x| = 1.$$

This implies

$$(F'q)(\theta) = e^{-\frac{\pi i}{4}} \sqrt{\frac{2}{\pi k}} \frac{2i}{\pi} \frac{1}{H_0^{(1)}(k)} \frac{1}{i^n H_n^{(1)}(k)} \cos n\theta, \quad 0 \leq \theta \leq 2\pi,$$

whence

$$(G'q)(\theta) = \frac{8}{\pi^2 k} \frac{J_0(k)}{|H_0^{(1)}(k)|^2} \frac{1}{\mathrm{Re}(i^{n+1}H_n^{(1)}(k))} \cos n\theta, \quad 0 \leq \theta \leq 2\pi,$$

follows. Thus here we simply have a diagonal matrix which is regular, but which shows again the drastic change of order when k is small for n odd. This is exactly as we discussed above.

4 Numerical Implementation

For the numerical implementation of these ideas we need to incorporate some regularisation in order to stabilise the ill-posedness of the inverse scattering problem. We also must obtain data which was obtained by solving the integral equation representation described in [2], p. 66. Since the same algorithm was used in the direct solver component of our iterative schemes, we made sure that the stepsizes and values of the coupling parameter controlling the combination of the double- and single-layer potentials were different for the data generating program and for that utilised in the inverse code.

The data consisted of N equally-spaced values of the amplitude of the far field for the target obstacle. Typically we took N = 64. Noise was then added to these values. By 1% noise we mean that for each data point with value v, a value $\delta v = 0.01\epsilon v$ was added where ϵ is a random number in the interval $[-1, 1]$.

We will try to approximate the boundary curve $r = r(\theta)$ by a trigonometric polynomial of the form

$$r(\theta) = \sum_{m=0}^{M} \alpha_m \cos m\theta + \sum_{m=1}^{M} \beta_m \sin m\theta \tag{39}$$

for some index M. The coefficients α_m and β_m are related to the $2M+1$ complex numbers a_m defined in (18) and (26) for $-M \leq m \leq M$. Clearly, we cannot recover more information than we put in, so the number of Fourier coefficients to be recovered cannot exceed the number of data values given. Thus, at the very least, $2M + 1 \leq N$.

The basic iterative scheme has the form

$$r_{n+1} = r_n - A_n[G(r_n) - |u_\infty|^2], \quad n = 0, 1, 2, \ldots. \tag{40}$$

where A_n is a linear operator.

The classical Newton scheme uses $A_n = [G'(r_n)]^{-1}$. Due to the severe ill-posedness of the inverse scattering problem it is clear that we cannot use this directly for there is no possibility of $G'(r_n)$ having a bounded inverse in any reasonable function space. Even in the case when full far field data is given (modulus and phase) the associated Fréchet derivative, although locally one to one, cannot have this property. Of course, in any numerical implementation of the Newton-scheme we would choose A_n to be some finite dimensional approximation to $[G'(r_n)]^{-1}$. However, there is no guarantee that the associated matrix representation will be invertible. For arbitrary q this statement remains true for the case of full far field data [12].

The ill-posedness of the inverse scattering problem will in fact guarantee the finite $(2M + 1) \times (2M + 1)$ matrix representing $G'(r_n)$ will have a condition number that grows with increasing M, that is, as the approximation to the actual derivative improves. Again, for the case of full far field data it was shown in [12] that the condition number actually grows exponentially with M.

The most common way of resolving this difficulty is by using Tikhonov regularisation. Here we let G'_n denote a finite-dimensional approximation to $G'(q_n)$ and define

$$A_n = [\alpha I + (G'_n)^* G'_n]^{-1} (G'_n)^*$$

for some positive constant α. The choice of this regularisation parameter is somewhat ad hoc. Although there is a well developed theory surrounding the issue, particularly for linear ill-posed problems, the associated conditions are often impossible to verify in any given example.

Another approach is to choose the finite dimensional approximant G'_n "sufficiently far" from G' that the associated linear system can be inverted in a stable manner. If we expand the boundary curve r as a finite dimensional Fourier series as in (39), then consider G_n to be the map from such a finite Fourier series to the $2M+1$ cosine and sine Fourier coefficients of the modulus of the far field pattern, then for M sufficiently small we might expect that G'_n would be invertible. This is the central idea to regularisation by spectral cut-off; we simply eliminate all frequencies higher than a given value M and we choose this value in order that the condition of the linear system be small enough for a stable inversion. The number M serves as a regularisation parameter for the iteration scheme.

The Landweber iteration method sets $A_n = c_n [G'(r_n)]^*$ for some constant c_n chosen so that $\|A_n\| < 1$. Here there is no question of invertibility of $G'(r_n)$ to consider, but the ill-conditioning of the problem cannot be resolved by mathematical tricks. Instead, we find that the residual $R_n := \||G(r_n) - |u_\infty|^2\|_{L^2(\Omega)}$ initially decreases, but then at a value n_0 increases once again. Implementation of the method requires the residual be monitored at each step to detect the value of n_0 at which point the scheme is terminated and r_{n_0} is the reconstruction. Thus the Landweber scheme is regularised by imposing a suitable stopping condition on the iteration process itself, namely that obtained by minimising the residual. The method is notoriously slow, indeed for linear problems it can be shown to be equivalent to the method of steepest descent with fixed step size applied to the least square functional. For certain nonlinear problems where the computational effort of the best schemes is relatively high, the Landweber method can be an effective tool.

An analysis of the Landweber method for a nonlinear operator in a Hilbert space setting has been given by Hanke, Neubauer and Scherzer [5]. They derive a discrepancy principle by suggesting an appropriate stopping criterion and analyse the rate of convergence of the scheme. The key condition for convergence is that locally the linearisation of the operator G should satisfy

$$\|G(q) - G(r) - G'(q)(q - r)\| \leq \eta \|G(q) - G(r)\| \qquad (41)$$

for some η with $0 < \eta < 1/2$. As shown in [5], the most straightforward means of establishing this inequality is by verifying a uniformity condition on the derivative G': for each q and r there exists a bounded invertible operator $R_{q,r}$ with

$$G'(r) = R_{q,r} G'(q). \qquad (42)$$

However verifying either of these conditions is often exceedingly difficult.

In the case that G' is a bounded invertible operator the equation (42) is easily shown to be valid. However, such boundedness is never the case for an ill-posed problem in an infinite dimensional space. If we can pose the problem in a suitable finite dimensional space and if the matrix representing G' is invertible then we can invoke these conditions and thereby obtain convergence estimates. As we have indicated in the previous sections, this invertibility condition is not easy to prove. In [7] an inverse problem seeking the recovery of an interior obstacle from Cauchy data was investigated. Condition (41) was shown to hold and an analysis of the Landweber scheme made. In [4] the authors considered the Landweber method for inverse obstacle scattering from full far field data. An explicit representation for the corresponding adjoint operator $(G')^*$ was obtained and then used in a numerical reconstruction algorithm. However, the authors were unable to verify condition (41) for this problem.

The computational cost of implementing the iteration scheme (40) consists mostly of two parts: a single direct solve to compute $G(r_n)$, and the cost of computing A_n (or more exactly that of computing the associated matrix representation). The first of these is independent of the choice of A_n and is the same for all such iteration schemes. The computation of A_n depends strongly on the choice of this operator and whether a matrix inversion is required. The use of the characterisation (7)–(8) allows considerable simplification in this computation (see [10, 11]) but is always at least the cost of a further direct solve. Both the Landweber and Newton schemes requires an evaluation of the Fréchet derivative at each stage. The Newton schemes require an additional matrix inversion to update r.

For these reasons a quasi-Newton scheme which uses the computation of the derivative at a fixed solution offers an attractive alternative. As we showed in Theorem 2, an explicit computation can be made of the derivative map at a circle of constant radius, which by an easy scaling can, without loss of generality, be taken to be the unit circle. Since any matrix inversions required can be performed prior to the start of the scheme, the computational cost of this approach is the number of iterations required for numerical convergence multiplied by the cost of a single direct scattering computation.

In the case of obstacle scattering from full far field data this approach gave excellent results and the final reconstructions were only marginally poorer than that obtained from the full-Newton scheme [12]. These considerations motivated a similar approach for amplitude-only data.

The central part of the numerical implementation requires the computation of the matrix T defined in Theorem 2, or more precisely, its finite dimensional version. In the spectral cut-off approach we shall represent the data $|u_\infty|^2(\theta_i)$, $1 \leq i \leq N$, as a finite Fourier series

$$|u_\infty|^2(\theta) = \sum_{m=0}^{M} u_m^c \cos m\theta + \sum_{m=1}^{M} u_m^s \sin m\theta$$

and consider the inverse problem to be the inversion of the mapping from $\mathbb{R}^{2M+1} \to \mathbb{R}^{2M+1}$ which takes the Fourier coefficients of $q_n = r_{n+1} - r_n$ onto the

Fourier coefficients of $|u_\infty|^2$. It should be noted that this integration, at least for low frequency Fourier modes, performs a filtering of the noise in the data. The update step of the scheme (40) will in this case require the computation the solution of the matrix equation

$$T_M \, q_n = d_n \tag{43}$$

where d_n is a vector of size $2M + 1$ representing the cosine and sine Fourier coefficients of the quantity $G(r_n) - |u_\infty|^2$. Here the Jacobian matrix T_M is of size $(2M+1) \times (2M+1)$ and is given in terms of the operator T defined in Theorem 2 through

$$T_M = \begin{bmatrix} T_M^c & 0 \\ 0 & T_M^s \end{bmatrix}. \tag{44}$$

The submatrices T_M^c and T_M^s are of size $(M+1) \times (M+1)$ and $M \times M$ respectively and are given by the corresponding principal subminors of the infinite matrices T^c and T^s.

Equation (43) was solved using the singular value decomposition of T_M. This allowed us to take into account the known degeneracies in the directions $q(\theta) = \cos \theta$ and $q(\theta) = \sin \theta$. We must expect that the maximum size of this system, and hence the dimension of the basis set for q that can be inverted in a stable manner, is rather small. Even with very accurate data we could not take M to be more than 6 and even at this value the reconstruction was quite poor. In fact, the optimum value, as measured by the best L^2 approximation to the actual curve, was obtained for $M = 4$.

Figure 1 shows reconstructions for various values of M for the bean-shaped curve

$$r_{\text{actual}}(\theta) = \frac{1 + 0.9 \cos \theta + 0.1 \sin 2\theta}{1 + 0.75 \cos \theta} \tag{45}$$

for the wave number $k = 1$. These results are quite in keeping with the reconstructions found from full far field data [12]. The actual data was computed as we described earlier and contained 1% added noise. The stopping condition for the algorithm consisted of verifying that the residual was reduced by at least 10^{-5} from the previous step. In these reconstructions the initial approximation was the unit circle and the values of the Fourier modes in the directions $\cos \theta$ and $\sin \theta$ were set to be the actual values, although this is simply a convenience for the purposes of comparison with the actual curve. The update procedure neglected these two modes. The incident field had the direction shown in the figures.

There is a further point to be made here in regards to the amount of data required. If we indeed wish to recover cosine and sine coefficients of the boundary curve r up to order M then, because of the translation invariance difficulty, we cannot recover the first cosine and sine modes. This leaves only $2M-1$ coefficients to be determined as we pointed out in the remark following Theorem 5. Thus if we use the pointwise data to obtain the first $2M + 1$ Fourier modes of $|u_\infty|^2$ the inversion problem is really overdetermined. However, this is exactly the procedure used to obtain Figure 1. One can easily modify the algorithm to accept only the first $2M-1$ Fourier coefficients of the data and the resulting system was uniquely invertible for all cases we considered. There was very little difference in the reconstructions, but that using less data was marginally superior, at least for the cases where $M \leq 5$. The reason for this is not hard to see; the ill conditioning of the problem manifests itself in the fact that the algorithm can utilise information in low frequency modes better than that in high frequency ones. If $2M+1$ are used and weighted equally, then the presence of the additional $\cos M\theta$ and $\sin M\theta$ modes "pollutes" the more reliable information encoded in the lower modes.

Figure 1. Quasi-Newton Method using spectral cut-off

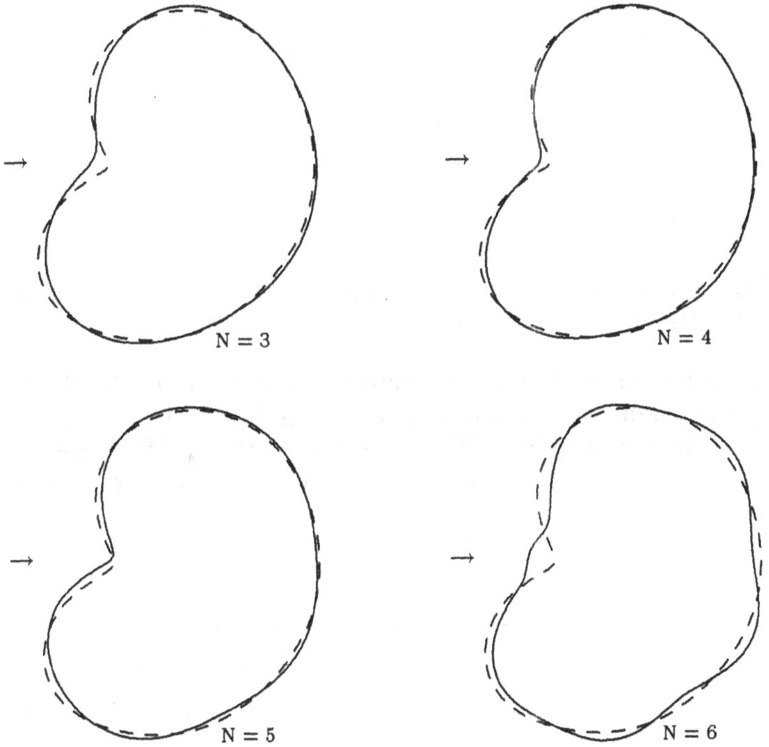

Reconstructions using spectral cut-off with $N = 3,4,5,6$. Data contains 1% error and approximately 15 iterations were needed.

For the case of inversion of the quasi-Newton scheme by Tikhonov regularisation we choose $A_n = A = \left[\alpha I + (G')^\star G'\right]^{-1}(G')^\star$ where G' means the derivative evaluated at the unit circle. We can again obtain the Jacobian matrix for G' from Theorem 2 via (44). Unlike the previous example using spectral cut-off regularisation, we are not restricted to using small values of M. In the numerical reconstructions shown below we used $M = 12$, so that the dimension of the matrix T_M was 25×25. Given the accuracy of the forward solver used, 25 Fourier modes are sufficient to approximate the quantities we must calculate. The regularisation parameter α was chosen by trial and error to obtain the smallest overall residual $\|G(r_n) - |u_\infty|^2\|_{L^2(\Omega)}$. For the problem at hand this turned out to be $\alpha \approx 0.4$. As in the previous case, the update procedure neglected the two modes corresponding to the directions $\cos\theta$ and $\sin\theta$. The results for two reconstructions of the same bean-shaped object, one with data error 1% the other with 5%, is shown in Figure 2.

Figure 2. Quasi-Newton Method using Tikhonov regularization

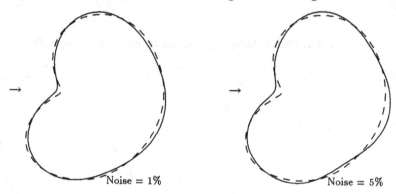

Reconstructions using Tikhonov regularization with 1% and 5% noise in the data. Approximately 12 iterations were needed.

In our implementation of the Landweber method we simply set $A_n = \mu T_M^*$ where the parameter μ was chosen so that $\|\mu T_M^*\| < 1$. As in the previous Newton scheme we used M $= 12$ in our representation T_M^* of the operator $(G')^*$. As should be expected from the Landweber method, the convergence rate was much slower than obtained using the Newton schemes. Two reconstructions for different levels of noise in the data are shown in Figure 3.

Figure 3. Landweber Scheme.

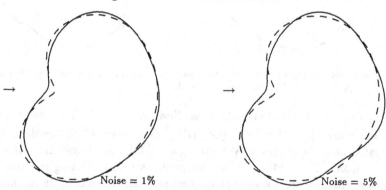

Reconstructions using Landweber scheme. Figure to the left was using data with 1% error and the stopping condition was invoked after 75 iterations. That on the right was with 5% data error and required 69 iterations.

The use of a quasi-Newton, or to continue the modifier, a quasi-Landweber, iteration scheme, gives clear computational cost advantages at each step. This will translate into an overall reduction in the number of computational steps only if the number of iterations required is not considerably less for the full Newton scheme. For this particular problem the quasi-Newton scheme does require more iterations, but this was never more than twice the number required for the full Newton scheme,

One disadvantage of using an approximation to the derivative held fixed at a known solution was discovered. In the case of the quasi-Newton method using spectral cut-off we took "accurate data," that is numerically computed data to which no noise had been added. When the quasi-Newton scheme was run with M = 4 the method was stopped after 20 iterations after the residual, which had always decreased, reached the value 0.00191 and the stopping condition was invoked. The value of $\|r_{20} - r_{actual}\|$ was 0.026. However, the values of $\|r_n - r_{actual}\|$ were not monotonic, but after an initial decrease, started to increase once more. At iteration 9 the value of $\|r_9 - r_{actual}\|$ was 0.009, but the residual was 0.00941. The explanation, no doubt, lies in the fact that the derivative direction chosen, which is never updated, actually drives the solution away from the correct value as the algorithm attempts to minimise the residual. Indeed, if we give data corresponding to the unit circle but use the bean-shaped obstacle as initial guess, then both the residual and the norm difference $\|r_n - r_{actual}\|$ decrease monotonically until the stopping condition is invoked.

A similar phenomenon was found for the other two methods used. In the case of the Landweber method with 1% data error the residual was 0.00305 at the stopping condition which took place after 75 iterations. The final error in r was 0.05909. However, after 17 iterations this result had already been achieved and a minimum norm difference of 0.04609 was obtained after 33 iterations (when the residual was 0.01184).

There is nothing to prevent us using a combination of some or all of the above ideas and thereby form a multiple-approach regularisation scheme. This can often lead to a robust algorithm able to reconstruct a wide variety of curves; the difficulty is, of course, in the proper choice of the various parameters. For example, the Landweber scheme often obtains a rough but usable approximation after a few iterations. Thereafter the convergence of r_n to the actual curve slows considerably. On the other hand, Newton-type schemes typically require the initial approximation to be close to the actual solution. In the case of ill-posed problems they also tend to overshoot the actual solution before the residual is minimised completely. One known cure is to use stepsize control on the Newton step, (see for example [7]). Another is to switch to a second update method, or more precisely, a different search direction, if the residual increases. Of course, combining two schemes with properties such as these to minimise residuals is far from new, and in our situation using a combination of quasi-Landweber and quasi-Newton schemes leads to a version of the Marquardt–Levenberg approach.

References

1. Colton, D., and Kress, R.: *Integral Equation Methods in Scattering Theory.* Wiley-Interscience Publication, New York 1983.
2. Colton, D., and Kress, R.: *Inverse Acoustic and Electromagnetic Scattering Theory.* Springer-Verlag, Berlin Heidelberg New York 1992.
3. Colton, D., and Sleeman, B.D.: Uniqueness theorems for the inverse problem of acoustic scattering. IMA J. Appl. Math. **31**, 253–259 (1983).
4. Hanke, M., Hettlich, F. and Scherzer, O.: The Landweber Iteration for an Inverse Scattering Problem. In: *Proceedings of the 1995 Design Engineering Technical Conferences, Vol.3 Part C, Vibration Control, Analysis, and Identification,* (Wang et. al., eds) 909-915. The American Society of Mechanical Engineers, New York, 1995.
5. Hanke, M., Neubauer, A. and Scherzer, O.: A convergence analysis of the Landweber iteration for nonlinear ill-posed problems. Numer. Math. **72**, 21–37 (1995).
6. Hettlich, F.: An iterative method for the inverse scattering problem from sound-hard obstacles. In: *Proceedings of the ICIAM 95, Vol. II, Applied Analysis,* (Mahrenholz & Mennicken, eds), Akademie Verlag, Berlin, 1996.
7. Hettlich, F., and Rundell, W.: A quasi-Newton method in inverse obstacle scattering. Inverse Problems **12**, 251–266 (1996).
8. Kirsch, A.: The domain derivative and two applications in inverse scattering theory. Inverse Problems **9**, 81–96 (1993).
9. Kirsch, A.: Numerical algorithms in inverse scattering theory, In: *Ordinary and Partial Differential Equations, Vol. IV,* (Jarvis & Sleeman, eds) Pitman Research Notes in Mathematics **289**, 93–111, Longman, London 1993.
10. Kress, R.: A Newton method in inverse obstacle scattering, In: *Inverse Problems in Engineering Mechanics,* (Bui et al, eds) 425–432, Balkema, Rotterdam 1994.
11. Kress, R.: Integral equation methods in inverse obstacle scattering, Engineering Anal. with Boundary Elements **15**, 171–179 (1995)
12. Kress, R., and Rundell, W.: A quasi-Newton method in inverse obstacle scattering, Inverse Problems **10**, 1145–1157 (1994).
13. Mönch, L.: A Newton method for solving the inverse scattering problem for a sound-hard obstacle. Inverse Problems **12**, 309–323 (1996).
14. Potthast, R.: Fréchet differentiability of boundary integral operators in inverse acoustic scattering. Inverse Problems **10**, 431–447 (1994).

Applied Inversion in Nondestructive Testing

K.J. Langenberg, M. Brandfaß, S. Klaholz, R. Marklein,
K. Mayer, A. Pitsch, R. Schneider

Department of Electrical Engineering, Electromagnetic Theory, University of Kassel,
34109 Kassel, Germany

1 Introduction

The explicit inverse problems in nondestructive testing range from material characterization to defect imaging, and, as such, they exhibit a large bandwidth of complexity: Material characterization should be *quantitative*, thus accounting for nonlinearities of the underlying physical phenomena as well as for the nonlinearity of the inverse problem, whereas defect imaging might already be sufficiently solved if the location, the size and the orientation of a defect has been determined. As a matter of fact, the latter task can be accomplished with rather simple inverse algorithms, which rely on the linearization of the elastic and/or electromagnetic wave inverse scattering problem. Nevertheless, in particular in safety relevant applications like nuclear power generation, aircraft and/or bridge testing, one is interested to extract the maximum amount of information from the data utilizing all a priori knowledge of the physical model under concern, for instance with regard to the propagation characteristics of the defect embedding medium or with regard to the polarization of the wave mode. In that sense, some recent fundamental improvements of linear diffraction tomographic inverse scattering have been made, which will be summarized and commented upon in the present article. In addition, a novel philosophy of computer aided nondestructive testing will be discussed, which comes under the alias ULIAS: Ultrasonic Inspection Applying Simulation. The key idea is to support the assessment of the output of existing imaging algorithms with simulations applying numerical techniques to compute wave propagation and scattering for the testing problem under concern; the resulting synthetic data supply a testbed for the inverse problem.

Of course, the solid part to be tested nondestructively allows for the exploitation of a large variety of physical effects ranging from static electromagnetics through eddy currents and electromagnetic waves to X-rays. Here, we will concentrate upon waves, and, of course, not only on the electromagnetic species but also on elastodynamics, in particular in the ultrasonic frequency regime. As far as numerical wave propagation simulations are concerned we rely on the Finite Integration Technique (FIT), which is very successful either for electromagnetics or elastodynamics [1, 2]. In three spatial dimensions (3D), numerical codes

94

for electromagnetic waves (EMFIT), acoustic waves (AFIT) and elastic waves (EFIT) have been independently developed, wheres in 2D, the interrelations given in Figure 1 make an acoustic code ready for applications to the shear-horizontal mode (SH) of elastodynamics and the TE- and TM-polarizations of electromagnetics. Even the — coupled — pressure-shear-vertical modes (P-SV) of elastodynamics can be — at least approximately — "scalarized" if time gating techniques are applied to the pressure and shear waves on behalf of their different wave speeds [3]. These interrelations of numerical modeling are equally relevant

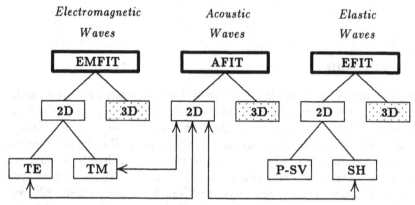

Fig. 1. Numerical codes for 2D and 3D wave simulation with the Finite Integration Technique

for the evaluation of imaging algorithms; for instance, the Synthetic Aperture Focusing Technique (SAFT), as it is addressed below, is instantaneously applicable in acoustics, electromagnetics and elastodynamics. Of course, the output is an "image" and *not* a quantitative solution of the inverse scattering problem, but, as already pointed out, this is very often sufficient.

2 Synthetic Aperture Focusing

Let $\Phi(\underline{R}, t)$ denote a scalar quantity — for instance, a voltage as output of a receiver — as function of the vector of position $\underline{R}$ and time t. In ultrasonic non-destructive testing the data are produced by an impulsive transducer excitation in the time domain, i.e. the scattered "field" $\Phi_s(\underline{R}, t)$ is supposed to be known for $\underline{R}$ varying on an appropriate measurement surface S_M. Of course, the ultrasonic pulses are bandlimited, and S_M is rarely a closed surface surrounding the test piece with the defect completely. Therefore, the data are generally incomplete. Another specific feature of ultrasonic testing is the simultaneous use of the transducer as transmitter and receiver, which is possible due to the time delay of the scattered signal with regard to the incident pulse. This transmitter-receiver is scanned along the measurement surface producing data $\Phi_s^{mo}(\underline{R}, t)$

in an impulse-echo or monostatic mode, the latter characterization originating from the electromagnetic radar community. As a matter of fact, electromagnetic nondestructive testing with microwaves becomes more and more popular for poorly conducting materials as the available frequency bandwidth gets higher and higher making the average wavelength comparable to the defect sizes under concern. Notice: In contrast to ultrasonics, microwave experiments are often made as swept frequency experiments within a finite bandwidth, but, as it is true for the ground probing radar, impulsive excitation is also applied. In any case, the monostatic mode is again the usual mode of operation.

Now, for the above characterized aperture- and frequency-bandlimited monostatic data $\Phi_s^{mo}(\mathbf{R}, t)$, a heuristic imaging scheme called SAFT for Synthetic Aperture Focusing Technique has been proposed for ultrasonic inspection, i.e. applying it to the scalar output of a transducer, which has somehow transformed the elastodynamic vector wavefield into a scalar voltage. The embedding of this scheme into scalar inverse scattering theory is discussed in [4] and the heuristic arguments for its "invention" are presented in [3] in some detail. Its extensive use and success in practical applications is documented in [5, 6, 7, 8, 9].

The SAFT scheme is simply given by the equation

$$o(\mathbf{R}) = \int\int_{S_M} \Phi_s^{mo}\left(\mathbf{R}', t = \frac{2|\mathbf{R} - \mathbf{R}'|}{c}\right) dS' \ . \tag{1}$$

Here, $o(\mathbf{R})$ is an image produced via integration of measured impulse-echo data over a two-dimensional measurement surface S_M, where the time argument

$$t = \frac{2|\mathbf{R} - \mathbf{R}'|}{c} \tag{2}$$

accounts for the monostatic backpropagation of the data with c, the wave speed of the homogeneous defect embedding medium, i.e. the wave speed of the test piece material. Since the solid test piece is able to support both pressure and shear waves with different phase velocities, an appropriate choice has to be made according to the selection of the wave mode for the experiment under concern. Very often, data collection over a two-dimensional aperture is too time consuming, and, hence, L-SAFT reduces the SAFT scheme to an integration along a single measurement line. Even though simple by nature, SAFT is presently considered to be the front end of sophisticated ultrasonic nondestructive testing, and, as a matter of fact, it has proven its usefulness and success in numerous applications.

Of course, there is no argument forbidding the application of (1) to a scalar physical quantity of monostatic electromagnetic scattering, and we will discuss some features of SAFT for these kind of data because results for ultrasonics are already widespread in the literature. In addition, this will give rise to a slight extension of (1) to a two-media problem.

The geometry under concern is displayed in Figure 2: An acrylic test specimen of size $35\times15\times7$ cm^3 contains a series of circular cylindrical side drilled holes with equal diameters of 0.3 cm in different depths; its surface is scanned along

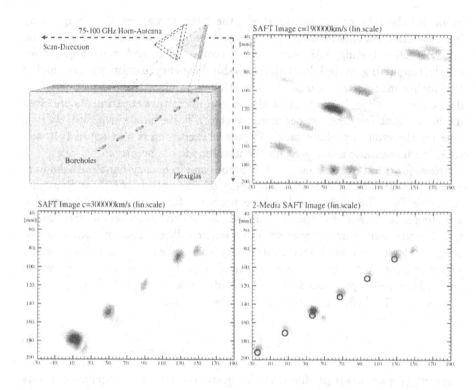

Fig. 2. Geometry of microwave experiment and various SAFT images

a linear x-aperture by a horn antenna in a pulse-echo mode, i.e. the antenna is simultaneously used as transmitter and receiver at 513 scan positions, the swept frequency range being 75-100 GHz. The microwave device is a Hewlett Packard network analyzer. Notice, the horn antenna is tilted with regard to the surface normal in order to avoid the reception of the surface reflected signal. Fourier transforming the received complex frequency data into the time domain results in xt-data. Feeding these data into the algorithm (1), an appropriate wave speed of a *homogeneous* medium has to be chosen. We have tried two alternatives, concentrating either on the air (vacuum) or on the acrylic wave speed, and, obviously, both microwave SAFT results are more or less garbage: Figure 2 exhibits "scattering centres" for both cases, but at the wrong locations. It seems necessary to formulate a two-media SAFT, which accounts for the wave propagation in air (vacuum) *and* acrylic. Since the surface of the specimen is known, a SAFT version based on Fermat's principle, thus accounting for the diffraction at the surface, could be implemented. Figure 3 explains, that for every image point $\mathbf{R}$ and every aperture point $\mathbf{R}'$ a point $\mathbf{R}''$ on the specimen

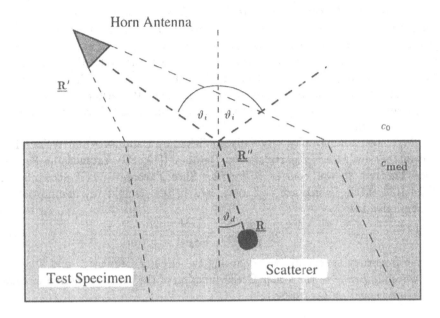

Fig. 3. Two-media microwave SAFT based on Fermat's principle.

surface is found via minimization of the travel time along the corresponding ray; then, (2) is replaced by

$$t = \frac{2|\underline{R}' - \underline{R}''|}{c_0} + \frac{2|\underline{R}' - \underline{R}|}{c_{med}} \ . \tag{3}$$

Of course, this is a *heuristic* argument built into a *heuristic* algorithm, amplitudes, for instance, are not considered. Nevertheless, the pertinent two-media microwave SAFT result as given in Figure 2 together with the — known — geometry of the holes, obviously exhibits the correct defect location now. A careful investigation of this result, however, reveals the presence of ghost images originating from multiple reflections between the single holes, i.e. the heuristic SAFT algorithm does not appropriately account for these multiple reflections, it actually linearizes the inverse problem, a fact, which becomes more obvious if SAFT is considered within the framework of diffraction tomography.

3 Scalar Diffraction Tomography

SAFT results from scalar inverse scattering theory via linearization and various subsequent additional approximations ([4]), and *linear* inverse wave scattering is best formulated as diffraction tomography.

A fundamental result of computerized X-ray tomography is the Fourier Slice Theorem, which states that the one-dimensional Fourier transform of the projection of a two-dimensional object taken under the angle θ is equal to the two-dimensional Fourier transform of the object along a line under the same angle. Therefore, varying θ fills up the Fourier space of the object, which is then recovered via a two-dimensional inverse Fourier transform ([10]). Alternatively, a backprojection operator can be applied to the differentiated and Hilbert-transformed projection data.

Diffraction tomography, originally published by Dändlicker und Weiss ([11]) and further evaluated in particular by Devaney ([12, 13]), extends the Fourier Slice Theorem to the Fourier *Diffraction* Slice Theorem, i.e. it accounts for diffraction effects, which are not considered in the straight ray assumption of tomography. Let

$$G(\mathbf{R}, \omega) = \frac{e^{jkR}}{4\pi R} \tag{4}$$

be the frequency spectrum — ω denoting the circular frequency[1] and $k = \omega/c$ the wavenumber — of the scalar Green function of the three-dimensional scalar Helmholtz equation according to

$$\Delta G(\mathbf{R}, \omega) + k^2 G(\mathbf{R}, \omega) = -\delta(\mathbf{R}) \tag{5}$$

for a homogeneous k-medium of infinite extent. An incident wavefield $\phi_i(\mathbf{R}, \omega)$ having its sources outside a scatterer with variable wavenumber $k(\mathbf{R})$ and compact support V_c produces a scattered field $\Phi_s(\mathbf{R}, \omega)$ having the equivalent sources

$$q_c(\mathbf{R}, \omega) = -k^2 \left[1 - \frac{k^2(\mathbf{R})}{k^2} \right] \Gamma_c(\mathbf{R}) \Phi(\mathbf{R}, \omega) \ , \tag{6}$$

where $\Phi(\mathbf{R}, \omega)$ is the total field as the superposition of the incident and the scattered field and $\Gamma_c(\mathbf{R})$ accounts for the finite support of the scatterer. An appropriate representation of the scattered field is the following

$$\Phi_s(x, y, z, \omega) = \tag{7}$$

$$\int_{-\infty}^{+\infty} \int_{-\infty}^{+\infty} \int_{-\infty}^{+\infty} q_c(x', y', z', \omega) \frac{e^{jk\sqrt{(x-x')^2+(y-y')^2+(z-z')^2}}}{4\pi\sqrt{(x-x')^2+(y-y')^2+(z-z')^2}} \, dx'dy'dz' \ ,$$

where we have used cartesian coordinates x, y, z. "Burying" the scatterer in the halfspace $z < d$ and considering the xy-plane at $z = d$ as measurement plane S_M, we find the Fourier Diffraction Slice Theorem via two-dimensional Fourier transform of the "measurements" $\Phi_s(x, y, d, \omega)$

$$\hat{\Phi}_s(K_x, K_y, d, \omega) = \frac{j}{2} \frac{e^{jd\sqrt{k^2-K_x^2-K_y^2}}}{\sqrt{k^2 - K_x^2 - K_y^2}} \tilde{q}_c(K_x, K_y, K_z = \sqrt{k^2 - K_x^2 - K_y^2}, \omega) \ , \tag{8}$$

---

[1] Notice: The *frequency* f in the engineering sciences as given in Hertz is related to the circular frequency via $f = \omega/2\pi$.

where the Fourier variables with regard to x and y are denoted by K_x and K_y; $\tilde{q}_c$ is the three-dimensional Fourier transform of the equivalent sources, where the restriction of K_z to the Ewald-sphere $|\mathbf{K}| = k$ reflects the relationship with the Fourier Slice Theorem: The Fourier-transformed data have to be arranged along *spheres* of radius k instead along lines. Unfortunately, varying the illumination as in X-ray tomography does not readily fill up Fourier space because the equivalent sources depend upon the *total* field and not upon the incident field alone. The remedy is in terms of linearization: Neglect the scattered field within V_c, i.e. apply the Born approximation to the model (6) of the equivalent sources! Assuming the incident field to be a plane wave

$$\Phi_i(\underline{\mathbf{R}}, \omega) = F(\omega) \exp(jk\hat{\underline{\mathbf{k}}}_i \cdot \underline{\mathbf{R}}) \tag{9}$$

with frequency spectrum $F(\omega)$ and unit phase vector $\hat{\underline{\mathbf{k}}}_i$ leaves us with two parameters to be varied to fill up Fourier space: $\hat{\underline{\mathbf{k}}}_i$ and ω, hence, an angular diversity or a frequuency diversity mode can be chosen as experimental operation. Fixed frequency and varying $\hat{\underline{\mathbf{k}}}_i$ is close to X-ray tomography, but it is not a big issue in NDT. Instead, varying ω with fixed $\hat{\underline{\mathbf{k}}}_i$ is called a bistatic arrangement in contrast to the monostatic arrangement that we already considered. As a matter of fact, it is also possible to derive a monostatic version of the Fourier Diffraction Slice Theorem ([4, 14]), but, in contrast to (8), linearization has to be introduced from the beginning. In [14], this monostatic Fourier Diffraction Slice Theorem — termed FT-SAFT for reasons to be discussed below — has been implemented as a 3D imaging scheme in NDT for an equivalent source model

$$q_c(\underline{\mathbf{R}}, \omega) = -\gamma_c(\underline{\mathbf{R}})\underline{\mathbf{n}} \cdot \boldsymbol{\nabla}\Phi(\underline{\mathbf{R}}, \omega) \ , \tag{10}$$

which holds for perfectly soft scatterers with a Dirichlet boundary condition approximatiing cracks and voids in solids; in (10), $\underline{\mathbf{n}}$ is the outward normal of V_c, and $\gamma_c(\underline{\mathbf{R}})$ is the distributional derivative of the support function $\Gamma_c(\underline{\mathbf{R}})$, the so-called singular function of the surface of the scatterer. The linearization $\Phi(\underline{\mathbf{R}}, \omega) \sim \Phi_i(\underline{\mathbf{R}}, \omega)$ in (10) is termed the physical optics or Kirchhoff approximation. For NDT purposes, it is valid with sufficient accuracy, accounting for the success of diffraction tomography in this field. In the FT-SAFT system, additional attempts have been made to improve the axial resolution as well as the lateral resolution of the images through signal processing techniques: The axial resolution depends upon the bandwidth of $F(\omega)$, and, therefore, deconvolution techniques do well to enhance it, but lateral resolution is difficult to improve because it depends upon the size of the transducer and the aperture, and, as it is the case in NDT, the aperture is mostly chosen to contain already the maximum amount of information; therefore, one can live with the missing data!

Embedding the Fourier Diffraction Slice Theorem within the concept of generalized holography ([15]) defining a generalized holographic field $\Theta_H(\underline{\mathbf{R}}, \omega)$ in terms of measurements $\Phi_s(\underline{\mathbf{R}}, \omega)$ and their corresponding normal derivatives $\underline{\mathbf{n}} \cdot \boldsymbol{\nabla}\Phi_s(\underline{\mathbf{R}}, \omega)$ — for planar measurement surfaces, the latter can be computed from the former —

$$\Theta_H(\underline{\mathbf{R}}, \omega) = \tag{11}$$

$$-\iint_{S_M} [\phi_s(\underline{\mathbf{R}}',\omega)\boldsymbol{\nabla}'G^*(\underline{\mathbf{R}}-\underline{\mathbf{R}}',\omega) - G^*(\underline{\mathbf{R}}-\underline{\mathbf{R}}',\omega)\boldsymbol{\nabla}'\Phi_s(\underline{\mathbf{R}}',\omega)]\cdot\underline{\mathbf{n}}'\,\mathrm{d}S'$$

allows for a generalization of diffraction tomography. In (11), the complex conjugate G^* of the Green function (4) accounts for the backpropagation of the data from a closed measurement surface; manipulation of (11) with Green's theorem results in the Porter-Bojarski integral equation

$$\Theta_H(\underline{\mathbf{R}},\omega) = 2\mathrm{j}\int_{-\infty}^{+\infty}\int_{-\infty}^{+\infty}\int_{-\infty}^{+\infty} q_c(\underline{\mathbf{R}}',\omega)G_I(\underline{\mathbf{R}}-\underline{\mathbf{R}}',\omega)\,\mathrm{d}^3\underline{\mathbf{R}}' \qquad (12)$$

with the imaginary part of the Green function as kernel; equ. (12) relates the measurements in terms of Θ_H to various models of equivalent sources. After linearization of the equivalent sources and integration with regard to either the diversity parameter $\underline{\mathbf{k}}_i$ or ω, (12) is *the* fundamental equation of linear scalar inverse scattering, because every algorithm, including the Fourier Diffraction Slice Theorem — FT-SAFT! — and SAFT can be conveniently derived from it ([4, 16]). As a matter of fact, in the frequency diversity mode, (12) can be "deconvolved" to yield a — bistatic — time domain backpropagation scheme[2], which, after introduction of several additional approximations, reduces to the bistatic version of SAFT. On the other hand, for planar measurement surfaces, (12) is only a marginal disguise of the Fourier Diffraction Slice Theorem, thus assessing a *quantitative* relationship between SAFT and FT-SAFT, and, indeed, the monostatic case can be treated along the same guidelines ([4]). Now the term FT-SAFT is justified, as the pertinent algorithm performs a SAFT data processing applying Fourier transforms only, which makes it fast and convenient for 3D. We will give an example in section 6, when we discuss the ULIAS system, which contains an implementation of FT-SAFT.

A comparison of SAFT and FT-SAFT processing for experimental ultrasonic data is given in [3], and for experimental electromagnetic data in [17].

4 Synthetic Aperture Focusing in an Anisotropic Host Medium

Recently, complex media with complicated wave propagation phenomena have found considerable attention in NDT: austenitic (corrosion-free) steel and fiber-reinforced composites. These materials behave anisotropically with regard to elastic wave propagation, and in order to develop an imaging scheme for these host media, the propagation of ultrasound has to be physically understood, which is not yet completely the case. Apart from analytical methods, which actually do not reach very far, numerical modeling methods play an important role: We have developed the EFIT-code for that purpose.

---

[2] In the farfield, it reduces to a back*projection* scheme, revealing a close relationship with X-ray tomography.

4.1 Elastic Wave Propagation

It is well-known that Maxwell's equations of electromagnetics either come in differential or in integral form, the first one is best suited to apply analytical vector analysis, whereas the latter gave rise to the invention of the numerical Finite Integration Technique (FIT: [18]). The basic idea is simple: Apply the line and surface integrals of Maxwell's equations to every single cell of a discretization of the underlying problem and compute the integrals approximately under the assumption of constant field components along the lines and on the surfaces. It has been shown that the resulting algebraic equations — Maxwell's grid equations — have the same physical property than the continuous equations, i.e., for example, the electric and magnetic flux densities are divergence-free in source-free regions. The numerical MAFIA-code (MAxwell's equations by Finite Integration Algorithms), which is based upon FIT, covers all applications from statics through quasistatics, frequency dependent and time varying problems ([19]).

The success of FIT and MAFIA initiated the development of its elastodynamic counterpart, the EFIT-code ([1, 20]). Assuming that the reader may not be *that* familiar with elastodynamics we give the fundamental equations, i.e. the Cauchy-Newton-Hooke equations, below. The Cauchy-Newton equation of motion for a "volume element" in a solid reads

$$\rho(\underline{R})\frac{\partial^2\underline{u}(\underline{R},t)}{\partial t^2} = \nabla \cdot \underline{\underline{T}}(\underline{R},t) + \underline{f}(\underline{R},t) \ . \tag{13}$$

Here, $\underline{u}(\underline{R},t)$ is the displacement vector, $\underline{\underline{T}}(\underline{R},t)$ the second rank stress tensor and $\rho(\underline{R})$ the mass density; $\underline{f}(\underline{R},t)$ accounts for volume force densities. Hooke's law of *linear* elastodynamics relates the stress to the strain via the fourth rank stiffness tensor:

$$\underline{\underline{T}}(\underline{R},t) = \underline{\underline{c}}(\underline{R}) : \underline{\underline{S}}(\underline{R},t) \ . \tag{14}$$

The colon means double contraction of neighboring indices. The second rank strain tensor is related to $\underline{u}(\underline{R},t)$ through

$$\underline{\underline{S}}(\underline{R},t) = \frac{1}{2}\left\{\nabla\underline{u}(\underline{R},t) + [\nabla\underline{u}(\underline{R},t)]^{21}\right\} \ , \tag{15}$$

where the upper indicial notation indicates transposition of elements.

For homogeneous isotropic media with

$$\underline{\underline{c}} = \lambda\underline{\underline{I}}\,\underline{\underline{I}} + \mu(\underline{\underline{I}}\,\underline{\underline{I}}^{1342} + \underline{\underline{I}}\,\underline{\underline{I}}^{1324}) \ , \tag{16}$$

λ and μ denoting Lamé's constants, and $\underline{I}$ being the dyadic idemfactor, insertion of (14) and (15) into (13) results in a Navier equation for the displacement

$$(\lambda + 2\mu)\nabla\nabla \cdot \underline{u}(\underline{R},t) - \mu\nabla \times \nabla \times \underline{u}(\underline{R},t) - \rho\frac{\partial^2\underline{u}(\underline{R},t)}{\partial t^2} = -\underline{f}(\underline{R},t) \ , \tag{17}$$

which, in terms of *plane* waves, allows for uncoupled pressure and shear waves with phase velocities $c_P = \sqrt{(\lambda + 2\mu)/\rho}$, and $c_S = \sqrt{\mu/\rho}$, respectively, where $c_P > c_S$.

In order to apply FIT to elastodynamics, we integrate (13) with regard to a "voxel" V with surface S of the discrete mesh and use Gauss' theorem:

$$\iiint_V \left[\rho(\underline{\mathbf{R}})\frac{\partial \underline{\mathbf{v}}(\underline{\mathbf{R}},t)}{\partial t} - \underline{\mathbf{f}}(\underline{\mathbf{R}},t)\right] \mathrm{d}^3\underline{\mathbf{R}} = \iint_S \underline{\mathbf{n}}\cdot\underline{\underline{\mathbf{T}}}(\underline{\mathbf{R}},t)\,\mathrm{d}S \ . \qquad (18)$$

Instead of $\underline{\mathbf{u}}(\underline{\mathbf{R}},t)$ we have introduced the particle velocity $\underline{\mathbf{v}} = \partial\underline{\mathbf{u}}/\partial t$, which changes (14) and (15) after integration over V into

$$\iiint_V \underline{\underline{\mathbf{s}}}(\underline{\mathbf{R}}) : \frac{\partial \underline{\underline{T}}(\underline{\mathbf{R}},t)}{\partial t}\,\mathrm{d}^3\underline{\mathbf{R}} = \iint_S \frac{1}{2}[\underline{\mathbf{n}}\underline{\mathbf{v}}(\underline{\mathbf{R}},t) + \underline{\mathbf{v}}(\underline{\mathbf{R}},t)\underline{\mathbf{n}}]\,\mathrm{d}S \ . \qquad (19)$$

For inhomogeneous anisotropic media it is appropriate to use the compliance tensor $\underline{\underline{\mathbf{s}}}(\underline{\mathbf{R}})$ as inverse of the stiffness tensor ([21]).

The discrete approximation of (18) and (19) over a staggered grid yields the EFIT-code, whose consistency, convergence, and stability has been proven in [20]. In [3, 22, 23] a number of successful applications in NDT have been reported.

There are reasons to model the anisotropic materials mentioned before — austenitic steel and fiber-reinforced composites — with *some* isotropic symmetry, i.e. transverse isotropy. We assume an axis with unit-vector $\hat{\mathbf{a}}$, perpendicular to which the medium behaves isotropically. The stiffness tensor of such materials is given in terms of 4 independent elastic constants replacing Lamé's constants:

$$\begin{aligned}
\underline{\underline{\mathbf{c}}}^{\mathrm{TI}} = {} & (c_{22} - 2c_{44})\underline{\underline{\mathbf{I}}}\,\underline{\underline{\mathbf{I}}} + c_{44}(\underline{\underline{\mathbf{I}}}\,\underline{\underline{\mathbf{I}}}^{1324} + \underline{\underline{\mathbf{I}}}\,\underline{\underline{\mathbf{I}}}^{1342}) + \\
& + [c_{11} + c_{22} - 2(c_{12} + 2c_{55})]\hat{\mathbf{a}}\,\hat{\mathbf{a}}\,\hat{\mathbf{a}}\,\hat{\mathbf{a}} + \\
& + (c_{12} - c_{22} + 2c_{44})(\underline{\underline{\mathbf{I}}}\,\hat{\mathbf{a}}\,\hat{\mathbf{a}} + \hat{\mathbf{a}}\,\hat{\mathbf{a}}\,\underline{\underline{\mathbf{I}}}) + \\
& + (c_{55} - c_{44})(\underline{\underline{\mathbf{I}}}\,\hat{\mathbf{a}}\,\hat{\mathbf{a}}^{1324} + \underline{\underline{\mathbf{I}}}\,\hat{\mathbf{a}}\,\hat{\mathbf{a}}^{1342} + \hat{\mathbf{a}}\,\hat{\mathbf{a}}\,\underline{\underline{\mathbf{I}}}^{1324} + \hat{\mathbf{a}}\,\hat{\mathbf{a}}\,\underline{\underline{\mathbf{I}}}^{1342}) \ . \quad (20)
\end{aligned}$$

To illustrate the time domain Green function of a homogeneous transversely isotropic solid of infinite extent, we compute the — two-dimensional — displacement, precisely $|\underline{\mathbf{v}}(\underline{\mathbf{R}},t)|$, for an impulsive line force with parallel orientation to $\hat{\mathbf{a}}$ using EFIT. The result is given in Figure 4 (top) where it is compared to the isotropic case (bottom). In an isotropic solid an impulsive line force creates *two* cylindrical wave fronts representing a pressure and a shear wave front, which travel with c_P, and c_S, respectively. The impulse time history of $\underline{\mathbf{f}}(\underline{\mathbf{R}},t)$ is reflected in the spatial cross-section of the wave fronts, and their amplitude distribution is non-homogeneous due to an angular dependent Green's tensor relating $\underline{\mathbf{f}}$ and $\underline{\mathbf{u}}$. Figure 4 reveals that a material with only transverse isotropy has a much more complicated behavior of its Green function: The pressure wave front is elliptical, and the shear wave front (SV-polarization, or, more precisely, quasi-SV-polarization) even exhibits cusps. As it is well-known in seismics ([24]) — a viewpoint, that has recently been realized in electromagnetic and elastodynamic NDT ([20, 25]) — the time domain Green function wave fronts reflect the energy or group velocities diagrams of *plane* waves.

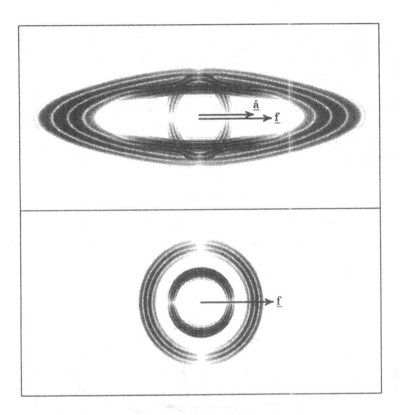

Fig. 4. Time domain wave fronts from an impulsive line force in an isotropic (bottom) and transversely isotropic (top) material as computed with the EFIT-code; the material parameters are those of a fiber-reinforced composite

Let us consider the source-free equation of motion for $\underline{u}(\underline{R}, t)$ in an arbitrarily homogeneous anisotropic material, which results from (13), (14) and (15) if general symmetry properties of $\underline{\underline{c}}$ are considered:

$$\nabla \cdot \underline{\underline{c}} \cdot \nabla \underline{u}(\underline{R}, t) - \rho \frac{\partial^2 \underline{u}(\underline{R}, t)}{\partial t^2} = 0 \quad . \tag{21}$$

Applying the fourdimensional Fourier transform

$$\underline{u}(\underline{K}, \omega) = \int_{-\infty}^{+\infty} \int_{-\infty}^{+\infty} \int_{-\infty}^{+\infty} \int_{-\infty}^{\infty} \underline{u}(\underline{R}, t) \exp\left[-j(\underline{K} \cdot \underline{R} - \omega t)\right] d^3\underline{R}\, dt \tag{22}$$

we obtain from (21)

$$\underline{\underline{W}}(\underline{K}, \omega) \cdot \underline{u}(\underline{K}, \omega) = 0 \tag{23}$$

with the wave tensor

$$\underline{\underline{W}}(\underline{K}, \omega) = \underline{K} \cdot \underline{\underline{c}} \cdot \underline{K} - \rho \omega^2 \underline{\underline{I}} \quad . \tag{24}$$

Equating the determinant of the wave tensor to zero results in a polynomial in K, its zeroes determining the wave numbers of possible plane wave solutions of (21) with propagation directions prescribed by the components of the unit-vector $\hat{\mathbf{K}} = \mathbf{K}/K$. That way, a *directional dependence* — anisotropy! — of the *phase velocity* is obtained: For transversely isotropic media, a possible factorization of the phase velocity polynomial allows for its analytical solution ([26]) in terms of two quasi-shear wave modes and one quasi-pressure wave mode. Therefore, for that particular case, the directional dependence of the energy or group velocity $\underline{c}_g$ as defined by

$$\underline{c}_g^\eta = \left(\frac{\partial \omega(\mathbf{K})}{\partial \underline{\mathbf{K}}} \right)_{\underline{\mathbf{K}} = \underline{\mathbf{K}}_\eta} , \tag{25}$$

where η denotes the wave mode under concern, can also be computed analytically. Figure 5 shows an example. Obviously, comparing Figures 4 and 5, one

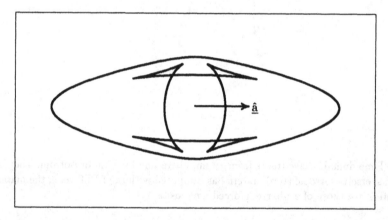

Fig. 5. Energy or group velocity diagram of the quasi-pressure and the quasi-SV-shear wave mode of a transversely isotropic material with the same elastic constants as in Fig. 4

recognizes that the directional dependence of the group veloctiy for *plane* waves is physically realized by time domain wave fronts of line (or point) sources, i.e. the *group* velocity has to appear in the *phase* term of the Green function in $\mathbf{R}\omega$-space. The consequences for NDT are rather dramatic. Suppose, for instance, that a 45°-shear wave transducer from the shelf, i.e. designed for conventional applications in isotropic materials like ferritic steel (Figure 6: top), is applied to the surface of a material with a particular $\hat{\underline{a}}$-anisotropy, it may result in a main beam, which is considerably skewed with regard to the intended energy direction (Figure 6: bottom), i.e. a weld in *austenitic* steel to be inspected with this transducer, might not even be "hit" by the ultrasound. The explanation for Figure 6 is given in Figure 7: Here, a geometrical construction of ultrasonic beams according to Huygens' principle is given; the top figure shows the isotropic case, where the transducer aperture is indicated by the black bar. In order to

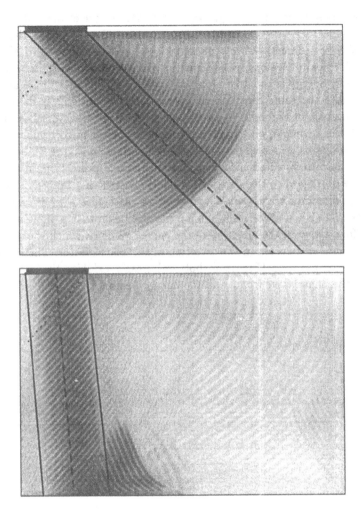

Fig. 6. 2D EFIT computation of the beams of a 45°-shear wave transducer applied to isotropic ferritic (top) and to transversely isotropic austenitic steel (bottom); an impulsive time variation of the transducer excitation as in Figure 4 has been chosen, and the resulting single time domain wave front frames have been superimposed

obtain a tilted beam — 45° in the present case — a time delay between the single "elementary line sources" representing the radiating aperture has to be properly adjusted, which has been indicated on top of the black bar. In Figure 7 two time frames of the wave fronts emanating from the left and right corner of the aperture have been superimposed, and, in the isotropic case, they are circles. Following Huygens, the tangent to these wave fronts — the envelope of all elementary "wavelets" — represents the *phase* wave front of the resulting beam, which, as foreseen, makes an angle of 45° with the surface of the specimen. Tracing the elementary wave fronts in time and space and constructing the envelope for every time moment — two representatives have been drawn in Figure 7 — a finite size beam develops, which has the same direction as the normal to the phase front: Energy is radiated along an angle of 45° because phase and energy velocity have the same direction in isotropic materials. This is in contrast to the bottom part of Figure 7: In an anisotropic — here: transversely isotropic — material, the elementary wavelets have to be replaced by corresponding group velocity diagrams — recognize the shear wave cusps in Figure 7! —, which, in addition, have to be tilted according to the assumed $\underline{a}$-direction, in the present case 60° with regard to the specimen surface; constructing tangents (envelopes) yields the direction of the *phase* vector — 45° as before —, but tracing these tangents in time and space results in a finite size beam with a different direction than before, i.e. with the direction of the energy velocity, which is orthogonal to the wavenumber diagram in the direction of the phase vector. The corresponding EFIT-computation (Figure 6, bottom) clearly exhibits the skewing angle between the phase wave fronts and the energy beams.

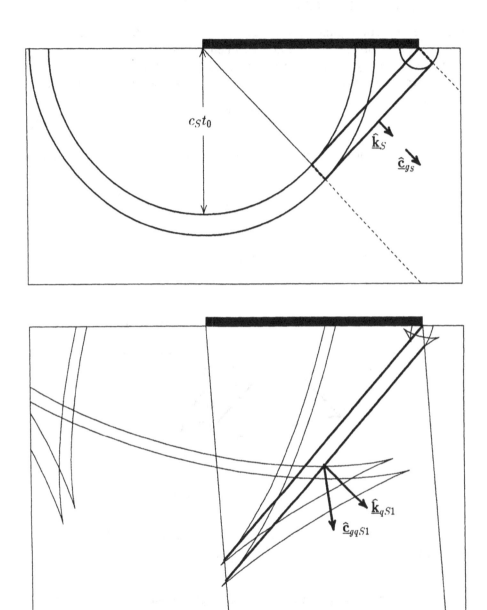

Fig. 7. Huygens-type construction of transducer beams in isotropic (top) and transversely isotropic (bottom) materials

4.2 Energy Velocity SAFT

With the heuristic arguments leading to the monostatic SAFT algorithm (1) and (2), it is no problem to extend it to a homogeneous anisotropic background medium: We simply replace the wave speed c in (2) by the magnitude of the direction dependent energy velocity c_g^η for the particular wave mode under concern according to

$$t = \frac{2|\underline{R} - \underline{R}'|}{c_g^\eta(\underline{R} - \underline{R}')} \quad , \tag{26}$$

where, of course, the c_g^η-diagram has to be tilted with the $\underline{\hat{a}}$-axis (Figure 8). This

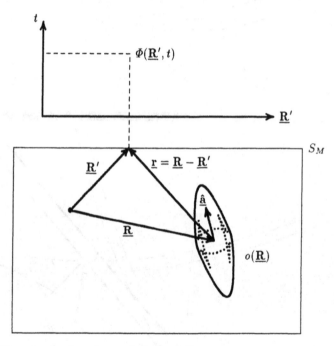

Fig. 8. SAFT processing in anisotropic host media

way, we "invert" the energy skewing as described in Figures 6 and 7. Again, as in the two-media SAFT of section 2, amplitudes are not considered.

In the following, we give an example for the performance of this anisotropic SAFT (in 2D). Figure 9 shows three time frames of EFIT-simulations: A homogeneous transversely isotropic host medium with $\underline{\hat{a}}$-direction as in Figure 8 contains two backwall drilled flat-bottom holes acting as scatterers and simulating defects. A transducer, which would primarily radiate a pressure wave normal to the surface into an *isotropic* medium, obviously shows the already addressed skewing of energy versus phase in the *transversely isotropic* medium. Figure 10 shows the resulting monostatic xt-data within the bar-indicated scanning aper-

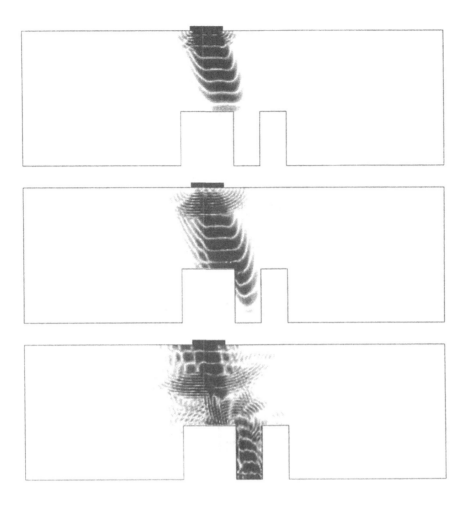

Fig. 9. EFIT wave fronts in transversely isotropic material (fiber-reinforced composite) with "defects"

ture and three SAFT images: The first two — from the top — play around with averaged wave speeds in a conventional SAFT, but only the third one (bottom) exhibits the correct location and size of the "defects", because we applied the anisotropic SAFT with (26).

5 Polarimetric Microwave Diffraction Tomography

Of course, *scalar* diffraction tomography, if applied in electromagnetics either to a voltage or to a single component of the electromagnetic field, neglects important polarization information. Hence, it seemed appropriate to develop an

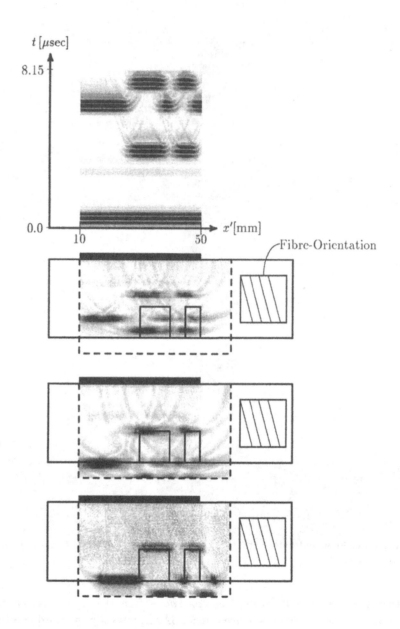

Fig. 10. Synthetic monostatic xt-data for the scattering problem of Figure 9 (top); SAFT images are obtained with conventional SAFT and "guessed" wave speeds (top and middle), and with anisotropic SAFT (bottom)

electromagnetic vector diffraction tomography, and, as a matter of fact, a dramatic improvement has been observed in various simulations ([27]).

The natural starting-point of a vector diffraction tomography is the electromagnetic counterpart to (11), i.e. the definition of a vector holographic field based, for instance, on the electric field representation

$$\Theta_H^E(\underline{R}, \omega) = - \int\int_{S_M} \{j\omega\mu[\underline{n}' \times \underline{H}_s(\underline{R}', \omega)] \cdot \underline{\underline{G}}^*(\underline{R} - \underline{R}', \omega)+$$

$$+[\underline{n}' \times \underline{E}_s(\underline{R}', \omega)] \cdot \nabla' \times \underline{\underline{G}}^*(\underline{R} - \underline{R}', \omega)\} \, dS' \quad , \tag{27}$$

where $\underline{E}_s$, $\underline{H}_s$ denotes the electromagnetic scattered field, and $\underline{\underline{G}}$ is the dyadic Green function

$$\underline{\underline{G}}(\underline{R} - \underline{R}', \omega) = \left(\underline{\underline{I}} + \frac{1}{k^2}\nabla'\nabla'\right) G(\underline{R} - \underline{R}', \omega) \quad ; \tag{28}$$

μ is the permeability of the host medium. Manipulation of (27) with the vector Green theorem results in the vector version of the Porter-Bojarski integral equation

$$\Theta_H^E(\underline{R}, \omega) = -2\omega\mu \int_{-\infty}^{+\infty} \int_{-\infty}^{+\infty} \int_{-\infty}^{+\infty} \underline{J}_c(\underline{R}', \omega) \cdot \underline{\underline{G}}_I(\underline{R} - \underline{R}', \omega) \, d^3\underline{R}' \quad , \tag{29}$$

where the equivalent current density $\underline{J}_c(\underline{R}, \omega)$ as source of the scattered field appears. Now, appropriate models for $\underline{J}_c(\underline{R}, \omega)$ have to be introduced; for perfectly conducting scatterers we have

$$\underline{J}_c(\underline{R}, \omega) = \gamma_c(\underline{R})\underline{n} \times \underline{H}(\underline{R}, \omega) \tag{30}$$

as a "vectorization" of (10). Linearization is now in terms of the Kirchhoff approximation

$$\underline{J}_c^{PO}(\underline{R}, \omega) = \begin{cases} 2\underline{\gamma}(\underline{R}) \times \underline{H}_i(\underline{R}, \omega) & \text{on the illuminated side} \\ 0 & \text{on the shadow side} \end{cases} \tag{31}$$

with the vector singular function $\underline{\gamma}_c(\underline{R}) = \gamma_c(\underline{R})\underline{n}$. Assuming plane wave illumination

$$\underline{E}_i(\underline{R}, \omega) = \hat{\underline{E}}_0 F(\omega) \exp(jk\hat{\underline{k}}_i \cdot \underline{R}) \tag{32}$$

with linear polarization $\hat{\underline{E}}_0$ we obtain

$$\underline{J}_c^{PO}(\underline{R}) = \underline{\gamma}_u(\underline{R}) \times (\hat{\underline{k}}_i \times \hat{\underline{E}}_0)$$
$$= \hat{\underline{k}}_i(\underline{\gamma}_u \cdot \hat{\underline{E}}_0) - \hat{\underline{E}}_0(\underline{\gamma}_u \cdot \hat{\underline{k}}_i) \quad , \tag{33}$$

where the physical optics vector singular function $\underline{\gamma}_u(\underline{R}) = \underline{\gamma}_c(\underline{R}) u(-\hat{\underline{k}}_i \cdot \underline{n})$ includes the unit-step-function u accounting for the physical optics shadow region. Notice: Equ. (33) is a decomposition of $\underline{J}_c^{PO}$ in terms of two unit-vectors $\hat{\underline{k}}_i, \hat{\underline{E}}_0$, where the scalar components are projections of $\underline{\gamma}_u$ on these vectors; hence, choosing the polarization as diversity parameter, we can establish an orthonormal set $\hat{\underline{k}}_i, \hat{\underline{E}}_0, \hat{\underline{E}}_{orth}$ with a polarization $\hat{\underline{E}}_{orth}$ orthogonal to $\hat{\underline{E}}_0$ giving rise to *three* components of $\underline{\gamma}_u$. That means, as soon as we recover these components from an appropriate algorithm, we can determine the magnitude of the "visible" singular function of the scatterer. Of course, the pertinent "experiment" has to be bistatic, because a monostatic arrangement does not yield any depolarization of the incident field within the Kirchhoff approximation, i.e., a *real* — linearized — polarimetric monostatic algorithm cannot be formulated.

Again, the most obvious deconvolution of the vector Porter-Bojarski integral equation (29) is via frequency diversity, and, as a matter of fact, the resulting dyadic time domain backpropagation algorithm has been derived in [28], where it was validated with analytical data for a perfectly conducting sphere. The comparison against pertinent results with *scalar* backpropagation proved stimulating, therefore, a geometrically more complicated scatterer — an air-plane model — was chosen ([27]), where synthetic data could be generated with the MAFIA-code ([19]). The results of the polarimetric scheme are overwhelmingly better than the ones of the scalar algorithm. What remained was the formulation of the complete set of linearized algorithms along the guidelines in [4]: frequency diversity within the Born approximation, angular diversity within the Kirchhoff and Born approximations, and, in particular, the vector version of the Fourier Diffraction Slice Theorem. This unified treatment of linearized electromagnetic inverse scattering is presented in [29]. Figures 11 and 12 give an example of the application of the vector Fourier Diffraction Slice Theroem to a civil engineering NDT problem: MAFIA data have been computed for the geometry of Figure 11, namely, a metallic tendon duct in an unbounded host medium (vacuum) partly covered by metallic rebars. The question to be answered was: Can a Ground Probing Radar "see" the duct below the reinforcement? The answer, given by Figure 12, is: Yes, at least with a polarimetric bistatic experiment, and applying the vector Fourier Diffraction Slice Theorem.

Of course, an unbounded host medium is not realistic for this application; therefore, a two-media vector FT-SAFT, where the surface of the specimen is accounted for by an approximation similar to section 2, has been formulated, and it was found, that the resulting image is only marginally deteriorated ([29]), the reason for the loss of lateral resolution being the relatively high relative permittivity of concrete (around seven).

6 Ultrasonic Inspection Applying Simulation: ULIAS

The success of SAFT related imaging for practical NDT applications required the development of ULIAS[3] ([30]), a user-oriented software package combining modeling and imaging algorithms, whence the name: ULtrasonic Inspection Applying Simulation. Modeling techniques have basically been implemented for two reasons: To provide a better physical understanding of elastic wave scattering

---

[3] BRITE/EURAM: BREU-CT91-0508 (RZJE), project no. BE-4574

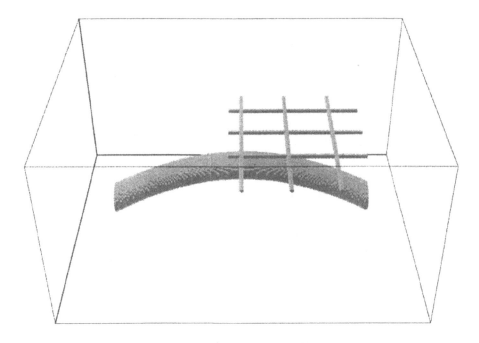

Fig. 11. MAFIA-modeled tendon duct in concrete together with reinforcement bars

— in particular in complex host media — and to serve as a testbed for imaging algorithms via synthetic data.

ULIAS has been developed by a European consortium, where the single partners provided different modules. We will focus on our own contributions, namely the EFIT- and the FT-SAFT-modules; Figure 13 displays their interrelations. The heart of ULIAS is the UDEF file (Ultrasonic Data Exchange Format), a binary file, which contains all relevant NDT information to build a realistic computer model. The UDEF file is handled by an editor; all modules have read/write access to a selected UDEF file using input/output functions of the LLL (Low Level Library). Further: All modules use the 1D/2D/3D capabilities of the VIS-LIB (Visualization Library) to display 1D-plots, 2D-raster images, or to display the ultrasonic data within the 3D geometry given by the CAD file in IGES format; the CAD/IGES file contains quantitative geometry and material information about the test specimen and prescribed defects. The 3D window of the VISLIB allows, for example, for light transformation, object transformation, volume and surface rendering, and voxel grid slicing.

For automatic user-oriented applications the EFIT-module requires a Voxel Grid Generator (VGG), which gets the necessary information from the IGES file. Primary results to be displayed with the VISLIB are time frames of the ultrasonic wave field and/or 1D/2D data fields, which are stored in an UDEF file to be read again, for instance, by the FT-SAFT-module.

FT-SAFT is implemented in 2D and 3D together with a variety of signal

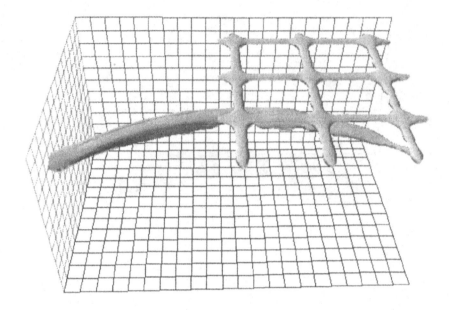

Fig. 12. Application of the electromagnetic Fourier Diffraction Slice Theorem to synthetic MAFIA data combining two orthogonal polarizations of the normally incident plane wave to recover the magnitude of the singular function

processing techniques like filtering, correlation, convolution and deconvolution. Due to the availability of the VISLIB within the FT-SAFT-module, the resulting images can be displayed within the CAD geometry. Figure 14 gives an example for a 3D FT-SAFT image using ULIAS; it has already been provided earlier ([3]) as a result of diffraction tomography, but this time, the image information is *quantitatively* related to the known geometry.

Figures 15 and 16 illustrate the EFIT-module: Figure 15 shows its main window displaying the test specimen, the transducer and the — linear — scanning path in a solid mode; Figure 16 shows 2D EFIT wave fronts in a selected cross-section of the 3D geometry, where, in addition, a striplike defect has been assumed.

ULIAS is supported by standard commercial UNIX based workstations with sufficient main memory (>128 MByte).

EFIT Modeling Module

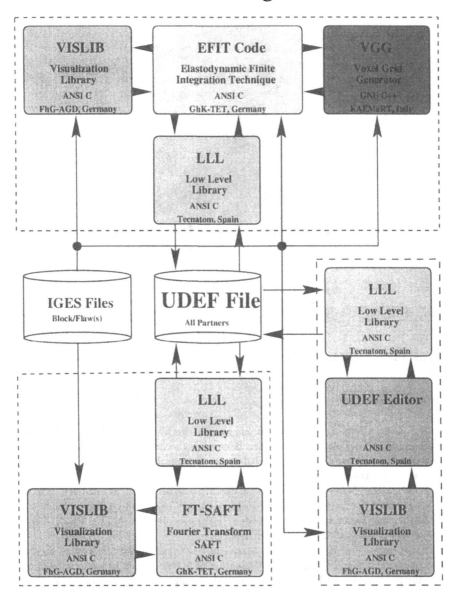

FT-SAFT Imaging Module   UDEF Editor

Fig. 13. EFIT- and FT-SAFT-modules within ULIAS

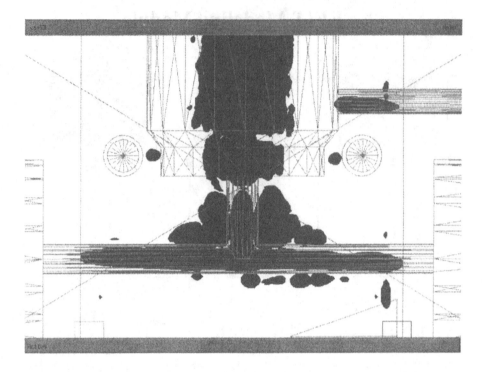

Fig. 14. FT-SAFT image of defected region next to a T-shaped drilling in a steel block

References

1. K.J. Langenberg, T. Weiland: Direkte numerische Lösung der Maxwellschen Gleichungen und der elastodynamischen Bewegungsgleichungen, Anlage 1 und 2. Final Report of a Research Project funded by the German Research Foundation (DFG), Kassel and Darmstadt 1996
2. R. Marklein: Numerische Verfahren zur Modellierung von akustischen, elektromagnetischen, elastischen und piezoelektrischen Wellenausbreitungsproblemen im Zeitbereich basierend auf der Finiten Integrationstechnik (FIT). Ph.D. Thesis, University of Kassel, Kassel, Germany 1997
3. K.J. Langenberg, P. Fellinger, R. Marklein, P. Zanger, K. Mayer, T. Kreutter: Inverse Methods and Imaging. In: Evaluation of Materials and Structures by Quantitative Ultrasonics (Ed.: J.D. Achenbach). Springer-Verlag, Vienna 1993
4. K.J. Langenberg: Applied Inverse Problems. In: Basic Methods of Tomography and Inverse Problems (Ed.: P.C. Sabatier). Adam Hilger, Techno House, Bristol 1987
5. V. Schmitz, M. Kröning, K.J. Langenberg: Quantitative NDT by Three-Dimensional Image Reconstruction. In: Proc. 22nd International Symposium on Acoustical Imaging (Eds.: P. Tortoli, L. Masotti). Plenum Press, New York 1996
6. J. Pitkänen, P. Kauppinen, H. Jeskanen, V. Schmitz: Evaluation of Ultrasonic Indications by Using PC-Based Synthetic Aperture Focusing Technique (PC-SAFT). International Conference on Computer Methods and Inverse Problems in Nondestructive Testing and Diagnostics, 21.-24.11.1995, Minsk, Belarus

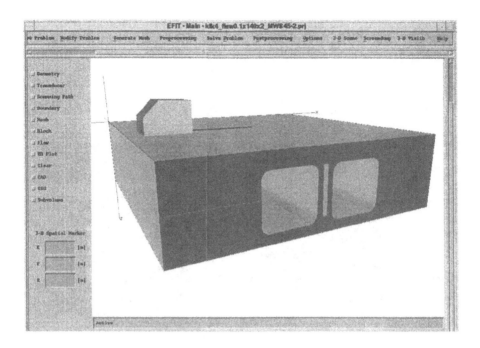

Fig. 15. EFIT main window: CAD geometry

7. W. Müller, G. Schäfer, K. Hoppstädter: European Stainless Steel Round Robin Test Inspection of 15 CCSS Samples Using the Line Synthetic Aperture Focusing Technique (L-SAFT) at the IzfP. Report 851115-E of the Fraunhofer Institute for Nondestructive Testing (IzfP), Saarbrücken 1985

8. W. Müller: Untersuchung eines Turbinenwellenstückes mit LSAFT. Report 860112-E of the Fraunhofer Institute for Nondestructive Testing (IzfP), Saarbrücken 1986

9. W. Müller: Wiederkehrende Prüfung ausgesuchter Schweißnahtbereiche am NH_3-Reaktor C702 mit SAFT. Report 940107-E of the Fraunhofer Institute for Nondestructive Testing (IzfP), Saarbrücken 1994

10. A. Rosenfeld, A.C. Kak: Digital Picture Processing, Vol. 1 and 2. Academic Press, Orlando 1982

11. R. Dändlicker, K. Weiss: Reconstruction of the Three-dimensional Refractive Index from Scattered Waves. Optics Comm. 1 (1970) 323

12. A.T. Devaney: A Filtered Backpropagation Algorithm for Diffraction Tomography. Ultrasonic Imaging 4 (1982) 336

13. A.T. Devaney: A Computer Simulation Study of Diffraction Tomography. IEEE Trans. Biomed. Eng. **BME-30** (1983) 377

14. K. Mayer, R. Marklein, K.J. Langenberg, T. Kreutter: Three-dimensional Imaging System based on Fourier Transform Synthetic Aperture Focusing Technique. Ultrasonics **28** (1990) 241

15. R.P. Porter: Diffraction-Limited Scalar Image Formation with Holograms of Ar-

118

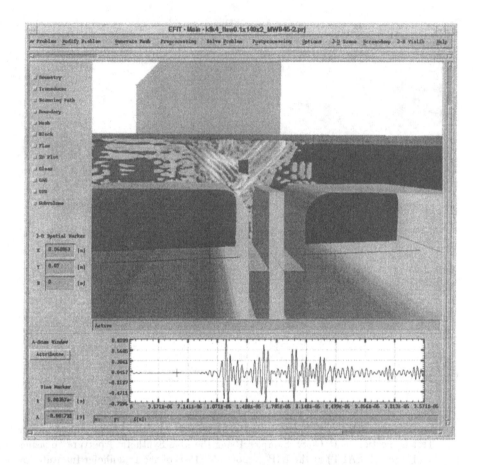

Fig. 16. EFIT wave fronts within CAD geometry

bitrary Shape. J. Opt. Soc. Am. **60** (1970) 1951

16. K.J. Langenberg: Introduction to the Special Issue on Inverse Problems. Wave Motion **11** (1989) 99

17. K.J. Langenberg, M. Brandfaß, K. Mayer, T. Kreutter, A. Brüll, P. Fellinger, D. Huo: Principles of Microwave Imaging and Inverse Scattering. EARSeL Advances in Remote Sensing **2** (1993) 163

18. M. Bartsch et al.: Solution of Maxwell's Equations. Computer Physics Communications **72** (1992) 22

19. MAFIA User Guide, Release 3.1, CST GmbH, Darmstadt, Germany 1991

20. P. Fellinger, R. Marklein, K.J. Langenberg. S. Klaholz: Numerical Modeling of Elastic Wave Propagation and Scattering with EFIT — Elastodynamic Finite Integration Technique. Wave Motion **21** (1995) 47

21. A.T. de Hoop: Handbook of Radiation and Scattering of Waves. Academic Press, London 1995

22. R. Marklein, K.J. Langenberg, S. Klaholz, J. Kostka: Ultrasonic Modeling of Real-Life NDT Situations: Applications and Further Developments. In: Review of Progress of Quantitative NDE, Vol. 15 (Eds.: D.O. Thompson, D.E. Chimenti). Plenum Press, New York 1996, pp. 57-64

23. R. Marklein, K.J. Langenberg, R. Bärmann, M. Brandfaß: Ultrasonic and Electromagnetic Wave Propagation and Inverse Scattering. In: Review of Progress of Quantitative NDE, Vol. 15 (Eds.: D.O. Thompson, D.E. Chimenti). Plenum Press, New York 1996, pp. 1839-1846

24. K. Helbig: Foundations of Anisotropy for Exploration Seismics. Pergamon, Trowbridge 1994

25. R. Marklein, K.J. Langenberg, T. Kaczorowski: Electromagnetic and Elastodynamic Point Source Excitation of Unbounded Homogeneous Anisotropic Media. Radio Science (1996) (accepted for publication)

26. M. Spies: Elastic Waves in Homogeneous and Layered Transversely Isotropic Media: Plane Waves and Gaussian Packets. A General Approach. J. Acoust. Soc. Am. 95 (1994) 1748

27. K.J. Langenberg, M. Brandfaß, A. Fritsch, B. Potzkai: Linearized 3D Electromagnetic Vector Wave Inversion. In: Three-Dimensional Electromagnetics (Eds.: M. Oristaglio, B. Spies). Investigations in Geophysics Series, Society of Exploration Geophysicists, 1996 (to be published)

28. K.J. Langenberg, M. Brandfaß, P. Fellinger, T. Gurke, T. Kreutter: A Unified Theory of Multidimensional Electromagnetic Vector Inverse Scattering within the Kirchhoff or Born Approximation. In: Radar Target Imaging (Eds.: W.-M. Boerner, H. Überall). Springer-Verlag, Berlin 1994

29. M. Brandfaß: Inverse Beugungstheorie elektromagnetischer Wellen: Algorithmen und numerische Realisierung. Ph.D. Thesis, University of Kassel, Kassel, Germany 1996

30. R. Marklein, K. Mayer, K.J. Langenberg: Modeling and Imaging with ULIAS: Ultrasonic Inspection Applying Simulation. In: Review of Progress of Quantitative NDE, Vol. 16 (Eds.: D.O. Thompson, D.E. Chimenti). Plenum Press, New York 1997 (to be published)

Application of the Approximate Inverse to 3D X–Ray CT and Ultrasound Tomography

A. K. Louis

Fachbereich Mathematik, Universität des Saarlandes, D-66041 Saarbrücken

1 Introduction

We study operator equations $Af = g$ for operators between Hilbert spaces X and Y. Both the cases of linear operators A and of nonlinear A with a special structure are treated. Approximate inverse means a solution operator which maps the data g to a stable approximation of the solution of the ill – posed problem $Af = g$. This inversion operator is precomputed without using the data g, see [10].

The method is based on two ideas. First, the computation of moments of the solution is stable; i.e., we compute instead of f the approximation $\langle f, e_\gamma \rangle$ with a suitable mollifier e_γ reducing in that way the high frequency components in the solution which are mostly affected by the data noise. This can be reformulated as using a weaker topology in the space X, see [4], [7]. Examples for e_γ are given in the next section, e_γ can be a basis function for projection methods, it can be chosen such that $\langle f, e_\gamma \rangle$ approximates a derivative of f; in wavelet language it can be a scaling function or a wavelet. Second, in the case of linear operators the computation of $\langle e_\gamma, f \rangle$ is then achieved by approximating e_γ in the range of the adjoint operator A^* by the reconstruction kernel $\psi_\gamma : A^* \psi_\gamma \simeq e_\gamma$. Then

$$\langle f, e_\gamma \rangle \simeq \langle f, A^* \psi_\gamma \rangle = \langle Af, \psi_\gamma \rangle = \langle g, \psi_\gamma \rangle .$$

Definition 1. The operator $S_\gamma : Y \to X$ defined as

$$S_\gamma g(x) = \langle g, \psi_\gamma(x) \rangle \tag{1}$$

where ψ_γ solves for a given and sufficiently smooth mollifier e_γ either

$$A^* \psi_\gamma(x) = e_\gamma(x, \cdot) \quad \text{for} \quad e_\gamma(x, \cdot) \in \mathcal{R}(A^*) \tag{2}$$

or

$$AA^* \psi_\gamma(x) = Ae_\gamma(x, \cdot) , \tag{3}$$

where A acts on the second variable of e_γ, is called *approximate inverse* and $\psi_\gamma(x)$ is called the *reconstruction kernel* for the point x.

This is the mollifier method presented in [11]. It also has been used to accelerate convergence for finite element solutions in [6]. The recently introduced method in smoothed particle hydrodynamics is based on the same ideas.

We show that the approximate inverse is a regularization method. For nonlinear operators we combine these ideas with the results of Snieder [19] who generalized the Backus – Gilbert method to nonlinear problems. A detailed analysis of the method shows that the computational effort is much smaller than in [19]. Applications to 3D x–ray CT and ultrasound CT conclude the paper.

2 Approximative Inverse for Linear Problems

In the following we assume A to be a linear, continuous operator between the Hilbert spaces X and Y. Especially we think of X as a space of functions and Y as a finite dimensional space of measurements. Hence, if necessary, we use $X = L_2(\Omega)$ for a suitable set $\Omega \subset \mathbb{R}^d$. Examples for mollifiers are

$$e_\gamma(x, y) = \frac{d}{\text{vol}(S^{d-1})\gamma^d} \chi_\gamma(x - y) \tag{4}$$

where χ_γ is the characteristic function of the ball around 0 with radius γ and $\text{vol}(S^{d-1})$ is the measure of the surface of the unit ball in $\mathbb{R}^d$. Here local averages of the solution are computed. With the band limiting filter

$$e_\gamma(x, y) = \left(\frac{\gamma}{\pi}\right)^d \text{sinc}(\gamma(x - y)) \tag{5}$$

the high – frequency components in the solution are eliminated. Fast decaying is the kernel of the heat equation

$$e_\gamma(x, y) = (2\pi)^{-d/2} \gamma^{-d} \exp(-|x - y|^2/(2\gamma^2)) . \tag{6}$$

In all cases the parameter γ acts as a regularization parameter. The mollifier e_γ is not necessarily a function with mean value 1. When the essential information we need are discontinuities in f we can use as e_γ a function such that $\langle f, e_\gamma(x, \cdot)\rangle$ approximates a derivative of $f(x)$. This means that e_γ can also be a wavelet, see e.g. [13].

First we assume the equation $A^*\psi_\gamma = e_\gamma$ to be solvable. Then we put

$$\langle f, e_\gamma\rangle = \langle f, A^*\psi_\gamma\rangle = \langle Af, \psi_\gamma\rangle = \langle g, \psi_\gamma\rangle =: S_\gamma g . \tag{7}$$

This is the technique to derive inversion formulas in x – ray computer tomography resulting in the so – called filtered backprojection methods, see e.g. [9], [15]. If the equation $A^*\psi_\gamma = e_\gamma$ is not solvable we approximate ψ_γ by minimizing the defect $\|A^*\psi_\gamma - e_\gamma\|$ for sufficiently smooth e_γ leading to the equation

$$AA^*\psi_\gamma = Ae_\gamma . \tag{8}$$

Then we get

$$\langle f, e_\gamma\rangle \simeq \langle f, A^*\psi_\gamma\rangle = \langle Af, \psi_\gamma\rangle = \langle g, \psi_\gamma\rangle =: S_\gamma g .$$

It is important to mention that no artificial discretization of f is needed as introduced by projection methods, see e.g. [15], [16], [18]. For the numerical computation of ψ_γ the matrix AA^* needs a coarse stabilization, the fine tuning is then achieved by the choice of γ, compare [17].

3 Comparison with other Methods

Now let A be a compact operator between the Hilbert spaces X and Y. Then it has a singular value decomposition

$$\{v_n, u_n; \sigma_n\}_n$$

where v_n, u_n are normalized and

$$Av_n = \sigma_n u_n \quad \text{and} \quad A^* u_n = \sigma_n v_n \ .$$

Regularization methods, like Tikhonov – Phillips, truncated singular value decomposition or Landweber iteration, have the form

$$T_\gamma g = \sum_n F_\gamma(\sigma_n)\sigma_n^{-1}\langle g, u_n\rangle v_n \ , \tag{9}$$

see for example[2], [5], [7]. The following result shows that these methods are special cases of the approximate inverse.

Theorem 2. *Let the regularization method T_γ in (9) be given with a filter F_γ. Then this method can be written as an approximate inverse with mollifier*

$$e_\gamma(x, y) = \sum_n F_\gamma(\sigma_n)v_n(x)v_n(y) \ . \tag{10}$$

Proof: The definition of ψ_γ as solution of $AA^*\psi_\gamma = Ae_\gamma$ in (3) leads with

$$\psi_\gamma(x) = \sum_n \sigma_n^{-1}\langle e_\gamma(x, \cdot), u_n\rangle v_n$$

to

$$\psi_\gamma(x) = \sum_n F_\gamma(\sigma_n)\sigma_n^{-1}u_n v_n(x) \ .$$

Then

$$S_\gamma g(x) = \langle g, \psi_\gamma(x)\rangle = T_\gamma g(x) \ .$$

In contrast to the Backus – Gilbert method, see [1], [18], the matrix for computing the reconstruction kernel does not depend on the reconstruction point. Also there is a the possibility to pattern the reconstruction kernel in almost any desirable way, one is not forced to approximate the delta distribution with a kernel like $|x - y|^{-2}$.

4 Regularization Properties of the Approximate Inverse

In the following we show that the approximate inverse is a regularization method. This means the following.

Definition 3. A *regularization* of $A^\dagger$ is a family of operators

$$\{R_\gamma\}_{\gamma > 0} , \quad R_\gamma : Y \to X$$

with the following properties:
there exists a mapping $\gamma : \mathbb{R}_+ \times Y \to \mathbb{R}_+$ such that for all $g \in \mathcal{R}(A)$ and for all $g^\varepsilon \in Y$ with $\|g^\varepsilon - g\| \leq \varepsilon$

$$\lim_{\varepsilon \to 0} R_{\gamma(\varepsilon, g^\varepsilon)} g^\varepsilon = A^\dagger g . \tag{11}$$

There are different methods to compare regularizations. In order to do this we need some notion. We define the Hilbert spaces

$$X_\nu = \mathcal{R}(A^* A)^{-\nu/2}$$

equipped with the norm

$$\|f\|_\nu = \left(\sum_n \sigma_n^{-2\nu} |\langle f, v_n \rangle|^2 \right)^{1/2}$$

for real ν. In a similar way we define norms on Y. For $\nu = 0$ we simply write X and $\| \cdot \|$. Note that

$$\|Af\|_\nu = \|f\|_{\nu-1} \quad \text{and} \quad \|A^\dagger g\|_\nu = \|g\|_{\nu+1} .$$

We use the following definition.

Definition 4. A regularization method is called *order-optimal* of order ν if there exists a constant c such that

$$\|R_\gamma g^\varepsilon - A^\dagger g\| \leq c \varepsilon^{\nu/(\nu+1)} \rho^{1/(\nu+1)} \tag{12}$$

for all $g \in Y_\nu$ with $\|A^\dagger g\|_\nu \leq \rho$.

Now we show that the approximate inverse is a regularization in the above mentioned sense. In order to avoid technical difficulties we assume in the following that for each x the mollifier $e_\gamma(x, \cdot)$ is in the range of A^*. Then we can represent

$$e_\gamma(x, \cdot) = \sum_n e_{\gamma, n}(x) v_n$$

with

$$e_{\gamma, n}(x) = \langle e_\gamma(x, \cdot), v_n \rangle .$$

From this we get with (2) the reconstruction kernel

$$\psi_\gamma(x) = \sum_n \sigma_n^{-1} e_{\gamma, n}(x) u_n$$

resulting in

$$S_\gamma g(x) = \sum_n \sigma_n^{-1} \langle g, u_n \rangle e_{\gamma,n}(x) .$$

Hence we decompose the operator S_γ into $E_\gamma A^\dagger$ where $A^\dagger$ is the generalized inverse given as

$$A^\dagger g = \sum_n \sigma_n^{-1} \langle g, u_n \rangle v_n$$

and

$$E_\gamma : \mathcal{N}(A)^\perp \to X$$

with

$$E_\gamma f(x) = \sum_n \langle f, v_n \rangle e_{\gamma,n}(x)$$

Theorem 5. *Let $E_\gamma : X \to X_{-1}$ be continuous for each γ; i.e., there exists a constant $c(\gamma) > 0$ such that*

$$\|E_\gamma f\| \le c(\gamma)\|f\|_{-1} \quad \text{for all} \quad f \in \mathcal{N}(A)^\perp \tag{13}$$

and

$$\lim_{\gamma \to 0} \|E_\gamma f - f\| = 0 \tag{14}$$

for all $f \in \mathcal{N}(A)^\perp$. Then $S_\gamma = E_\gamma A^\dagger$ is a regularization of $A^\dagger$.

Proof. Let $g \in \mathcal{R}(A)$ and $g^\epsilon \in Y$ with $\|g^\epsilon - g\| \le \epsilon$, then

$$\begin{aligned}
\|S_\gamma g^\epsilon - A^\dagger g\| &\le \|S_\gamma (g^\epsilon - g)\| + \|(S_\gamma - A^\dagger)g\| \\
&= \|E_\gamma A^\dagger (g^\epsilon - g)\| + \|(E_\gamma - I)A^\dagger g\| \\
&\le c(\gamma)\|A^\dagger (g^\epsilon - g)\|_{-1} + \|(E_\gamma - I)A^\dagger g\| \\
&\le c(\gamma)\epsilon + \|(E_\gamma - I)A^\dagger g\|
\end{aligned}$$

which completes the proof.

In a similar manner we can show the order–optimality of the approximate inverse.

Theorem 6. *Let $E_\gamma : X \to X_{-1}$ be continuous with*

$$\|E_\gamma f\| \le c\gamma^{-\alpha}\|f\|_{-1} \quad \text{for all} \quad f \in \mathcal{N}(A)^\perp \tag{15}$$

and

$$\|E_\gamma f - f\| \le c_\nu \cdot \gamma^{\alpha\nu^*}\|f\|_{\nu^*} \tag{16}$$

for all $f \in X_{\nu^*}$ and a $\alpha \in \mathbb{R}$. Then the method is order–optimal for all $0 \le \nu \le \nu^*$.

The proof follows the ideas of the above theorem and techniques given for example in [7].

For the classical regularization methods we have

$$E_\gamma v_n = F(\sigma_n)v_n \tag{17}$$

and then the order–optimality follows from conditions for the filter F_γ given for example in [7]. Again we see that this is a special case of the approximate inverse where

$$E_\gamma v_n = \langle e_\gamma(x, \cdot), v_n \rangle \ .$$

For the approximate inverse we can use results for mollifiers to prove order–optimality.

5 Efficient Implementation

If the problem shares some invariance properties they can be used for a fast realisation of the method. Let in the following E_γ be a function of the variable y only. We can think of $E_\gamma(y) = e_\gamma(0, y)$; i.e., a mollifier concentrated around 0 which then may be shifted to arbitrary points as $e_\gamma(x, y) = E_\gamma(x - y)$.

Theorem 7. Let $A : X \to Y$ and let T_1^x be a linear operator on X and T_2^x, T_3^x be linear operators on Y such that

$$AT_1^x = T_2^x A \tag{18}$$

and

$$T_2^x AA^* = AA^* T_3^x \ . \tag{19}$$

Let w_γ be the minimum norm solution of

$$AA^* w_\gamma = AE_\gamma \ . \tag{20}$$

Then the minimum norm solution of

$$AA^* \psi_\gamma(x) = AT_1^x E_\gamma$$

is

$$\psi_\gamma(x) = T_3^x w_\gamma \ . \tag{21}$$

Proof: From the invariance properties follows

$$AT_1^x E_\gamma = T_2^x AE_\gamma$$
$$= AA^* T_3^x w_\gamma$$

which completes the proof.//[2mm] This means that only the solution w_γ has to be computed and stored, the kernels for other reconstruction points x are found by the action of T_1^x on E_γ and by T_3^x on w_γ.

In the case of a finite number of data where $(Af)_n = Af(x_n)$, $n = 1, \ldots, N$

for suitable points x_n the reconstruction kernel w_γ is a vector in $\mathbb{R}^N$ with $(w_\gamma)_n = w_\gamma(x_n)$. Then $w_\gamma(x_n - x)$ can be evaluated by linear interpolation between $(w_\gamma)_m$ and $(w_\gamma)_{m+1}$ with $x_m \leq x_n - x < x_{m+1}$.

For $Y = \mathbb{R}^N$ and M reconstruction points the storage needs is $M \times N$ real numbers. If the problem has invariance properties this can be dramatically reduced. If translation invariance for example holds only N real numbers have to be stored!

As an example consider the Radon transform in two dimensions,

$$Rf(\omega, s) = \int f(s\omega + t\omega^\perp)dt$$

for real s and a unit vector ω. In order to reduce the high amount of storage needs we profit from invariance properties of the Radon transform. Shift and rotation invariances have already been used by Davison – Grunbaum, [3], in order to find a series expansion of the reconstruction kernel. In that way they were able to simplify the normal equation. But here we are using the invariances for finding the corresponding properties of the reconstruction kernel. For details see [14].

Now consider the translation T_1^x

$$T_1^x f(y) = f(y - x) \ .$$

Then a simple change of variable shows that

$$RT_1^x f(\omega, s) = Rf(\omega, s - x^\top \omega)$$

or

$$RT_1^x = T_2^x R$$

where $T_2^x g(\omega, s) = g(\omega, s - x^\top \omega)$. If we now chose the mollifier e_γ as shifted version of a fixed mollifier $\bar{e}_\gamma$, namely $e_\gamma(x, y) = T_1^x \bar{e}_\gamma(y)$, then we get as a consequence of Theorem 7 that

$$\psi_\gamma(x; \omega, s) = \bar{\psi}_\gamma(\omega, s - x^\top \omega) \ ,$$

which means that the storage needs for the new reconstruction kernel $\bar{\psi}_\gamma$ is reduced to the number of data.

Next we rotate the object. Let U be a unitary matrix and T_1^U be the rotation $T_1^U f(x) = f(Ux)$. Then

$$RT_1^U f(\omega, s) = Rf(U\omega, s)$$

hence

$$RT_1^U = T_2^U R$$

with $T_2^U g(\omega, s) = g(U\omega, s)$. Again, $T_2^U RR^* = RR^* T_2^U$. Now we choose $\bar{e}_\gamma$ as a circular symmetric mollifier which means that $T_1^U \bar{e}_\gamma = \bar{e}_\gamma$. Then the same result holds for the reconstruction kernel which is then independent of ω :

$$w_\gamma(s) = \bar{\psi}_\gamma(\omega, s) \ .$$

Finally we use the invariance with respect to dilations. Let $\gamma > 0$ and

$$T_1^\gamma f(x) = \gamma^2 f(\gamma x) \ .$$

Then

$$RT_1^\gamma f(\omega, s) = \gamma^2 \int_{\mathbb{R}} f(\gamma s \omega + \gamma t \omega^\perp) dt = \gamma Rf(\omega, \gamma s) \ ,$$

hence

$$RT_1^\gamma = T_2^\gamma R$$

with

$$T_2^\gamma g(\omega, s) = \gamma g(\omega, \gamma s) \ .$$

Furthermore, let

$$T_3^\gamma g(\omega, s) = \gamma^2 g(\omega, \gamma s) \ ,$$

then

$$R^* T_3^\gamma g(x) = \gamma^2 \int_{S^1} g(\omega, \gamma x^\top \omega) d\omega$$
$$= T_1^\gamma R^* g(x)$$

and so

$$RR^* T_3^\gamma = RT_1^\gamma R^* = T_2^\gamma RR^* \ .$$

So, if

$$e_\gamma(x) = T_1^\gamma e(x) = \gamma^2 e(\gamma x)$$

then

$$w_\gamma(s) = \gamma^2 w(\gamma s) \ .$$

This means that the reconstruction kernel can be determined independently of γ, and a simple scaling leads to the correct values of w_γ.

6 Nonlinear Problems

We start the presentation of the approach for the nonlinear problem

$$A : L_2(\Omega) \to \mathbb{R}^N$$

by considering for the sake of simplicity only a quadratic problem. Let the operator A be given as

$$Af = A_1 f + A_2 f$$

where A_1 is linear,

$$(A_1 f)_n = \int_\Omega k_n^1(y) f(y) dy$$

and A_2 is a quadratic operator defined as

$$(A_2 f)_n = \int_\Omega \int_\Omega k_n^2(y_1, y_2) f(y_1) f(y_2) dy_1 dy_2 \ .$$

With k^1 we denote the vector of the N components of k_n^1 and similarly with k^2 the vector of the N components of k_n^2. For the approximate inverse we follow Snieder [19] and make the following ansatz

$$f_\gamma(x) = \langle g, \psi_\gamma(x) \rangle + \langle g, V_\gamma(x) g \rangle$$

where $V_\gamma(x)$ is an $N \times N$ matrix. We replace g by Af and get

$$f_\gamma(x) \simeq \langle A_1 f, \psi_\gamma(x) \rangle + \langle A_2 f, \psi_\gamma(x) \rangle + \langle A_1 f, V_\gamma(x) A_1 f \rangle \qquad (22)$$

where we omitted the higher order terms.

In the following we always use $x \in \Omega$ as the reconstruction point which is arbitrarily fixed; and with y_1, y_2 and so on we denote the integration variables in the integral operators.

Of course we can attempt to approximate with the right – hand side an expression like $\langle f, e_\gamma(x, \cdot) \rangle$. But then the approximate inverse is not independent of the data, this does not lead to an approximate inverse as aimed for. We therefore follow [19] and consider the terms separately. We approximate the mollified solution with the linear term as well as possible which means

$$\langle A_1 f, \psi_\gamma(x) \rangle \simeq \langle f, e_\gamma(x, \cdot) \rangle \ ,$$

hence

$$A_1 A_1^* \psi_\gamma = A_1 e_\gamma \ .$$

The computation of ψ_γ thus follows exactly the lines as in the linear case. When this term presents the solution it only remains to make the rest as small as possible. Denoting the remainder by

$$R(x)(y_1, y_2) = \psi_\gamma(x)^\top k^2(y_1, y_2) + k^1(y_1)^\top V_\gamma(x) k^1(y_2) \qquad (23)$$

where $a^\top b$ is the scalar product in the image space $\mathbb{R}^N$, we can write the rest in (22) as

$$\int_\Omega \int_\Omega R(x)(y_1, y_2) f(y_1) f(y_2) dy_1 dy_2 \ .$$

In order to make this term as small as possible we minimize with respect to $V_\gamma(x)$ for each reconstruction point x the norm

$$\|R(x)(\cdot, \cdot)\|^2_{L_2(\Omega \times \Omega)} \to \min \ .$$

We get

$$\|R(x)\|^2 = \int_{\Omega \times \Omega} \left(\psi_\gamma^\top(x) k^2(y_1, y_2) + k^1(y_1)^\top V_\gamma(x) k^1(y_2) \right)^2 dy_1 dy_2$$

$$= \int_{\Omega \times \Omega} \left((\psi_\gamma(x)^\top k^2(y_1, y_2))^2 \right.$$

$$+ 2\psi_\gamma(x)^\top k^2(y_1, y_2) k^1(y_1)^\top V_\gamma(x) k^1(y_2)$$

$$\left. + (k^1(y_1)^\top V_\gamma(x) k^1(y_2))^2 \right) dy_1 dy_2 \ .$$

Differentiating this expression with respect to the fixed matrix element $(V_\gamma)_{ij}(x)$ and equating the derivative to zero we find

$$\int_\Omega k_i^1(y_1) k^1(y_1)^\top dy_1 \ V_\gamma(x) \int_\Omega k_j^1(y_2) k^1(y_2)^\top dy_2$$

$$= - \int_{\Omega \times \Omega} \psi_\gamma^\top(x) k^2(y_1, y_2) k_i^1(y_1) k_j^1(y_2) dy_1 dy_2 \ , i, j = 1, \ldots, N \ .$$

In matrix notion this is simply

$$(A_1 A_1^*) V_\gamma(x)(A_1 A_1^*) = - \sum_{n=1}^N \psi_{\gamma,n}(x) B_n \ , \tag{24}$$

where the matrices B_n on the right – hand side are

$$B_n = \int_{\Omega \times \Omega} k^1(y_1) k_n^2(y_1, y_2) k^1(y_2)^\top dy_1 dy_2 \ .$$

This means that with $C_n = (A_1 A_1^*)^{-1} B_n (A_1 A_1^*)^{-1}$ the function $k^{1^\top}(y_1) C_n k^1(y_2)$ is the orthogonal projection of the function $k_n^2(y_1, y_2)$ on the linear space

$$\text{span}\{k_i^1(y_1) k_j^1(y_2) : i, j = 1, \ldots, N\} \ .$$

Hence, if the k_n^1 are linearly independent, the matrix V_γ is simply

$$V_\gamma(x) = - \sum_{n=1}^N \psi_{\gamma,n}(x) C_n$$

and we get

$$f_\gamma(x) = \langle g, \psi_\gamma(x) \rangle - \sum_{n=1}^{N} \psi_{\gamma,n}(x) \langle g, C_n g \rangle \ .$$

It is important for the implementation that the matrices C_n are independent of the reconstruction points x. Hence the complexity is determined by the linear part. An example for identifying a vibration string from relative shifts in the eigenvalues is reported in [10].

7 3D X-Ray CT

In [12] we presented a method to reconstruct contours from 3D x–ray data when the x–ray source is moved on a circle around the object. It is fired at 400 positions and the cone of rays is detected at an array of 512×512 detectors resulting in more than 100 million data.

As mollifier we chosed a wavelet such that

$$\hat{e}(\xi) = \|\xi\| h(\xi)$$

for a suitable h resulting in a formula of filered backprojection type

$$f_\gamma(x) \simeq \Delta_x \int_\Gamma \|x - a\|^{-2} Df\left(a, \frac{x-a}{\|x-a\|}\right) da \tag{25}$$

where Γ denotes the curve where the x–ray source is moved and $Df(a, \theta)$ is the data from source position a and direction $\theta \in S^2$.

a

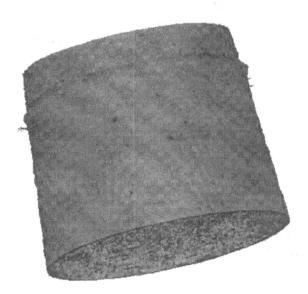

b

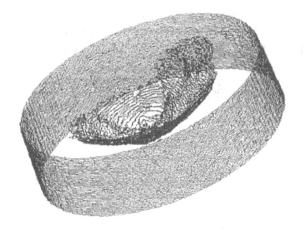

Reconstruction from 10^8 x–ray data, measured at the Fraunhofer Institut für zerstörungsfreie Prüfverfahren, Saarbrücken
Fig. a: Ceramical valve, Fig. b: Display of the interior inclusion of air caused by the production, invisible from the outside.

8 Ultrasound Tomography

We present a technique to apply the approximate inverse to an inverse scattering problem for the Helmholtz equation. In the following we first consider the case of just one incident plane wave in direction Θ. We define the mapping

$$A : L_2(\Omega) \to L_2(\Gamma)$$

where we first put $\Omega = \Gamma = \mathbb{R}^3$, that means we make no use of the fact that f is compactly supported. Let G be the Greens function for the Helmholtz equation, then

$$A\Phi(\eta) = \int_\Omega G(|\eta - y|)\Phi(y)dy \qquad (26)$$

which is a convolution equation. From the last section we know that also the reconstruction is of displacement type using $T_1 = T_2 = T_3 = D^z$ where $D^z f(x) = f(x - z)$ in Theorem 7 if $e_\gamma(x, y) = D^x E_\gamma(y) = E_\gamma(y - x)$. The mapping AA^* is generated by the kernel

$$G_2(\eta - \xi) = \int_{\mathbb{R}^3} G(|\eta - x|)G(|\xi - x|)dx .$$

Defining with the unitary matrix U the operator D^U as $D^U f(x) = f(Ux)$ we compute that $AD^U = D^U A$ and $AA^* D^U = D^U AA^*$, leading to another invariance and a simplification of the reconstruction kernel ψ_γ for circular symmetric $E_\gamma(|y|)$.

After solving $AA^*\psi_\gamma(x, \cdot) = Ae_\gamma(x, \cdot)$ for the reconstruction point x we put for the data given on Γ

$$\Phi_\gamma(x) = \langle u^s, \psi_\gamma(x, \cdot)\rangle_{L_2(\Gamma)} = \int_\Gamma u^s(\eta)\psi_\gamma(|x - \eta|)d\eta . \qquad (27)$$

Evaluating the integral in (26) at the point $x \in \Omega$ we find an approximation for the scattered field inside the scatterer as

$$u^s_\gamma(x) := \int_{\mathbb{R}^3} G(|x - y|)\Phi_\gamma(y)dy$$

$$= \int_\Gamma u^s(\eta) \int_{\mathbb{R}^3} G(|x - y|)\psi_\gamma(|y - \eta|)dyd\eta$$

$$= \int_\Gamma K_\gamma(x - \eta)u^s(\eta)d\eta .$$

We observe that also the kernel K_γ can be precomputed independant of the data. Then we put

$$f_\gamma(x) := \Phi_\gamma(x)/(u^i(x) + u^s(x))$$

$$= \frac{\int_\Gamma u^s(\eta)\psi_\gamma(|x - \eta|)d\eta}{e^{i\Theta x} + \int_\Gamma u^s(\eta)K_\gamma(x - \eta)d\eta} .$$

For multiple incoming plane waves we average over these values, resulting in a discretization of

$$f_\gamma(x) = \frac{1}{4\pi} \int_{S^2} \frac{\int_\Gamma u^s(\Theta,\eta)\psi_\gamma(|x-\eta|)d\eta}{e^{i\Theta x} + \int_\Gamma u^s(\Theta,\eta)K_\gamma(x-\eta)d\eta} d\Theta \; . \tag{28}$$

The solution of the ill-posed linear problem is achieved by precomputing the reconstruction kernel ψ_γ and based on this also the kernel K_γ. Hence the reconstruction is realized by a fast implementation of this formula of filtered backprojection type used in x-ray tomography, compare [9], [15].

Acknowledgement

The research of the author has been supported by BMBF, grant 20M360 - 03LO7SAA - 8, and DFG, grant Lo 310/4-1.

References

[1] Backus G and Gilbert F 1967 *Geophys. J. R. Astron. Soc.* **13** 247-76
[2] Bertero M, de Mol C and Viano C 1980 in *Inverse scattering in optics* ed H P Baltes (Berlin:Springer) pp 161-214
[3] Davison M E and Grunbaum F A 1981 Tomographic reconstruction with arbitrary directions *Comm Pure Appl Math* **34** p77-119
[4] Eckhardt U 1976 *Computing* **17** 193-206
[5] Engl H W 1993 *Surveys on Mathematics for Industry* **3** 71-143
[6] Louis, A K 1979 *Numerische Mathematik* **33** 43-53
[7] Louis A K 1989 *Inverse und schlecht gestellte Probleme* (Stuttgart: Teubner)
[8] Louis A K 1984 *Mathematische Zeitschrift* **185** 429–440
[9] Louis A K 1992 *Inverse Problems* **8** 709-738
[10] Louis A K 1996 *Inverse Problems* **12** 175-190
[11] Louis A K and Maaß P 1990 *Inverse Problems* **6** 427-440
[12] Louis A K and Maass P 1993 *IEEE Trans. Med. Imaging* **12** 764-769
[13] Louis A K, Maaß P, Rieder A 1994 *Wavelets* (Stuttgart:Teubner)
[14] Louis A K and Schuster Th 1996 *Inverse Problems* **12** 686-696
[15] Natterer F 1986 *The mathematics of computerized tomography* (Stuttgart: Teubner-Wiley)
[16] Parker R L 1994 *Geophysical Inverse Theory* (Princeton: U Press)
[17] Plato R and Vainikko G 1990 *Numerische Mathematik* **57** 63-79
[18] Sabatier P C 1987 in *Tomography and inverse problems* ed P C Sabatier (Bristol:Hilger) pp 471-667
[19] Snieder R 1991 *Inverse Problems* **7** 409-433

Wavelet-Accelerated Tikhonov-Phillips Regularization with Applications

Peter Maaß[1]* and *Andreas Rieder*[2]**

[1] Fachbereich Mathematik, Universität Potsdam, Postfach 601553,
  D-14415 Potsdam, Germany
[2] Fachbereich Mathematik, Universität des Saarlandes, Postfach 151150,
  D-66041 Saarbrücken, Germany

1 Introduction

1.1 Tikhonov-Phillips Regularization of Ill-Posed Problems

Many technical and physical problems can be mathematically modeled by operator equations (1) of the first kind,

$$Ax = y, \tag{1}$$

where x is the searched-for information under observed data y. We mention only a few typical examples: medical imaging, see e.g. [16, 20], and inverse scattering problems, see e.g. [6].

To fix the mathematical setup we consider A (throughout the paper) as a compact non-degenerate linear operator acting between the real Hilbert spaces X and Y. In this setting the problem (1) is *ill-posed*, that is, its minimum norm solution x^+ does not depend continuously on the right hand side y. Small perturbations in y may cause dramatic changes in x^+. This instability has to be taken into account by any solution technique for (1). The more as only a perturbation y^δ of the exact but unknown data y is available in general. The perturbation of y is caused by noise which can not be avoided in real-life applications due to the specific experiment and due to the limitations of the measuring apparatus. The perturbed data y^δ are assumed to satisfy $\| y - y^\delta \|_Y \leq \delta$ with an a-priori known *noise level* $\delta > 0$.

One of the theoretically best understood and most often used stabilization techniques for (1) is *Tikhonov-Phillips regularization* where the linear equation (1) is replaced by the minimization problem

$$
\begin{aligned}
&\text{find } x_\alpha^\delta \in X \text{ which minimizes} \\
&T_\alpha(x) = \| Ax - y^\delta \|_Y^2 + \alpha \|x\|_X^2 \ .
\end{aligned}
\tag{2}
$$

* partially supported by a grant of the Deutsche Forschungsgemeinschaft under grant number Ma 1657/1–1
** partially supported by a grant of the Bundesministerium für Bildung, Wissenschaft, Forschung und Technologie under grant number 03–LO7SAA

Here, $\alpha > 0$ is the *regularization parameter*. The idea of Tikhonov-Phillips regularization (2) is to control the influence of the data error in the regularized solution x_α^δ by adding a penalty term. The unique minimizer of (2) is given as the unique solution of the regularized normal equation

$$(A^*A + \alpha I)\, x_\alpha^\delta \,=\, A^*y^\delta \ . \tag{3}$$

The high art of regularization is the determination of the regularization parameter $\alpha = \alpha(\delta, y^\delta)$ such that x_α^δ converges to x^+ as $\delta \to 0$. Examples for such parameter selection strategies are presented in Section 3.

In this paper we introduce two methods to speed up the solution process of (3) which even can be combined. Both methods employ wavelet techniques. For the reader's convenience we therefore give a brief overview on the wavelet theory in the next subsection.

In Section 2 we present a fast multilevel iteration for the solution of a discrete version of the normal equation (3). The theoretical results we achieve are illustrated by numerical examples where the abstract operator equation (1) will be an integral equation. Finally, we discuss the potential of our multilevel method for solving the $3D$-reconstruction problem in computerized tomography.

Any iterative scheme for solving (3) requires the multiplication of a vector by the operator $A^*A + \alpha I$ (resp. a matrix version thereof). Typically, this operator (matrix) will be dense. Therefore, operator compression techniques will speed up any iterative solver. Such methods are considered in Section 3. First, we study compression schemes from a theoretical point of view and then we discuss two ways of computing such compressions. We report on results obtained by applying this approach to hyperthermia treatment planning.

1.2 A Compact Course to Wavelets

We give a brief overview to the univariate theory. Multivariate wavelets, for instance, can be generated from univariate ones by tensor products. We refer to e.g. [10, 17] for a comprehensive introduction to wavelets.

The starting point is the concept of a *refinable* or *scalable* function $\varphi \in L^2(\mathbb{R})$ which is compactly supported and satisfies the following *refinement* or *scaling* equation

$$\varphi(\cdot) = \sqrt{2} \sum_{k \in \mathbb{Z}} h_k \, \varphi(2 \cdot - k) \ . \tag{4}$$

The finite sequence $\{h_k\}_{k \in \mathbb{Z}}$ of real numbers is called mask or filter corresponding to φ. Taking the Fourier transform on both sides of (4) we realize that any non-trivial scaling function has a non-vanishing mean value. Without loss of generality we therefore assume

$$\int_{\mathbb{R}} \varphi(t) \, dt = 1 \ . \tag{5}$$

Further, we require that the integer translates of φ generate a Riesz system in $L^2(\mathbb{R})$, i.e. we have the norm equivalence

$$\left\| \sum_{k \in \mathbb{Z}} a_k \, \varphi(\cdot - k) \right\|_{L^2} \sim \|a\|_{\ell^2} \quad \text{for all } a \in \ell^2(\mathbb{Z}) . \tag{6}$$

We use the notation $f \sim g$ to indicate the existence of two positive constants c_1 and c_2 such that $c_1 f \leq g \leq c_2 f$.

Typical examples for scaling functions with the above requirements are B-splines, several kinds of box-splines and the Daubechies scaling functions whose integer translates are even orthonormal.

Using the scaling function φ we define subspaces V_l of $L^2(\mathbb{R})$ by

$$V_l := \overline{\text{span}\{ \varphi_{l,k} \mid k \in \mathbb{Z} \}}, \quad l \in \mathbb{Z}, \tag{7}$$

where

$$f_{l,k}(\cdot) := 2^{l/2} \, f\!\left(2^l \cdot - k\right)$$

for any $f \in L^2(\mathbb{R})$. The closure in (7) is taken with respect to the L^2-norm. The spaces V_l are nested by (4), $V_l \subset V_{l+1}$, and $\{ \varphi_{l,k} \mid k \in \mathbb{Z} \}$ is a Riesz basis of V_l by (6). By (4), (5) and (6) it follows that

$$\bigcap_{l \in \mathbb{Z}} V_l = \{0\} \quad \text{and} \quad \overline{\bigcup_{l \in \mathbb{Z}} V_l} = L^2(\mathbb{R}) .$$

To any scaling function φ satisfying (5) and (6) there exists a function ψ such that

$$W_l := \overline{\text{span}\{ \psi_{l,k} \mid k \in \mathbb{Z} \}}, \quad l \in \mathbb{Z},$$

coincides with the orthogonal complement of V_l in V_{l+1}: $V_{l+1} = V_l \oplus W_l$. Moreover,

$$\{ \psi_{l,k} \mid l \in \mathbb{Z}, \, k \in \mathbb{Z} \} \tag{8}$$

is an orthonormal basis of $L^2(\mathbb{R})$. The function ψ is called *orthogonal wavelet*. In general ψ does not inherit the compact support from φ. This disadvantage can be avoided by relaxing the requirements. We speak of *pre-wavelets* if the spaces W_l are mutually orthogonal and the wavelet system (8) is only a Riesz basis in $L^2(\mathbb{R})$.

There exists a family, the Daubechies family, of compactly supported orthogonal wavelets, see [10]. The smoothness of the Daubechies wavelets increases monotonically with their support. Also, there exists a family, the Chui-Wang family, of compactly supported pre-wavelets, see [4]. The Chui-Wang wavelets are spline functions. Their corresponding scaling functions are the B-splines.

Both wavelet families can be adapted to bounded intervals, see [4, 5].

The wavelet space W_l is a subspace of V_{l+1}. Therefore, the wavelet ψ can be expanded with respect to the Riesz basis $\{ \varphi_{1,k} \mid k \in \mathbb{Z} \}$ of V_1. Consequently, there exists a unique sequence $g \in \ell^2(\mathbb{Z})$ of real numbers such that

$$\psi(\cdot) = \sqrt{2} \sum_{k \in \mathbb{Z}} g_k \, \varphi(2 \cdot - k) \tag{9}$$

holds true. The sequence g is finite if ψ has a compact support.

Any $f \in L^2(\mathbb{R})$ can be represented by

$$f = \sum_{k \in \mathbb{Z}} c_k(f)\, \varphi_{0,k} + \sum_{l \in \mathbb{N}_0} \sum_{k \in \mathbb{Z}} d_{l,k}(f)\, \psi_{l,k} . \tag{10}$$

If the scaling function φ is q-times continuously differentiable then we have the norm equivalence, see [19, 7],

$$\|f\|_{H^s}^2 \sim \sum_{k \in \mathbb{Z}} |c_k(f)|^2 + \sum_{l \in \mathbb{N}_0} 2^{2sl} \sum_{k \in \mathbb{Z}} |d_{l,k}(f)|^2, \quad 0 \le s \le q, \tag{11}$$

where $\|f\|_{H^s}^2 = \int_{\mathbb{R}} (1+|\xi|^2)^s\, |\hat{f}(\xi)|^2\, d\xi$ is the norm of the Sobolev space $H^s(\mathbb{R}) = \{f \in L^2(\mathbb{R}) \,|\, \|f\|_{H^s} < \infty\}$. Here, $\hat{f}$ denotes the Fourier transform of f.

2 A Multilevel Iteration for Tikhonov-Phillips Regularization

When it comes to a numerical realization of the Tikhonov-Phillips regularization one has to project the normal equation (3) to a finite dimensional subspace of X. The most commonly used projection technique in combination with Tikhonov-Phillips regularization is the method of least squares, see e.g. [15] and [24]. Here we get the finite dimensional regularized normal equation

$$(A_l^* A_l + \alpha I)\, x_l = A_l^* y^\delta, \tag{12}$$

with $A_l = AP_l$ where $P_l : X \to V_l$ is the orthogonal projection onto a finite dimensional subspace $V_l \subset X$.

We require two essential properties of the sequence $\{V_l\}_l$ of finite dimensional approximation spaces: it should be expanding, that is, $V_l \subset V_{l+1}$, and it should be dense in X, that is, $\overline{\cup_l V_l} = X$. With these properties at hand the solution $x_l^{\delta,\alpha}$ of (12) converges to the minimum norm solution x^+ of (1) as $l \to \infty$ and $\delta \to 0$, provided α is determined according to the parameter choice strategies introduced in [24].

In the remainder of this section we will present an efficient multilevel iteration for the resolution of (12) *under the general assumption of a fixed noise level δ.*

2.1 Multilevel Splitting

The basis of all multilevel iterations is the decomposition of the approximation space into subspaces. Therefore, we introduce the splitting $V_{l+1} = V_l \oplus W_l$ where W_l is the X-orthogonal complement of the approximation space V_l with respect to the larger space V_{l+1}. Here, $\oplus$ denotes the X-orthogonal sum. Inductively, we yield the multilevel splitting (13) of V_l,

$$V_l = V_{l_{\min}} \oplus \bigoplus_{j=l_{\min}}^{l-1} W_j, \quad l_{\min} \le l-1, \tag{13}$$

where $l_{\min}$ is called the coarsest level of the splitting. By Q_j we denote the X-orthogonal projection from X onto W_j.

The convergence behavior of the multilevel iteration will depend on the decay rate of the quantity

$$\gamma_l = \|A - A_l\| = \|A(I - P_l)\| \tag{14}$$

as $l \to \infty$. For a proof of $\gamma_l \to 0$ as $l \to \infty$ see e.g. [14].

In the next lemma we show that compact operators vanish asymptotically on the complement spaces W_l.

Lemma 1. *Let V_l and W_l be the spaces defined above and let $A : X \to Y$ be a compact linear operator. Then,*

$$\|AQ_l\| \le \gamma_l \to 0 \quad as \quad l \to \infty$$

with γ_l defined in (14).

Proof. The orthogonality of V_l and W_l yields $P_l Q_l = 0$. Therefore, $\|AQ_l\| = \|A(I - P_l)Q_l\| \le \|A(I - P_l)\| = \gamma_l$. $\qquad\square$

For our further considerations and for the description of the iteration it will be convenient to reformulate (12) as a variational problem

$$\text{find } x_l^{\delta,\alpha} \in V_l : \quad a\big(x_l^{\delta,\alpha}, v_l\big) = \big\langle A_l^* y^\delta, v_l \big\rangle_X \quad \text{for all } v_l \in V_l \tag{15}$$

with the bilinear form $a : X \times X \to \mathbb{R}$,

$$a(u, v) := \langle Au, Av \rangle_Y + \alpha \langle u, v \rangle_X$$

which is symmetric and positive definite. The form a induces the energy norm $\|\cdot\|_a^2 = a(\cdot, \cdot)$ on X.

The operators $\mathcal{A}_l := A_l^* A_l + \alpha P_l : V_l \to V_l$ and $\mathcal{B}_l := Q_l A^* A Q_l + \alpha Q_l : W_l \to W_l$ are related to the bilinear form a via $a(u_l, v_l) = \langle \mathcal{A} u_l, v_l \rangle$ for all $u_l, v_l \in V_l$ and $a(w_l, z_l) = \langle \mathcal{B} w_l, z_l \rangle$ for all $w_l, z_l \in W_l$, respectively.

The strengthened Cauchy inequalities we present now are crucial for the later convergence analysis. Basically, they indicate that the spaces V_l and W_l as well as W_l and W_m are not only X-orthogonal but also asymptotically orthogonal with respect to the inner product on X induced by a.

Theorem 2. *Let V_l and W_m be defined as above and let $m \ge l$. The strengthened Cauchy inequality*

$$|a(v_l, w_m)| \le \min\{1, \gamma_m/\sqrt{\alpha}\} \, \|v_l\|_a \, \|w_m\|_a \tag{16}$$

holds true for all $v_l \in V_l$ and for all $w_m \in W_m$. Further, let $j \ne l$. Then,

$$|a(w_j, w_l)| \le \min\{1, \gamma_l/\sqrt{\alpha}\} \, \min\{1, \gamma_j/\sqrt{\alpha}\} \, \|w_j\|_a \, \|w_l\|_a \tag{17}$$

for all $w_j \in W_j$ and for all $w_l \in W_l$.

Proof. Since v_l and w_m are X-orthogonal we have that $a(v_l, w_m) = \langle Av_l, Aw_m \rangle_Y$. Further,

$$
\begin{aligned}
|a(v_l, w_m)| &= |\langle A_l A_l^{-1/2} A_l^{1/2} v_l, AQ_m B_m^{-1/2} B_m^{1/2} w_m \rangle_Y| \\
&\leq \|A_l A_l^{-1/2}\| \, \|A_l^{1/2} v_l\|_X \, \|AQ_m B_m^{-1/2}\| \, \|B_m^{1/2} w_m\|_X \\
&\leq \|A_l A_l^{-1/2}\| \, \|v_l\|_a \, \|AQ_m\| \, \|B_m^{-1/2}\| \, \|w_m\|_a.
\end{aligned}
$$

Using arguments from spectral theory it is easy to verify that $\|A_l A_l^{-1/2}\| \leq 1$ and $\|B_m^{-1/2}\| \leq \alpha^{-1/2}$. Thus, (16) is proved by $\|AQ_m\| \leq \gamma_m$ (Lemma 1). The second inequality (17) can be proved in the very same way. $\square$

2.2 The Multilevel Iteration

Motivation and Definition. The general idea of multilevel methods is to approximate the original large scale problem (in our situation: (12)) by a sequence of related auxiliary problems on smaller scales which can be solved very cheaply. If the auxiliary problems are designed in a proper way their combination should result in a fair approximation to our original problem, see e.g. [29].

Now, we introduce the concept of subspace corrections, see [29]. Suppose that we have a given approximation u_l^{old} to the solution $x_l^{\delta,\alpha}$ of (12). If the residue $r_l^{\text{old}} = A_l u_l^{\text{old}} - A_l^* y^\delta$ is small we are done. Otherwise, we consider the equation

$$
A_l e_l = r_l^{\text{old}} \tag{18}
$$

for the error $e_l := u_l^{\text{old}} - x_l^{\delta,\alpha}$. Instead of the large scale problem (18) we solve restricted equations with respect to each of the subspaces of the splitting (13):

$$
B_j e_j = Q_j r_l^{\text{old}}, \quad \text{for } l_{\min} \leq j \leq l-1, \tag{19}
$$

$$
A_{l_{\min}} e_{l_{\min}} = P_{l_{\min}} r_l^{\text{old}} .
$$

We observe that

$$
\alpha \|w_j\|_X^2 \leq \langle B_j w_j, w_j \rangle_X = a(w_j, w_j) \leq (1 + \gamma_j^2/\alpha) \, \alpha \, \|w_j\|_X^2 \tag{20}
$$

for all $w_j \in W_j$ which is an immediate consequence of Lemma 1. Hence, B_j can be approximated well by αI on W_j and

$$
\tilde{e}_j = \alpha^{-1} Q_j r_l^{\text{old}}, \quad \text{for } l_{\min} \leq j \leq l-1,
$$

may be viewed as reasonable approximations to the e_j's defined in (19). Finally we are in a position to define the *subspace correction* of u_l^{old} relative to W_j by

$$
u_{W_j}^{\text{new}} := u_l^{\text{old}} - \tilde{e}_j = u_l^{\text{old}} - \alpha^{-1} Q_j \left(A_l u_l^{\text{old}} - A_l^* y^\delta \right)
$$

and relative to $V_{l_{\min}}$ by

$$
u_{V_{l_{\min}}}^{\text{new}} := u_l^{\text{old}} - e_{l_{\min}} = u_l^{\text{old}} - A_{l_{\min}}^{-1} P_{l_{\min}} \left(A_l u_l^{\text{old}} - A_l^* y^\delta \right) .
$$

Starting with an approximation $u_l^\mu \in V_l$ the (Jacobi-like) *additive Schwarz iteration* produces a new iterate by performing the subspace corrections simultaneously, that is,

$$u_l^{\mu+1} = u_l^\mu - C_{l,l_{min}}^{add} \left(A_l u_l^\mu - A_l^* y^\delta \right), \quad \mu = 0, 1, 2, \ldots , \tag{21}$$

with an arbitrary starting guess $u_l^0 \in V_l$ and with

$$C_{l,l_{min}}^{add} = A_{l_{min}}^{-1} P_{l_{min}} + \alpha^{-1} \sum_{j=l_{min}}^{l-1} Q_j .$$

Algebraic Structure of the Iteration. Here we give a detailed description of the algebraic structure of the Schwarz iteration (21). Therefore, we assume that X is a function space over the compact interval $[a, b]$, $X = L^2(a, b)$ for example. The results obtained can easily be generalized to tensor product spaces, e.g. $X = L^2([a, b] \times [c, d])$.

Let φ be a compactly supported scaling function satisfying (4). For convenience, we neglect – just for now – necessary boundary modifications and suppose that

$$V_l = \text{span}\{\varphi_{l,k} \mid k = 0, \ldots, n_l - 1\} \subset X$$

for all $l \geq l^* > 0$. Further, let W_l be spanned by the pre-wavelet ψ, that is,

$$W_l = \text{span}\{\psi_{l,k} \mid k = 0, \ldots, m_l - 1\} .$$

Since the sum of two functions $f_l = \sum_k c_k^l \varphi_{l,k} \in V_l$ and $q_l = \sum_k d_k^l \psi_{l,k} \in W_l$ is in V_{l+1}, it can be expressed by $f_l + q_l = \sum_k c_k^{l+1} \varphi_{l+1,k}$. Applying both refinement equations (4) and (9) we get the relation

$$c_k^{l+1} = \sum_i h_{k-2i} c_i^l + \sum_j g_{k-2j} d_j^l$$

which we write in matrix notation as

$$c^{l+1} = H_{l+1}^t c^l + G_{l+1}^t d^l . \tag{22}$$

Clearly, $H_{l+1} : \mathbb{R}^{n_{l+1}} \to \mathbb{R}^{n_l}$ and $G_{l+1} : \mathbb{R}^{n_{l+1}} \to \mathbb{R}^{m_l}$.

The solution $x_l^{\delta,\alpha}$ of the variational problem (15) resp. of the normal equation (12) can be expanded in the basis of V_l as $x_l^{\delta,\alpha} = \sum_k (\xi_l)_k \varphi_{l,k}$. The vector $\xi_l \in \mathbb{R}^{n_l}$ of the expansion coefficients is the unique solution of the linear system

$$A_l \xi_l = \beta_l \tag{23}$$

where the entries of the positive definite matrix A_l and of the right-hand side β_l are given by

$$(A_l)_{i,j} = \langle A\varphi_{l,i}, A\varphi_{l,j} \rangle_Y + \alpha \langle \varphi_{l,i}, \varphi_{l,j} \rangle_X,$$

$$(\beta_l)_j = \langle y^\delta, A\varphi_{l,j} \rangle_Y .$$

The following lemma enables matrix representations of the operators $Q_j \mathcal{A}_l$, $l_{\min} \le j \le l-1$, and $\mathcal{A}_{l_{\min}}^{-1} P_{l_{\min}} \mathcal{A}_l$ which are the building blocks of the Schwarz iteration (21). For a proof see [25].

Lemma 3. *Define the restrictions*

$$\mathcal{H}_{l,j} := H_{j+1} H_j \cdots H_{l-1} H_l : \mathbb{R}^{n_l} \to \mathbb{R}^{n_j},$$

$$\mathcal{G}_{l,j} := G_{j+1} H_j \cdots H_{l-1} H_l : \mathbb{R}^{n_l} \to \mathbb{R}^{m_j}$$

for $j \le l-2$ and set $\mathcal{H}_{l,l-1} := H_l$ and $\mathcal{G}_{l,l-1} := G_l$.

For $v_l = \sum_k c_k^l \varphi_{l,k} \in V_l$ we have that

$$Q_j \mathcal{A}_l v_l = \sum_{k=0}^{n_l-1} \left(\mathcal{G}_{l,j}^t \, B_j^{-1} \mathcal{G}_{l,j} \, A_l \, c^l \right)_k \varphi_{l,k}, \quad l_{\min} \le j \le l-1,$$

where B_j is the Gramian matrix $(B_j)_{r,s} = \langle \psi_{j,r}, \psi_{j,s} \rangle_X$, and

$$\mathcal{A}_{l_{\min}}^{-1} P_{l_{\min}} \mathcal{A}_l v_l = \sum_{k=0}^{n_l-1} \left(\mathcal{H}_{l,l_{\min}}^t \, A_{l_{\min}}^{-1} \, \mathcal{H}_{l,l_{\min}} \, A_l \, c^l \right)_k \varphi_{l,k} \,.$$

Now, the abstract additive iteration (21) translated into an iteration acting on (23) reads

$$z_l^{\mu+1} = z_l^\mu - C_{l,l_{\min}}^{\text{add}} \left(A_l z_l^\mu - \beta_l \right), \quad \mu = 0, 1, 2, \ldots, \tag{24}$$

with an arbitrary starting guess $z_l^0 \in \mathbb{R}^{n_l}$ and where

$$C_{l,l_{\min}}^{\text{add}} = \mathcal{H}_{l,l_{\min}}^t \, A_{l_{\min}}^{-1} \, \mathcal{H}_{l,l_{\min}} + \alpha^{-1} \sum_{j=l_{\min}}^{l-1} \mathcal{G}_{l,j}^t \, B_j^{-1} \mathcal{G}_{l,j} \,.$$

Remark. In applying the iteration (24) one has to solve a linear system with band matrix B_j on each level j during the multilevel process. However, this does not slow down the iteration. Since the entries of B_j do not depend on j one can precompute a Cholesky decomposition of B_j independently of $j \ge l^*$.

Employing the additive structure of $C_{l,l_{\min}}^{\text{add}}$ the multiplication of the residue by $C_{l,l_{\min}}^{\text{add}}$ can be done in parallel. This leads to a significant speed up if the iteration is implemented on a parallel machine. Since the subspaces of the splitting (13) do not intersect the communication between processors is reduced to a minimum.

Convergence Analysis. Provided a mild decay assumption on γ_j (14) we have the convergence result stated in Theorem 4.

In general, an exact computation of γ_j is impossible. However, upper bounds are often available. In the sequel we will therefore work with such an upper bound.

Theorem 4. *Let η_l be an upper bound of γ_l ($\gamma_l \leq \eta_l$) satisfying*

$$\eta_l \leq \eta_{l-1} \quad and \quad \sum_{j=l_{min}}^{l-1} \eta_j \leq C_\eta\, \eta_{min} \tag{25}$$

with a positive constant C_η which does neither depend on l nor on l_{min}. Let $\{u_l^\mu\}_\mu$ be sequence generated by the Schwarz iteration (21). If $\sigma_{l_{min}} := \eta_{min}/\sqrt{\alpha} \leq 1$ then

$$\left\| u_l^\mu - x_l^{\delta,\alpha} \right\|_a \leq \rho^\mu \left\| u_l^0 - x_l^{\delta,\alpha} \right\|_a$$

with the convergence rate

$$\rho = 2\,C_\eta\,(C_\eta + 2)\,\sigma_{l_{min}} \ . \tag{26}$$

Proof. We roughly sketch the proof. For more details we refer to [25].

It is well known, see e.g. [13], that $\rho_a = \max\{|1 - \Gamma_1|, |1 - \Gamma_2|\}$ where Γ_1 and Γ_2 are positive constants such that

$$\Gamma_1 \,|||\, v_l \,|||^2 \leq \| v_l \|_a^2 \leq \Gamma_2 \,|||\, v_l \,|||^2 \tag{27}$$

holds true for all $v_l \in V_l$. Here, the norm $||| \cdot |||$ on V_l is given by $||| v_l |||^2 :=$ $\| P_{l_{min}} v_l \|_a^2 + \alpha \sum_{j=l_{min}}^{l-1} \| Q_j v_l \|_X^2$. Using the Cauchy inequalities (16), (17) and the estimate (20) one can show that (27) is satisfied with

$$\Gamma_1 = 1/\left(1 + 2\,C_\eta\,(1 + (C_\eta + 1)\,\sigma_{l_{min}})\,\sigma_{l_{min}} \right)$$

and

$$\Gamma_2 = \left(1 + \sigma_{l_{min}}^2 \right)\left(1 + 2\,C_\eta\,\sigma_{l_{min}} \right) \ .$$

$\square$

Numerical Examples. Here we present some numerical experiments to illustrate the theoretical result of Theorem 4.

The ill-posed problem under consideration is the integral equation

$$Af(\cdot) = \int_0^1 k(\cdot, t)\, x(t)\, dt = y(\cdot) \tag{28}$$

where $A : L^2(0,1) \to L^2(0,1)$ is the integral operator with the non-degenerate and square integrable kernel $k(x,y) = x - y$, if $x \geq y$ and $k(x,y) = 0$, otherwise.

As finite dimensional approximation space $V_l \subset L^2(0,1)$ we choose the space of piecewise linear functions with respect to the discretization step-size $s_l = 2^{-l}$. Then, the splitting (13) becomes just the pre-wavelet splitting of the linear spline space, see [3].

Remark. The numerical realization of (21) for the solution of (28) based on spline spaces and on the spaces of the Daubechies scaling functions can be found in some detail in [25]. Also, implementation issues as well as the computational complexity are discussed.

We provide numerical approximations to the convergence rate ρ (26). In the present situation the assumptions (25) are met with $\eta_l = C_k \, s_l^2$ and $C_\eta = 4/3$ resulting in

$$\rho \leq C_A \, s_{l_{\min}}^2 / \sqrt{\alpha} \qquad (29)$$

with a constant C_A independent of l, $l_{\min}$ and α.

By our first experiment we check the decay rate 2 of ρ as $l_{\min} \to \infty$. Figure 2.2 displays approximations to $\rho = \rho(l)$ and the quotient $q_l := \rho(l)/\rho(l-1)$ as functions of the approximation level l with $l_{\min} = l - 5$ and $\alpha = 10^{-4}$.

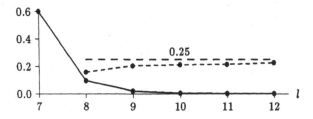

Fig. 1. Approximations to the convergence rate $\rho = \rho(l)$ (solid curve) and the quotient $q_l = \rho(l)/\rho(l-1)$ (dashed curve) for $l_{\min} = l - 5$ and $\alpha = 10^{-4}$. The theoretical bound 0.25 for q_l is drawn as a dashed straight line.

Now we show approximations to $\rho = \rho(l)$ where the coarsest level $l_{\min}$ is fixed to be 2, see Fig. 2.2. In the latter setting the iteration converges for $\alpha = 0.001$ and $\alpha = 0.005$ and Theorem 4 predicts convergence rates which are uniformly bounded in l.

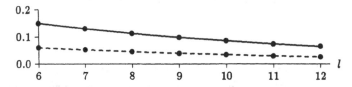

Fig. 2. Convergence rates $\rho = \rho(l)$ for $l_{\min} = 2$. Solid curve: $\alpha = 0.001$, dashed curve: $\alpha = 0.005$.

2.3 Multilevel Approach to Cone Beam Reconstruction

The ultimate goal is an implementation of the above introduced multilevel iteration for the reconstruction of a three-dimensional object from finitely many cone beam X-ray projections.

In the following we investigate what we may expect in this application from a theoretical point of view.

Speaking in mathematical terms the reconstruction problem can be formulated as the operator equation (30) of the first kind,

$$Df = g^\delta, \tag{30}$$

where the cone beam (or divergent beam) transform D is given as

$$Df(a, \omega) := \int_0^\infty f(a + t\omega) \, dt, \quad a \in \mathbb{R}^3, \ w \in S^2 \ .$$

Physically, one can think of a as the position of the X-ray source emitting an X-ray into the direction ω (S^2 denotes the unit sphere in $\mathbb{R}^3$). In the sequel we assume that the searched-for density function f has compact support in the unit box $\square = [0, 1]^3$ and is square integrable, i.e. $f \in L^2(\square)$.

If Γ, the set of all source points a, is compact and does not intersect $\square$ then D maps $L^2(\square)$ continuously to $L^2(\Gamma \times S^2)$, see e.g. [20].

Now we apply the method of least squares together with a Tikhonov-Phillips regularization to (30). As approximation space V_l we choose tensor product B-spline spaces with respect to the step-size $s_l = 2^{-l}$. Thus we have to solve

$$(D_l^* D_l + \alpha I) f_l = D_l^* g^\delta, \tag{31}$$

where $D_l = DP_l$ and P_l is the orthogonal projection from $L^2(\square)$ onto V_l.

To set up our multilevel iteration we need the complement spaces W_l, cf. Sect. 2.1. But these spaces are just the tensor product spline wavelet spaces, see [3]. Hence, the multilevel iteration (21) for solving (31) is well-defined.

Lemma 5. *Suppose that we have complete data, that is, $\Gamma = \partial B$ where ∂B is the boundary of an open Ball B containing the box: $\square \subset B$. Then, the convergence rate ρ (26) of the multilevel iteration (21) acting on (31) fulfills*

$$\rho \le C_D \sqrt{s_{l_{min}}/\alpha} \tag{32}$$

where l_{min} is the coarsest level in the underlying wavelet splitting of the tensor product B-Spline space V_l. The positive constant C_D does neither depend on l, l_{min} nor on α.

Consequently, the iteration converges if l_{min} is sufficiently large.

Proof. The assertion follows by Theorem 4 as soon as we are able to verify that $\gamma_l = \|D(I - P_l)\| \le C \sqrt{s_l}$.

To establish such an estimate we note a relation between the cone beam transform D and the parallel beam transform L defined by

$$Lf(x, \vartheta) := \int_{\mathbb{R}} f(x + t\vartheta) \, dt, \quad \vartheta \in S^2, \ x \in \vartheta^\perp \ .$$

Let the radius of B be r. Then,

$$\int_{S^2}\int_{\Gamma} |Df(a,\omega)|^2 \,|\langle a,\omega\rangle|\,da\,d\omega = 2r\int_{S^2}\int_{\omega^\perp} |Lf(x,\omega)|^2\,dx\,d\omega$$

which follows by a change of coordinates in the inner integral on the left-hand side: set $a = x + \langle a,\omega\rangle\omega$ where x is the orthogonal projection of a onto $\omega^\perp$ and where $|\langle a,\omega\rangle|\,da = r\,dx$. By our assumptions on B and $\square$ there is an $\epsilon > 0$ such that $Df(a,\omega) = 0$ for $|\langle a,\omega\rangle| < \epsilon$. Hence,

$$\|Df\|_{L^2(\Gamma\times S^2)} \le \sqrt{2r/\epsilon}\;\|Lf\|_{L^2(T)}$$

where T is the tangent bundle $T = \{(x,\vartheta)\,|\,\vartheta \in S^2,\; x \in \vartheta^\perp\}$.

As in the proof of Theorem 5.1 in [20] we show that

$$\|Lf\|_{L^2(T)} \le C_L\,\|f\|_{H^{-1/2}}\quad \text{for all}\;\; f \in C_0^\infty(\square),$$

where $\|f\|_{H^\beta}^2 = \int_{\mathbb{R}^3}\left(1+\|\xi\|^2\right)^\beta |\widehat{f}(\xi)|^2\,d\xi$. Here, $\widehat{f}$ is the Fourier transform of f. Denoting the closure of $C_0^\infty(\square)$ with respect to $\|\cdot\|_{H^{-1/2}}$ by $H_0^{-1/2}(\square)$, we finally have

$$\|Df\|_{L^2(\Gamma\times S^2)} \le \sqrt{2r/\epsilon}\;C_L\,\|f\|_{H^{-1/2}}\quad \text{for all}\;\; f \in H_0^{-1/2}(\square)\;.$$

The dual space to $H_0^{-1/2}(\square)$ is $H^{1/2}(\square) = \{v\,|\,\text{there is a } u \in L^2(\mathbb{R}^3) \text{ such that}$ $\|u\|_{H^{1/2}} < \infty$ and $u|_\square = v\}$ with norm $\|v\|_{H^{1/2}(\square)} = \inf\{\|u\|_{H^{1/2}}\,|\,u|_\square = v\}$, see e.g. [28, Chap. 17.2].

From the abstract theory of dual operators, see e.g. [26, Theorem 4.10], it is well known that D^*, the adjoint or dual of D, maps $L^2(\Gamma\times S^2)$ boundedly to $H^{1/2}(\square)$ with norm

$$\|D^*\| = \|D\| \le \sqrt{2r/\epsilon}\;C_L\;.$$

Now, relying on approximation results for tensor product B-splines, see e.g. [27], the proof ends by

$$\|(I - P_l)D^*g\|_{L^2(\square)} \le C_S\,\sqrt{s_l}\;\|D^*g\|_{H^{1/2}(\square)}$$

$$\le C_S\,\sqrt{2r/\epsilon}\;C_L\,\|g\|_{L^2(\Gamma\times S^2)}\,\sqrt{s_l}$$

which implies that $\gamma_l = \|(I - P_l)D^*\| \le C_S\,\sqrt{2r/\epsilon}\;C_L\,\sqrt{s_l}$. $\quad\square$

Remark. Compared to the decay rate 2 of ρ in (29) (as $s_{l_{\min}} \to 0$), the decay rate $1/2$ of ρ in (32) is poor. This difference comes from the different smoothing properties of the operators A (28) and D expressed in Sobolev scales.

The assumptions of Lemma 5 are somewhat unrealistic. In commercial scanners finitely many source positions are distributed on a curve Γ surrounding the object and at each source position only finitely many X-ray projections are taken. Mostly, Γ is a planar circle.

From now on we therefore consider the cone beam transform as a mapping with finite dimensional image space, i.e.

$$D : L^2(\square) \rightarrow \mathbb{R}^{p \cdot q},$$

where p is the number of source positions on Γ and q is the number of X-rays emitted at each source position.

In this setting the structure of the linear system being equivalent to (31), cf. (23), is suited in particular for applying an iterative solver. Let $\{\varphi_{l,k} \,|\, k \in \mathcal{I}_l\}$ be the B-spline basis of V_l. The system matrix $\mathbf{A}_l$ can be written as

$$\mathbf{A}_l = \mathbf{D}_l^t \mathbf{D}_l + \alpha \mathbf{G}_l$$

with

$$(\mathbf{D}_l)_{(i,j),k} = D\varphi_{l,k}(a_i, \omega_{i,j}) \quad \text{and} \quad (\mathbf{G}_l)_{m,k} = \langle \varphi_{l,m}, \varphi_{l,k} \rangle_{L^2(\square)} .$$

Here, a_i, $1 \le i \le p$, are the discrete source positions on Γ and $\omega_{i,j}$, $1 \le j \le q$, are the directions of the X-rays emitted at source position a_i. Since the basis functions in V_l have a local support (the width of the support is proportional to s_l), both matrices $\mathbf{D}_l$ and $\mathbf{G}_l$ are sparse, that is, almost all of their entries are zero. This is obvious for the Gramian $\mathbf{G}_l$. At the source position a_i only a few X-rays hit the support of $\varphi_{l,k}$ which explains the sparsity of $\mathbf{D}_l$.

So, we can employ sparse matrix techniques to store $\mathbf{D}_l$ as well as $\mathbf{G}_l$ and hence $\mathbf{A}_l$. Additionally, the evaluation of the residue, which has to be done at each iteration step, cf. (24), can be realized very efficiently.

Our theoretical results indicate that it might be worth to tackle the cone beam reconstruction problem by the introduced multilevel iteration. However, only an implementation on a parallel computer can finally settle the question whether this algorithm yields satisfactory results in a reasonable run-time.

3 The Use of Approximating Operators

Again we consider Tikhonov regularization for solving (1), i.e. we consider

$$x_\alpha^\delta = (A^* A + \alpha I)^{-1} A^* y^\delta , \tag{33}$$

where $\|y - y^\delta\| \le \delta$ and A is a compact operator between Hilbert spaces X, Y

$$A : X \rightarrow Y .$$

Now assume that a family of approximating operators $\{A_h\}$ is given with

$$\|A - A_h\| \le h \tag{34}$$

and that A is replaced by A_h in (33). Hence we study the approximation properties of

$$x_{\alpha,h}^\delta = (A_h^* A_h + \alpha I)^{-1} A_h^* y^\delta . \tag{35}$$

The introduction of the operators $\{A_h\}$ serves two purposes. First of all any numerical method for computing (33) always requires a finite dimensional approximation of the operator equation (1), cf. Section 2. Secondly we may aim at choosing a sparse or compressed approximation A_h which will yield faster algorithms – this is our main intention for introducing A_h.

The choice of α and h determine the approximation properties of $x_{\alpha,h}^\delta$. We will choose α according to a discrepancy principle of the form (or some modification thereof)

$$\|A_h x_{\alpha,h}^\delta - y^\delta\| = \tau\delta, \tag{36}$$

where $\tau > 1$. This still describes an idealized situation: in practice one never aims at solving (36) precisely, one rather chooses α from a sequence of test parameters and determines $\alpha_N \in \{\alpha_n = q^n\alpha_0 | n \in \mathbb{N}\}$ by requiring

$$\|A_h x_{\alpha_N,h}^\delta - y^\delta\| \leq \tau\delta \tag{37}$$

$$\|A_h x_{\alpha_n,h}^\delta - y^\delta\| > \tau\delta \quad \text{for} \quad n < N . \tag{38}$$

Hence the overall algorithm for computing $x_{\alpha,h}^\delta$ requires to solve $(N+1)$ operator equations

$$(A_h^* A_h + \alpha_n I)x = A_h^* y^\delta, \quad n = 0, 1, \ldots, N . \tag{39}$$

Thus an efficient procedure for obtaining sparse approximations A_h in connection with a reliable strategy for selecting the approximation level h will greatly reduce the numerical cost of the algorithm. Our main objective in this chapter is to determine an approximation level $h(\delta, \alpha)$ such that $x_{\alpha,h}^\delta$ exhibits optimal convergence rates. Note that the approximation level $h(\delta, \alpha)$ may change with α during the search process for the optimal regularization parameter α_N. This will later be used to choose coarser approximations for larger values of α.

As usual we assume that the generalized solution x^+ lies in the range of $(A^* A)^\nu$, that is,

$$x^+ = (A^* A)^\nu v, \quad \|v\| \leq \varrho . \tag{40}$$

Moreover we restrict ourselves to smoothness assumptions of the order

$$0 \leq \nu \leq \frac{1}{2} ,$$

since higher order regularity of x^+ does not further improve the convergence rate of $\|x_\alpha^{\delta,h} - x^+\|$. This is consistent with the theory of a posteriori parameter selection for classical Tikhonov regularization since – even when using the exact operator A – applying a discrepancy functional of type (36) limits optimal convergence rates to the range $0 \leq \nu \leq 1/2$. To avoid unnecessary notation we furthermore assume that A_h is a compact operator and that

$$\overline{\text{range}(A)} = Y, \quad \|y^\delta\| > \delta, \quad \|A\|, \|A_h\| \leq 1 . \tag{41}$$

Notation. A missing index of $x_{\alpha,h}^{\delta}$ indicates that the related quantity is zero, for instance, $x_{\alpha,h}$ denotes the solution of (35) with exact data y.

We will frequently use the singular value decomposition for a compact operator A, which is denoted by $\{u_n, v_n, \sigma_n\}$ where $u_n \in X$, $v_n \in Y$ are the singular vectors and $\sigma_n > 0$ are the singular values.

The starting for this investigation is a basic estimate which reveals the three error contributions in estimating $\|x_{\alpha,h}^{\delta} - x^+\|$. This result is – in principle – contained in Lemma 2.5 of [22]. However we include the full proof since we will need some intermediate steps again later.

Lemma 6. *Let x^+ be the generalized solution of $Ax = y$ and let $x_{\alpha,h}^{\delta}$ be defined by (35). Assume that $\|y - y^{\delta}\| \le \delta$ and that x^+ obeys (40). Then,*

$$\|x_{\alpha,h}^{\delta} - x^+\| \le \frac{\delta}{2\sqrt{\alpha}} + \frac{h\|x^+\|}{\sqrt{\alpha}} + \alpha^{\nu} c_{\nu,\alpha}(v)$$

where

$$c_{\nu,\alpha}^2(v) = \sum_{n \ge 0} \left\{ \frac{\alpha^{1-\nu}\sigma_n^{2\nu}}{(\sigma_n^2 + \alpha)} \langle v, u_n \rangle \right\}^2 \le \{(1-\nu)^{1-\nu}\nu^{\nu}\varrho\}^2 .$$

Proof. We follow the proof of Lemma 2.5 in [22]. Equation (40) and inserting the singular value decomposition yields

$$\|(A^*A + \alpha I)^{-1}x^+\| \le \tilde{c}_{\nu}\alpha^{\nu-1} \|v\| .$$

Moreover we need the following estimates for a compact operator T, they follow from standard estimates using the singular value decomposition of T:

$$\|(T^*T + \alpha I)^{-1}T^*\| \le \frac{1}{2\sqrt{\alpha}}, \qquad \|(T^*T + \alpha I)^{-1}\| \le \alpha^{-1},$$

$$\|T(T^*T + \alpha I)^{-1}T^*\| \le 1,$$

where $T = A$ or $T = A_h$. Now we have

$$\|x_{\alpha,h}^{\delta} - x^+\| \le \|x_{\alpha,h}^{\delta} - x_{\alpha,h}\| + \|x_{\alpha,h} - x_{\alpha}\| + \|x_{\alpha} - x^+\|$$

where those three terms can be estimated as follows

$$\|x_{\alpha} - x^+\| = \| (A^*A + \alpha I)^{-1}A^*Ax^+ - x^+\|$$

$$= \alpha\|(A^*A + \alpha I)^{-1}x^+\|$$

$$\le c_{\nu\alpha}(v)\alpha^{\nu}\|\rho\|,$$

$$\|x_{\alpha,h} - x_{\alpha}\| = \|(A_h^*A_h + \alpha I)^{-1}A_h^*y - (A^*A + \alpha I)^{-1}A^*y\| .$$

Now we observe that

$$\{(A_h^* A_h + \alpha I)^{-1} - (A^* A + \alpha I)^{-1}\}$$

$$= (A_h^* A_h + \alpha I)^{-1} [(A^* A) - (A_h^* A_h)] (A^* A + \alpha I)^{-1}$$

$$= (A_h^* A_h + \alpha I)^{-1} \{(A^* - A_h^*)A + A_h^*(A - A_h)\} (A^* A + \alpha I)^{-1} .$$

Inserting this identity and $y - A(A^* A + \alpha I)^{-1} A^* y = \alpha(AA^* + \alpha I)^{-1} y$ we obtain

$$\|x_{\alpha,h} - x_\alpha\| = \|(A_h^* A_h + \alpha I)^{-1}(A_h^* - A^*) [y - A(A^* A + \alpha I)^{-1} A^* y]$$

$$+ (A_h^* A_h + \alpha I)^{-1} A_h^*(A - A_h)(A^* A + \alpha I)^{-1} A^* y\|$$

$$\leq \frac{1}{\alpha} h \, \alpha \, \|(AA^* + \alpha I)^{-1} A x^+\| + \frac{1}{2\sqrt{\alpha}} h \, \|x^+\|$$

$$\leq h \, \|x^+\|/\sqrt{\alpha} .$$

Finally,

$$\|x_{\alpha,h}^\delta - x_{\alpha,h}\| = \|(A_h^* A_h + \alpha I)^{-1} A_h^*(y^\delta - y)\| \leq \frac{\delta}{2\sqrt{\alpha}}$$

concludes the proof. □

Remark. Lemma 6 describes the different contributions to the error $\|x_{\alpha,h}^\delta - x^+\|$. The approximation error $\alpha^\nu c_{\alpha\nu}(v)$ as well as the influence of the data error $\frac{\delta}{2\sqrt{\alpha}}$ are the same as for Tikhonov regularization with exact operator A. In addition the operator error introduces a new term of the order $\frac{h\|x^+\|}{\sqrt{\alpha}}$. Of course $\|x^+\|$ is not precisely known, but, since A has been scaled to $\|A\| \leq 1$, we have $\|x^+\| \leq \varrho$.

The total error $\| x_{\alpha,h}^\delta - x^+ \|$ depends on the choice of h and α. To begin with let us choose h to be fixed for all α and let us determine α according to a modified discrepancy principle:

$$\text{choose } \alpha \text{ s.t.} \quad \| A_h \, x_{\alpha,h}^\delta - y^\delta \| = \tau\delta + \sigma h . \tag{42}$$

Various types of discrepancy principles, both in terms of the functional on the left hand side and the expression on the right hand side have been investigated, see [11, 12, 15, 22].

Investigating a posteriori strategies of this sort always starts by proving that choosing α according to (42) is equivalent to a discrepancy principle with exact data and exact operator, see e.g. [21].

Lemma 7. *Let $\tau > 2$, $\sigma > \frac{9}{4}\|x^+\|$, and assume that α is chosen according to (42). Then, x_α satisfies a discrepancy principle*

$$\|Ax_\alpha - y\| = \tilde\tau\delta + \tilde\sigma h ,$$

where $|\tau - \tilde\tau| \leq 2$, $|\sigma - \tilde\sigma| \leq \frac{9}{4}\|x^+\|$, in particular $\tilde\tau > 0$, $\tilde\sigma > 0$.

Proof. The term $\|Ax_\alpha - y\|$ can be extended as follows:

$$\|Ax_\alpha - y\| = \|A(A^*A + \alpha I)^{-1}A^*y - y\|$$

$$= \|\underbrace{(A - A_h)(A^*A + \alpha I)^{-1}A^*y}_{= x_\alpha} + A_h(x_\alpha - x_{\alpha,h}) + A_h(x_{\alpha,h} - x_{\alpha,h}^\delta)$$

$$+ [A_h x_{\alpha,h}^\delta - y^\delta] + (y^\delta - y)\|.$$

These five terms have to be estimated separately,

$$\|(A - A_h)(A^*A + \alpha I)^{-1}A^*y\| \le h\,\|(A^*A + \alpha I)^{-1}A^*Ax^+\| \le h\,\|x^+\|.$$

Now we use the same modifications as in the proof of Lemma 6 for $\|x_\alpha - x_{\alpha,h}\|$.

$$\|A_h(x_\alpha - x_{\alpha,h})\| = \|A_h\left[(A^*A + \alpha I)^{-1}A - (A_h^*A_h + \alpha I)^{-1}A_h^*\right]y\|$$

$$\le \frac{1}{2\sqrt{\alpha}}\,h\,\alpha\|(AA^* + \alpha I)^{-1}Ax^+\| + h\,\|x^+\|$$

$$\le \frac{1}{4}h\|x^+\| + h\|x^+\|,$$

$$\|A_h(x_{\alpha,h} - x_{\alpha,h}^\delta)\| = \|A_h(A_h^*A_h + \alpha I)^{-1}A_h^*(y - y^\delta)\| \le \delta,$$

$$\|A_h x_{\alpha,h}^\delta - y^\delta\| = \tau\delta + \sigma h,$$

$$\|y^\delta - y\| \le \delta.$$

Combining these estimates yields

$$\|Ax_\alpha - y\| \le \tau\delta + \sigma h + \frac{9}{4}\,\|x^+\|\,h + 2\delta$$

and similarly by the inverse triangle inequality we have

$$\|Ax_\alpha - y\| > (\tau - 2)\delta + \left(\sigma - \frac{9}{4}\|x^+\|\right)h.$$

$\square$

Now we can deal with y and A instead of y^δ and A_h. This gives rise to an estimate for the a posteriori chosen regularization parameter α.

Lemma 8. *Let α be chosen according to (42) then*

$$(\bar\tau\delta + \bar\sigma h)^2 = \alpha^{2\nu+1}\,d_{\alpha,\nu}^2(v)$$

or equivalently

$$\alpha = (\bar\tau\delta + \bar\sigma h)^{\frac{2}{2\nu+1}}\,d_{\alpha,\nu}^{-\frac{2}{2\nu+1}}(v)$$

Proof. The proof is based on the same type of arguments as used in [21]. Applying the results of the previous lemmata yields

$$(\bar{\tau}\delta + \bar{\sigma}h)^2 = \|Ax_\alpha - y\|^2 = \|(A(A^*A + \alpha I)^{-1}A^* - I)Ax^+\|^2$$

$$= \sum_{n \geq 0} \left(\frac{\sigma_n^2}{\sigma_n^2 + \alpha} - 1\right)^2 (\sigma_n \sigma_n^{2\nu})^2 \, |\langle v, u_n \rangle|^2$$

$$= \alpha^{2\nu+1} \underbrace{\sum_{h \geq 0} \frac{\sigma_n^{4\nu+2}\alpha^{1-2\nu}}{(\sigma_n^2 + \alpha)^2} \, |\langle v, u_n \rangle|^2}_{= \, d_{\alpha,\nu}^2(v)} \;.$$

$\square$

Now we can combine the above estimate for α with Lemma 6. First one should note that inserting the singular value decomposition shows that $d_{\alpha,\nu}(v)$ is bounded for $0 \leq \nu \leq 1/2$ and by the Hölder inequality one obtains, see e.g. [21],

$$c_{\alpha,\nu}(v) \, d_{\alpha,\nu}^{\frac{-2\nu}{2\nu+1}}(v) \leq c \;.$$

Lemma 6 now be reformulated as

$$\|x_{\alpha,h}^\delta - x^+\| \leq \frac{\delta \cdot d_{\alpha,\nu}^{\frac{1}{2\nu+1}}(v)}{2(\bar{\tau}\delta + \bar{\varepsilon}h)^{\frac{1}{2\nu+1}}} + \frac{h\|x^+\| \, d_{\alpha,\nu}^{\frac{1}{2\nu+1}}(v)}{(\bar{\tau}\delta + \bar{\varepsilon}h)^{\frac{1}{2\nu+1}}} + \alpha^\nu c_{\alpha,\nu}(v)$$

$$\leq C(\delta + h)^{\frac{2\nu}{2\nu+1}} \;.$$

Theorem 9. *If $0 \leq \nu \leq 1/2$ and if α is chosen according to the discrepancy principle (42) then*

$$\|x_{\alpha,h}^\delta - x^+\| = O\left((\delta + h)^{\frac{2\nu}{2\nu+1}}\right) \;.$$

If the operator error h is linked to the data error by

$$h = O(\delta) \;,$$

then an order optimal convergence rate is achieved by the modified Tikhonov-regularization.

Remark. As always we can strengthen the estimate if $0 \leq \nu < 1/2$ to

$$\|x_{\alpha,h}^\delta - x^+\| = o\left((\delta + h)^{\frac{2\nu}{2\nu+1}}\right) \;.$$

Now we consider the algorithm where α is chosen by testing various parameters

$$\alpha \in \{\alpha_n \,|\alpha_n = q^n \alpha_0 \}$$

according to

$$\|A_h x^\delta_{\alpha_N,h} - y^\delta\| \le \tau\delta + \sigma h, \tag{43}$$

$$\|A_h x^\delta_{\alpha_n,h} - y^\delta\| > \tau\delta + \sigma h \quad \text{for} \quad n < N . \tag{44}$$

As we will see in the following, a little bit stronger assumptions on the choice of τ and σ insure the same convergence properties as in Theorem 9. As the main ingredient we need the equivalent of Lemma 7.

Lemma 10. *If α_N is chosen according to (43) with $\tau > 2/q$ and $\sigma > 9\|x^+\|/4q$ then there exist $\tilde\tau > 0$ and $\tilde\sigma > 0$ s.t. x_{α_N} satisfies the discrepancy principle*

$$\|A x_{\alpha_N} - y\| = \tilde\tau\delta + \tilde\sigma h .$$

Proof. We compare α_N with the parameter α^*, which stems from solving the discrepancy principle (42) exactly. Since the functional $\|A_h x^\delta_{\alpha,h} - y^\delta\|$ increases monotonically with α (this can be seen by expressing this functional in terms of the singular functions of A_h) we have

$$q\,\alpha^* < \alpha_N \le \alpha^*$$

and

$$\|A_h x^\delta_{q\alpha^*,h} - y^\delta\| \le \|A_h x^\delta_{\alpha_N,h} - y^\delta\| \le \tau\delta + \sigma h .$$

A lower estimate is obtained by $(q < 1)$

$$\|A_h x^\delta_{q\alpha^*,h} - y^\delta\| = \left(\sum \left(\frac{(\sigma^h_n)^2}{(\sigma^h_n)^2 + q\alpha^*} - 1 \right)^2 ((y^\delta, v^h_n))^2 \right)^{1/2}$$

$$\ge q \left(\sum \left(\frac{(\sigma^h_n)^2}{(\sigma^h_n)^2 + \alpha^*} - 1 \right)^2 ((y^\delta, v^h_n))^2 \right)^{1/2}$$

$$= q\|A_h x^\delta_{\alpha^*,h} - y^\delta\|$$

$$\ge q(\tau\delta + \sigma h) .$$

Combining both estimates therefore shows that $x^\delta_{\alpha_N,h}$ satisfies a discrepancy principle with (τ^*, σ^*) where $q\tau \le \tau^* \le \tau$ and $q\sigma \le \sigma^* \le \sigma$. In particular $\tau^* > 2$ and $\sigma^* > 9\|x^+\|/4$, hence Lemma 7 applies. $\qquad\square$

Remark. The above lemma implies that choosing α from a decreasing sequence $\alpha = q^n \alpha_0$, $(q < 1)$, yields optimal convergence rates in connection with the discrepancy principle (43).

So far we have discussed to which extend A may be replaced by an approximating operator A_h, where A_h is kept fixed for all possible values of the regularization parameter α. However since we choose α by testing different values of the regularization parameter we would also like to link the quality of the approximation $\|A - A_h\|$ to α. This will allow us to use coarser approximations for large values of α. The approximation only has to be refined as α gets small.

Let us consider approximation levels of the type

$$h = O(\delta^p \alpha^q) \tag{45}$$

where $0 \leq p, q \leq 1$ and the regularization parameter is assumed to be bounded above by $\alpha \leq \alpha_0$.

All the previous estimates remain valid in this case, in particular we obtain

$$\|x_{\alpha,h}^\delta - x^+\| = O\left((\delta + h)^{\frac{2\nu}{2\nu+1}}\right) . \tag{46}$$

But now h depends on α and we need an additional upper bound for the regularization parameter α. Simply using $\alpha \leq \alpha_0$ would yield a suboptimal convergence rate $O(\delta^{2\nu q/(2\nu+1)})$. But, since we expect that asymptotically the regularization parameter of our modified scheme behaves similar to the standard Tikhonov regularization where $(0 \leq \nu \leq 1/2)$

$$\alpha = O(\delta^{2/(2\nu+1)}) \leq c\delta ,$$

we anticipate asymptotically at least $\alpha = O(\delta)$. In order to make this statement precise let us reconsider the relation between δ, h and α as described in Lemma 8,

$$(\bar{\tau}\delta + \bar{\sigma}h)^2 = \alpha^{2\nu+1} (d_{\alpha,\nu}(v))^2 .$$

Up to here we have used this relation to obtain an upper bound on $1/\sqrt{\alpha}$ by proving that $d_{\alpha,\nu}(v)$ itself is bounded for $0 \leq \nu \leq 1/2$. Now we need an upper bound for α itself. The proof of Lemma 8 begins with

$$(\bar{\tau}\delta + \bar{\sigma}h)^2 = \alpha^2 \sum_{n>0} \frac{\sigma_n^{4\nu+2}}{(\sigma_n^2 + \alpha)^2} |\langle v, u_n \rangle|^2 .$$

Since $(\sigma_n^2 + \alpha)^2 \leq (\sigma_0^2 + \alpha_0)^2 \leq c_0$ is bounded we obtain a lower bound for the right hand side by

$$(\bar{\tau}\delta + \bar{\sigma}h)^2 \geq \alpha^2 c \sum_{n\geq 0} \sigma_n^{4\nu+2} |\langle v, u_n\rangle|^2 = \alpha^2 c \|A(A^*A)^\nu v\|^2 = \alpha^2 c \|Ax^+\|^2 .$$

Our assumptions on the computability of the discrepancy principle (41) stated $\|Ax^+\| = \|Ax^+ - y^\delta + y^\delta\| \geq \|y^\delta\| - \delta > 0$. Hence we obtain

$$(\bar{\tau}\delta + \bar{\sigma}h)^2 \geq c\alpha^2 . \tag{47}$$

Let us now insert the adaptive approximation level $h = O(\delta^p \alpha^q)$.

Lemma 11. *If $h = O(\delta^p \alpha^q)$, where we assume that*

$$0 < p, q, \quad p + q = 1,$$

and if $\|Ax^+\| > 0$ then

$$\alpha = O(\delta) .$$

Remark. We expect an even faster decay, namely $\alpha = O(\delta^{2/(2\nu+1)})$. However, this is not obvious for a posteriori parameter selection. Nevertheless applying the above estimate allows us to show optimal convergence rates.

Proof. We have to consider two cases. First assume that $\tilde{\tau}\delta \geq \tilde{\sigma}h$. Then we obtain directly by (47)

$$\alpha^2 \leq c\delta^2 .$$

Secondly, assume that $\tilde{\tau}\delta < \tilde{\sigma}h$. Then,

$$\alpha^2 \leq ch^2 = O(\delta^p \alpha^q)^2$$

which implies $(p + q = 1)$

$$\alpha^{2-2q} = O(\delta^{2p}) \quad \text{or} \quad \alpha = O(\delta) .$$

$\square$

Theorem 12. *If $h = O(\delta^p \alpha^q)$, with $0 < p, q$, $p + q = 1$, and if α is chosen by the modified discrepancy principle (42), then*

$$\|x^\delta_{\alpha,h} - x^+\| = O(\delta^{2\nu/(2\nu+1)}) .$$

Proof. Combining (46) and Lemma 11 gives the desired result. $\square$

Remark. The above theorem shows that we can e.g. chose $p = q = 1/2$ and still obtain optimal convergence rates. Such a choice is preferable for large values of α which is the case in the beginning of our iterative search for the optimal regularization parameter.

Optimal convergence rates cannot be achieved in general if $p + q < 1$.

3.1 Computing Approximating Families $\{A_h\}$

Replacing A by A_h serves two purposes: first of all any numerical implementation of Tikhonov regularization requires a finite dimensional approximation and secondly one may aim at approximations which have a sparse structure leading to accelerated algorithms. The conventional way of satisfying the first requirement is to replace A by AP_h, where P_h is a projector onto a finite dimensional subspace, see e.g. [24]. However this leads in general to dense matrices. An exception arises when using a singular function system of A, which leads to a diagonal matrix. But those singular functions are in general not known or difficult to construct.

In the following we will discuss two possibilities. Truncated singular value decompositions fall in the class $A_h = AP_h$. But – as usual – they are not recommended for practical applications, nevertheless they achieve optimal convergence rates for a wider range of discrepancy principles. As a second possibility we will apply wavelet techniques in a lazy fashion: we assume that A has been discretized and reduced to a matrix formulation by any standard discretization which might be suitable for the application at hand. Then this matrix is compressed by computing its two–dimensional discrete wavelet transform and discarding small coefficients. This yields an approximating operator which cannot be expressed as $A_h = AP_h$.

Truncated Singular Value Decomposition. Let us assume that the singular value decomposition of A is denoted by $\{u_n, v_n, \sigma_n\}$ and let $n(h)$ denote the index s.t. $|\sigma_n| \leq h$ for all $n \geq n(h)$. Then a family of approximating operators is defined by

$$A_h x := \sum_{n \leq n(h)} \sigma_n \langle x, u_n \rangle v_n \ .$$

Obviously we have $\|A - A_h\| \leq h$. In this situation we can describe the regularized solution explicitly by

$$x^\delta_{\alpha,h} = \sum_{n \leq n(h)} \frac{\sigma_n}{\sigma_n^2 + \alpha} \langle y^\delta, v_n \rangle u_n \ . \tag{48}$$

In the previous chapter we considered a discrepancy principle with a modified right hand side, namely $\tau\delta + \sigma h$. However this modification is not necessary when using the truncated singular value decomposition.

Theorem 13. *Let $\{A_h\}$ be defined by truncated singular decompositions, choose*

$$h = c_1 \delta^p \alpha^q, \quad 1/2 \leq q, \quad 1/3 < p,$$

and determine α by

$$\|A_h x^\delta_{\alpha,h} - y^\delta\| = \tau\delta \ .$$

If $\tau > 2$ and $0 \leq \nu \leq 1/2$ then

$$\|x^\delta_{\alpha,h} - x^+\| = O(\delta^{2\nu/(2\nu+1)}) \ .$$

Proof. The central part of the proofs in the previous section is contained in Lemma 7, which allows to deal with the exact data and the full operator A. The proof of this Lemma consists of estimating five terms. All of them can be expressed with the help of the singular value decomposition. The first term gives $(Ax^+ = y)$:

$$(A - A_h)(A^*A + \alpha I)^{-1}A^*Ax^+ = \sum_{n > n(h)} \sigma_n \frac{\sigma_n^2}{\sigma_n^2 + \alpha} \langle x^+, u_n \rangle v_n \ .$$

Hence its norm is bounded by a multiple of

$$h^3/\alpha = c_1 \delta^{3p} \alpha^{3q-1} .$$

Since $p > 1/3$ and $\alpha \leq \alpha_0$ this norm can be bounded by $c_2\delta$, where $c_2 = O(\delta^{3p-1})$ can be chosen arbitrarily small as δ tends to zero.

The second term vanishes since $x_\alpha - x_{\alpha,h}$ contains only contributions to singular values smaller than h which are in the kernel of A_h. The other terms remain the same. Hence $\tau > 2$ guarantees that x_α obeys the same discrepancy principle with a $\tilde{\tau} > 0$. This, via Lemma 8, gives the relation

$$\tilde{\tau}^2 \delta^2 = \alpha^{2\nu+1} d_{\alpha,\nu}^2 .$$

Now we have to revise the basic error estimate of Lemma 6 in the light of the truncated singular value decompositions. Here the second term, the operator error is given by

$$\|x_{\alpha,h} - x_\alpha\| \leq h^2/\alpha = c_1^2 \delta^{2/3} .$$

The remaining terms can be estimated in the standard fashion:

$$\|x_{\alpha,h}^\delta - x^+\| = O(\delta^{2\nu/(2\nu+1)}) .$$

$\square$

Wavelet Compression Techniques. Another possibility for constructing approximating operators arises from applying wavelet techniques. The theory of sparsifying or compressing general operators by wavelet techniques has been extensively studied in [2, 8], for applications to compact operators and inverse problems see e.g. [9, 23]. Wavelet–vaguelette decompositions are also considered in the last paper. They can be precomputed and serve as a good compromise between singular functions and finite elements: they also lead to diagonal matrices, moreover the wavelets may be chosen compactly supported.

There exist various ways of achieving a wavelet compression of integral operators with kernel $k(s,t)$. One can e.g. apply a two-dimensional discrete wavelet transform to k to obtain a two-dimensional version of the expansion (10). Discarding all coefficients on scales l smaller than h or using a threshold t, that is, discarding those $d_{l,k}$-coefficients on all scales which are smaller than t leads to compressed operators. In both cases one obtains error estimates by either applying Lemma 1 or the norm equivalence (11). For a more detailed analysis in the framework of ill–posed problems see [9].

A lazy method for accelerating the regularization method is to discretize the operator with an arbitrary Galerkin–type approach. This is rather suitable for many applications where e.g. a triangular model (or tetrahedral model) has been build with large effort and a volume integration technique has lead to a full matrix of large dimension. After computing the wavelet transform of this matrix one can easily either apply thresholding or truncation.

We will only shortly examplify the order of acceleration which can be achieved when this approach is used for optimizing hyperthermia treatment planning, see [18]. For an introduction to the mathematical problems of hyperthermia we refer to [1].

The related matrix has been compressed by thresholding using the Daubechies wavelet with 6 coefficients. The following table shows the number of zeroes obtained for various levels of thresholding.

t_h	n_h	e_h
0.01	47.7%	0.016
0.015	56.8%	0.026
0.05	81.2%	0.0826
0.1	90.93%	0.146
0.25	97.8%	0.27

Different choices t_h of the thresholding parameter t lead to different approximating operators A_h. In the above table n_h denotes the percentage of highpass-coefficients which were set to zero. The deviation e_h is computed by

$$e_h^2 = \frac{\sum_{i,j}(a_{ij} - a_{ij}^h)^2}{\sum_{i,j} a_{ij}^2}$$

which only gives a very rough upper bound to the approximation error. Here, a_{ij} and a_{ij}^h denote the entries of A and A^h, respectively. Typical values for the threshold (discarding about 90% of the wavelet coefficients) resulted – due to the overhead cost for computing the wavelet transforms – in a speed up factor of about 7, without distorting the result visibly.

Acknowledgement. The first author wants to thank A. Gruenbaum and C. Nefeli for their hospitality while staying at the University of California at Berkely in March 96 where this article was finished.

References

1. Böhm, M., Kremer, J., Louis, A. K.: Efficient algorithm for computing optimal control of antennas in hyperthermia. Surv. Math. Ind. **3** (1993) 233–251
2. Beylkin, B., Coifman, R.R., Rokhlin, V.: Wavelets in Numerical Analysis. In Ruskai, M. B., et al. (eds.), Wavelets and their Applications. Jones and Bartlett Pub., Boston (1992)
3. Chui, C. K., Quak, E.: Wavelets on a bounded interval. In Braess, D., Schumaker, L. L. (eds.), Numerical methods in approximation theory, vol. 9. Birkhäuser Verlag, Basel (1992) 53–75
4. Chui, C. K., Wang, J. Z.: On compactly supported spline wavelets. Trans. Amer. Math. Soc. **330** (1992) 903–915
5. Cohen, A., Daubechies I., Vial, P.: Wavelets on the interval and fast wavelet transforms. App. and Comp. Harm. Anal. **1** (1993) 54–81

158

6. Colton, D., Kress, R.: Inverse acoustic and electromagnetic scattering theory. Springer-Verlag, Berlin (1992)
7. Dahmen, W., Kunoth, A.: Multilevel preconditioning. Numer. Math. **63** (1992) 315-344
8. Dahmen, W., Prößdorf, S., Schneider, R.: Wavelet approximation methods for pseudo–differential operators II. Advances Comp. Math. **1** (1993) 259-335
9. Dicken, V., Maaß, P.: Wavelet–Galerkin methods for ill–posed problems. J. Inv. Ill–Posed Prob. (to appear)
10. Daubechies, I.: Ten lectures on wavelets. SIAM, Philadelphia (1992)
11. Engl, H.W.: Discrepancy principles for Tikhonov regularization of ill–posed problems leading to optimal convergence rates. J. Opti. Theory Appl. **52** (1987) 209-215
12. Gfrerer, H.: An a posteriori parameter choice for ordinary and iterated Tikhonov regularization of ill–posed problems leading to optimal convergence rates. Math. Comp. **49** (1987) 507-522
13. Griebel, M., Oswald, P.: On the abstract theory of additive and multiplicative Schwarz algorithms. Numer. Math. **70** (1995) 163-180
14. Groetsch, C. W.: The theory of Tikhonov regularization for Fredholm equations of the first kind. Pitman, Boston (1984)
15. King, J. T., Neubauer, A.: A variant of finite-dimensional Tikhonov regularization with a-posteriori parameter choice. Computing **40** (1988) 91-109
16. Louis, A. K.: Medical imaging – the state of the art and future developments. Inverse Problems **8** (1992) 709-738
17. Louis, A. K., Maaß, P., Rieder, A.: Wavelets – Theorie und Anwendungen. Teubner, Stuttgart (1994). English version: Wiley, Chichester (to appear 1997)
18. Maaß, P., Ramlau, R.: Wavelet accelerated regularization methods for hyperthermia treatment planning. submitted for publication, Preprint University of Potsdam (1995)
19. Meyer, Y.: Ondelettes et Opérateurs I – Ondelettes. Hermann, Paris (1990)
20. Natterer, F.: The mathematics of computerized tomography. Wiley, Chichester (1986)
21. Neubauer, A.: An a posteriori parameter selection choice for Tikhonov regularization in Hilbert scales leading to optimal convergence rates. SIAM J. Numer. Anal. **25** (1988) 1313-1326
22. Neubauer, A.: An a posteriori parameter choice for Tikhonov regularization in the presence of modeling error. Appl. Num. Math. **4** (1988) 507-519
23. Pereverzev, S.V.: Optimization of projection methods for solving ill-posed problems. Computing **55** (1995)
24. Plato, R., Vainikko, G. M.: On the regularization of projection methods for solving ill-posed problems. Numer. Math. **57** (1990) 73-79
25. Rieder, A.: A wavelet multilevel method for ill-posed problems stabilized by Tikhonov regularization. Numer. Math. **75** (1997) 501-522
26. Rudin, W.: Functional Analysis. Tata McGraw-Hill, New Delhi, 12th Ed. (1988)
27. Schumaker, L. L.: Spline functions: basic theory. Wiley, New York (1981)
28. Wloka, J.: Partielle Differentialgleichungen. Teubner, Stuttgart (1982)
29. Xu, J.: Iterative methods by space decomposition and subspace correction. SIAM Review **34** (1992) 581-613

An Initial Value Approach to the Inverse Helmholtz Problem at Fixed Frequency

Frank Natterer

Institut für Numerische und instrumentelle Mathematik, Universität Münster, D-48149 Münster, Germany

1 Introduction

The inverse Helmholtz problem calls for the determination of the function f in $\Omega \subseteq \mathbf{R}^n$ from the boundary values $g(\theta, x) = u(x)$, $x \in \partial\Omega$ of the solution u of the Helmholtz equation

$$\Delta u(x) + k^2(1 + f(x))u(x) = 0$$

$$u(x) = e^{ikx\cdot\theta} + w(x) \tag{1.1}$$

in $\mathbf{R}^n$, where w satisfies the Sommerfeld radiation condition. The number $k > 0$ is the frequency of the incident plane wave with direction $\theta \in S^{n-1}$. We assume $f = 0$ outside Ω. g is measured for a single fixed frequency k and all $\theta \in S^{n-1}$.

The mathematical theory of this inverse problem is fairly well developed [10]. There exists an extensive literature on numerical methods. If the Born or Rytov approximation is valid, the algorithms of diffraction tomography [3] can be used. For the general case, iterative ([1], [2], [4], [8]) and direct [13] methods have been suggested.

The purpose of the present paper is to give a rigourous mathematical justification of the method already described in [12] and to demonstrate its efficacy by computer simulations.

An essential feature in [12] is the use of initial value methods for the Helmholtz equation. Initial value methods, namely the parabolic equation approximation, are also used in [1]. In contrast to [1] we work with initial value problems of second order. The stability analysis is given in §2. In §3 we describe our method for the inverse problem in a continuous setting. The necessary discretizations have been described in [12]. In §4 we report the results of the reconstruction of a breast phantom from simulated data.

2 The Initial Value Problem for the Helmholtz Equation

We consider the $2D$ Helmholtz equation

$$\frac{\partial^2 u}{\partial x_1^2} + \frac{\partial^2 u}{\partial x_2^2} + k^2(1 + f)u = r \tag{2.1}$$

in the upper half plane $x_2 > 0$, subject to the initial conditions

$$u = g \;,\;\; \frac{\partial u}{\partial x_2} = h \tag{2.2}$$

on $x_2 = 0$. This problem is notoriously unstable. However, this instability is a purely high frequency phenomenon. As soon as we restrict everything to sufficiently low frequencies, this instability disappears. More precisely, let u_κ be a low pass filtered version of u with cut off frequency κ, i.e.

$$\hat{u}_\kappa(\xi_1, x_2) = \begin{cases} \hat{u}(\xi_1, x_2) \;,\; |\xi_1| < \kappa \;, \\ 0 \;\;\;\;, \; \text{otherwise} \end{cases}$$

where $\hat{u}$ is the Fourier transform

$$\hat{u}(\xi_1, x_2) = (2\pi)^{-1/2} \int\limits_{-\infty}^{+\infty} e^{-ix_1 \cdot \xi_1} u(x_1, x_2) dx_1$$

of u with respect to x_1, then u_κ admits a perfectly reasonable estimate in terms of the initial values g, h provided κ is chosen properly. For $f = 0$, $r = 0$ and $\kappa < k$ this follows easily from the explicit solution

$$\hat{u}(\xi_1, x_2) = \hat{g}(\xi_1) \cos(x_2 \sqrt{k^2 - \xi_1^2}) + \frac{\hat{h}(\xi_1)}{\sqrt{k^2 - \xi_1^2}} \sin(x_2 \sqrt{k^2 - \xi_1^2}) \;.$$

In the following we extend this stability result to the general case.
We need the following estimate:

Proposition 1. *Let $v \in C_2([0, \infty), H)$ be a solution to*

$$v'' + A(t)v = r \;,\;\;\;\; t > 0 \tag{2.3}$$

where $A(t)$ is a linear bounded operator in the Hilbert space H with the following properties: We have $A = A_1 + A_2$ with $A_1^* = A_1$ and

$$\alpha_1^2(v, v) \leq (v, A_1 v) \leq \beta_1^2(v, v) \;, \tag{2.4}$$
$$(v, A_1' v) \leq \gamma_1(v, v) \;, \tag{2.5}$$
$$\|A_2\| \leq \beta_2 \tag{2.6}$$

with $\alpha_1 > 0$. Let $\phi = (v', v') + (v, A_1 v)$. Then,

$$\phi(t) \leq \left(\phi(0) + \int\limits_0^t \|r(\tau)\|^2 d\tau \right) e^{(1 + 2\beta_2/\alpha_1 + \gamma_1/\alpha_1^2)t} \;. \tag{2.7}$$

Proof: We use the energy method see e.g. [5]. Multiplying (2.3) with v' we obtain

$$(v', v'') + (v', Av) = (v', r) . \tag{2.8}$$

Using

$$\frac{1}{2} \frac{d}{dt}(v', v') = Re(v', v'') ,$$

$$\frac{1}{2} \frac{d}{dt}(v, A_1 v) = Re(v', A_1 v) + \frac{1}{2}(v, A_1' v)$$

we can rewrite the real part of (2.8) as

$$\frac{1}{2} \frac{d}{dt}(v', v') + \frac{1}{2} \frac{d}{dt}(v, A_1 v)$$
$$= Re(v', r) + \frac{1}{2}(v, A_1' v) - Re(v', A_2 v) .$$

Integrating we obtain

$$\phi(t) = \phi(0) + 2 \int_0^t \left\{ Re(v', r) + \frac{1}{2}(v, A_1' v) - Re(v', A_2 v) \right\} dt .$$

Cauchy-Schwarz and (2.5), (2.6) yield

$$\phi(t) \leq \phi(0) + \int_0^t \left\{ 2\|v'\|\|r\| + \gamma_1\|v\|^2 + 2\beta_2\|v'\|\|v\| \right\} dt .$$

By an appropriate use of the inequality

$$ab \leq \frac{1}{2}(\delta^2 a^2 + \delta^{-2} b^2) , \quad \delta > 0$$

we obtain

$$\phi(t) \leq \phi(0) + \int_0^t \left\{ \|v'\|^2 + \|r\|^2 + \gamma_1\|v\|^2 + \frac{\beta_2}{\alpha_1}\|v'\|^2 + \beta_2\alpha_1\|v\|^2 \right\} dt$$

$$= \phi(0) + \int_0^t \|r\|^2 dt + \int_0^t \left\{ \left(1 + \frac{\beta_2}{\alpha_1}\right)\|v'\|^2 + (\gamma_1 + \beta_2\alpha_1)\|v\|^2 \right\} dt .$$

Using

$$\phi \geq \|v'\|^2 + \alpha_1^2\|v\|^2$$

we obtain

$$\phi(t) \leq c_1(t) + c_2 \int_0^t \phi(t) dt ,$$

$$c_1(t) = \phi(0) + \int_0^t \|r\|^2 dt , \quad c_2 = 1 + 2\frac{\beta_2}{\alpha_1} + \frac{\gamma_1}{\alpha_1^2} .$$

Now (2.7) follows from Gronwall's inequality (see e.g. [6], p. 24).

□

Now we can prove our stability estimate for u_κ.

Theorem 2. *Let $f \in C^1(\mathbf{R}^2)$ and $f = f_1 + \frac{i}{k}f_2$ with f_1, f_2 real, and let m_ν, M_ν be constants such that*

$$-1 < m_1 \le f_1 \le M_1\,, \quad \left|\frac{\partial f_1}{\partial x_2}\right| \le M_1\,, \quad |f_2| \le M_2\,.$$

Then, for $\kappa < k\sqrt{1+m_1}$, we have

$$\|u'_\kappa(\cdot,x_2)\|^2 \le e^{\alpha x_2}\left(\|h\|^2 + k^2(1+M_1)\|g\|^2 + 2\|r\|^2 + 2k^4\|f(u-u_\kappa)(\cdot,x_2)\|^2\right) \tag{2.9}$$

where

$$\alpha = 1 + \frac{2M_2}{\vartheta} + \frac{M_1}{\vartheta^2}\,, \quad \vartheta = \sqrt{1 + m_1 - \left(\frac{\kappa}{k}\right)^2}\,.$$

Proof: Taking in (2.1) the Fourier transform with respect to x_1 we obtain

$$(k^2 - \xi_1^2)\hat{u}(\xi_1,x_2) + \frac{\partial^2}{\partial x_2^2}\hat{u}(\xi_1,x_2) + (2\pi)^{-1/2}k^2 \int_{-\infty}^{+\infty} \hat{f}(\xi_1 - \eta_1, x_2)\hat{u}(\eta_1,x_2)d\eta_1$$

$$= \hat{r}(\xi_1,x_2)\,.$$

We consider this equation only for $|\xi_1| \le \kappa$ and decompose the integral accordingly, i.e.

$$(k^2 - \xi_1^2)\hat{u}_\kappa(\xi_1,x_2) + \frac{\partial^2}{\partial x_2^2}\hat{u}_\kappa(\xi_1,x_2) + (2\pi)^{-1/2}k^2 \int_{-\infty}^{+\infty} \hat{f}(\xi_1 - \eta_1, x_2)\hat{u}_\kappa(\eta_1,x_2)d\eta_1$$

$$= \hat{r}(\xi_1,x_2) + \hat{\varepsilon}(\xi_1,x_2)\,, \quad \hat{\varepsilon}(\xi_1,x_2) = -(2\pi)^{-1/2}k^2 \int_{|\eta_1|\ge\kappa} \hat{f}(\xi_1 - \eta_1, x_2)\hat{u}(\eta_1,x_2)d_2$$

Obviously,

$$\varepsilon = -k^2 f(u - u_\kappa)\,.$$

For fixed ξ_1 we rewrite the last equation for $\hat{u}_\kappa$ as

$$\hat{u}''_\kappa(x_2) + A(x_2)\hat{u}_\kappa(x_2) = \hat{r}(x_2) + \hat{\varepsilon}(x_2) \tag{2.10}$$

In order to apply Proposition 1 to (2.9) we only have to find the constants in (2.4 - 2.6) for the operator A from (2.10). We have

$$(A\hat{u}, \hat{v}) = ((k^2 - \xi_1^2)\hat{u}, \hat{v}) + (2\pi)^{-1/2}k^2 \int_{-\infty}^{+\infty} (\hat{f} \ast \hat{u})\bar{\hat{v}}d\xi_1$$

$$= ((k^2 - \xi_1^2)\hat{u}, \hat{v}) + k^2 \int_{-\infty}^{+\infty} \widehat{fu}\bar{\hat{v}}d\xi_1$$

$$= ((k^2 - \xi_1^2)\hat{u}, \hat{v}) + k^2 \int_{-\infty}^{+\infty} fu\bar{v}dx_1$$

where we have used Parseval's relation. Writing f as $f_1 + \frac{i}{k}f_2$ it readily follows that

$$(A_1\hat{u}, \hat{u}) = ((k^2 - \xi_1^2)\hat{u}, \hat{u}) + k^2 \int\limits_{-\infty}^{+\infty} f_1 |u|^2 dx_1 \,,$$

$$(A_2\hat{u})^{\sim} = ik f_2 u \,.$$

From these relations we easily read

$$\alpha_1^2 = k^2 - \kappa^2 + k^2 m_1 \,, \quad \beta_1^2 = k^2(1 + M_1) \,, \quad \gamma_1 = k^2 M_1 \,, \beta_2 = kM_2 \,.$$

Inserting this into (2.7) and using

$$\|\hat{u}_\kappa'(\cdot, x_2)\|^2 \le \phi(x_2) \le \|\hat{u}_\kappa'(\cdot, x_2)\|^2 + k^2(1 + M_1)\|\hat{u}_\kappa(\cdot, x_2)\|^2$$

yields (2.9).

$$\square$$

The estimate of Theorem 2 makes sense only if $u - u_\kappa$ is small in some sense. In the next theorem we show that this is in fact the case for the scattered wave w from (1.1) with $\theta = \binom{0}{1}$. For w we have the Lippmann-Schwinger equation

$$w(x) = \frac{-i}{4} k^2 \int\limits_{\mathbf{R}^2} H_0(k|x - x'|) f(x')(e^{ikx_2'} + w(x'))dx'$$

with the Hankel function of the first kind H_0. Taking the Fourier transform with respect to x_1 we obtain

$$\hat{w}(\xi_1, x_2)$$

$$= -\frac{i}{4\sqrt{2\pi}} k^2 \int\int\int H_0(k\sqrt{(x_1 - x_1')^2 + (x_2 - x_2')^2})e^{-i\xi_1 x_1} dx_1$$

$$(e^{ikx_2'} + w(x_1', x_2')) f(x_1', x_2') dx_1' dx_2' \,.$$

The x_1 integral can be evaluated as follows. With $a(\xi) = \sqrt{k^2 - \xi^2}$ we have

$$H_0(k\sqrt{u^2 + v^2}) = \frac{-i}{4\pi} \int e^{i(|u|a(\xi) + v\xi)} \frac{d\xi}{a(\xi)} \,,$$

see e.g. [9], p. 123. Hence

$$\int H_0\left(k\sqrt{(x_1 - x_1')^2 - (x_2 + x_2')^2}\right) e^{-i\xi_1 x_1} dx_1$$

$$= \frac{-i}{4\pi} \int\int e^{i(|x_2 - x_2'|a(\xi) + (x_1 - x_1')\xi) - i\xi_1 x_1} \frac{dx_1 d\xi}{a(\xi)}$$

$$= \frac{-i}{2} \int e^{i(|x_2 - x_2'|a(\xi) - x_1'\xi)} \delta(\xi - \xi_1) \frac{d\xi}{a(\xi)}$$

$$= -\frac{i}{2} e^{i(|x_2 - x_2'|a(\xi_1) - x_1'\xi_1)} \frac{1}{a(\xi_1)} \,.$$

It follows that

$$\hat{w}(\xi_1, x_2)$$

$$= \frac{k^2}{8a(\xi_1)} \int \int e^{i(|x_2 - x_2'|a(\xi_1) - x_1'\xi_1)} \left(e^{ikx_2'} + w(x_1', x_2') \right) f(x_1', x_2') dx_1' dx_2' .$$

Now assume that the straight line $x_2' = x_2$ misses $\text{supp}(f)$ by the quantity $\varepsilon > 0$ and $\xi_1 > k$. Then,

$$|\hat{w}(\xi_1, x_2)| \leq \frac{k^2}{8\sqrt{\xi_1^2 - k^2}} e^{-\varepsilon \sqrt{\xi_1^2 - k^2}} (1 + \|w\|_\infty) \|f\|_1 .$$

Hence we have for arbitrary θ:

Theorem 3. *Let w be the scattered wave for incident direction θ, and let L be a straight line perpendicular to θ which misses the support of f. Then, the Fourier transform of w along L decays exponentially beyond k.*

We shall apply Theorem 2 with m_1 negative but close to zero (typically $m_1 = -0.01$). Then, Theorem 2 requires κ to be slightly smaller than k, while, according to Theorem 3, $u - u_\kappa$ in Theorem 2 is small if κ is slightly bigger than k. In practice this conflict did not cause any problems. With $\kappa = 0.99k$ we observed both stability and accuracy.

3 The Inversion Method

We consider the case $n = 2$. Assume that Ω is the ball of radius ρ centered at the origin. Let the scattered field w_j be measured on $\partial\Omega$ for p directions θ_j. We first extend w_j to the exterior of Ω. Since w_j satisfies there the homogeneous Helmholtz equation $\Delta w_j + k^2 w_j = 0$, this is easily done by expanding $w_j(x)$ for $|x| > \rho$ as

$$w_j(r \cos \varphi, r \sin \varphi) = \sum_\ell c_\ell e^{i\ell\varphi} H_\ell(kr)$$

with H_ℓ the first kind Hankel function of order ℓ. The coefficients c_ℓ are readily obtained from the data by

$$c_\ell = \frac{1}{2\pi H_\ell(k\rho)} \int_0^{2\pi} w_j(\rho \cos \varphi, \rho \sin \varphi) d\varphi .$$

Now let Q_j be the square circumscribed to Ω, two of its edges, named Γ_j, parallel to θ_j. The other edges are denoted by Γ_j^-, Γ_j^+ with θ_j pointing from Γ_j^- to Γ_j^+. We define an operator $R_j : L_2(\Omega) \to L_2(\Gamma_j^+)$ by solving the initial value problem

$$\Delta w + k^2(1 + f)w = -k^2 f e^{ikx\cdot\theta} \quad \text{in } Q_j ,$$

$$w = w_j , \quad \frac{\partial w}{\partial \nu} = \frac{\partial w_j}{\partial \nu} \quad \text{on } \Gamma_j^- , \quad w = w_j \text{ on } \Gamma_j$$

and putting $R_j(f) = w$ on Γ_j^+. We also put $g_j = w_j\big|_{\Gamma_j^+}$.

Now we have to solve the nonlinear system

$$R_j(f) = g_j , \quad j = 1,\ldots,p$$

for f. We do this by an ART type algorithm.

With f^0 an initial approximation to f we compute a new approximation f^1 by

$$f_0 = f^0 ,$$
$$f_j = f_{j-1} + \gamma R_j'^*(f_{j-1})(g_j - R_j(f_{j-1})) , \quad j = 1,\ldots,p$$
$$f^1 = f_p .$$

γ is a relaxation parameter.

$R_j'^*$ can be evaluated by solving an initial value problem with initial values on Γ_j^+. This can done by the usual five point finite difference star, combined with filtering along the grid lines perpendicular to θ_j. For details see [12].

4 Numerical Experiment

We did reconstructions from data obtained from a computer generated breast phantom which has been patterned after a phantom created by Borup et al. [1]. With c the sound speed in the breast tissue, $c_0 = 1500\frac{m}{sec}$ the sound speed in the surrounding water, and α the attenuation coefficient in the breast tissue we have

$$f = \frac{c_0^2}{c^2} - 1 - i\frac{2\alpha c_0}{kc} , \quad w = c_0 k . \tag{4.1}$$

The phantom is made up of four different kinds of tissue: fat, glandular tissue, tumor, and cyst. The values of c and α (at 1MHZ) are

tissue	$c[\frac{m}{sec}]$	$\alpha[\frac{db}{m}]$	$Re f$	$Im f$
fat	1458	41	0.058	$-9.4/k$
glandular tissue	1519	80	-0.025	$-18.4/k$
tumor	1564	118	-0.080	$-27.2/k$
cyst	1568	10	-0.084	$-2.3/k$

The value of α in column 2 have to be converted to those in formula (4.1) by dividing with the factor $20\log_{10}(e)$, yielding α in units $[\frac{1}{m}]$. Therefore, k in column 4 is in units of $[\frac{1}{m}]$, too.

We generated data by solving the forward problem with the initial value method, assuming the backscatter to be zero. We worked on a 128×128 grid, using $p = 128$ equally spaced directions in $[0, 2\pi)$. The frequency of the irradiating plane waves was 1MHZ, i.e. $\omega = 2\pi \cdot 10^6$ sec^{-1}, hence $k = 4189m^{-1}$.

The condition for the Born approximation to hold is

$$R|f| \ll \frac{2\pi}{k}$$

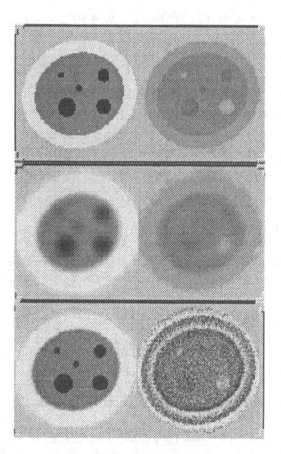

Figure captions

Fig. 1 (top): Breast phantom. Real part left, imaginary part right. Since the imaginary part is much smaller than the real part it has been scaled. The location of the 3 tumors and 2 cysts is clear from the real part, while they can be distinguished by looking at the imaginary part.

Fig. 2 (middle): Initial approximation which has been computed from data corresponding to $k = 1000 \ m^{-1}$ using 0 as initial approximation.

Fig. 3 (bottom): Reconstruction after 6 sweeps with $\gamma' = 0.5$.

where R is the Radon transform. This is a slight generalisation of the condition given by Kak and Slaney [7]. It is obviously far from being satisfied. As has been discussed in [12], we can't use 0 as initial approximation in this case. We used the reconstruction for the smaller value $k = 1000 \ m^{-1}$ instead which can be computed starting out from 0. A smoothed version of the initial approximation thus obtained is shown in Fig. 2.

The reconstruction after 6 sweeps is shown in Fig. 3. The total computation time on a SPARC 20 was 5 minutes. The value of γ has been chosen in the following way. First we determined in [11] the asymptotic value $1/(\rho k^2)$ of the operator $\left(R'_j(0)R'^*_j(0)\right)^{-1}$ for large k. Then we put $\gamma = \gamma'/(\rho k^2)$ where, in agreement with the convergence properties of the Kaczmarz procedure, $0 < \gamma' < 2$. We used $\gamma' = 0.5$.

References

1. Borup, D.T. - Johnson, S.A. - Kim, W.W. - Berggren, M.J.: Nonperturbative diffraction tomography via Gauss-Newton iteration applied to the scattering integral equation, *Ultrasonic Imaging* **14**, 69-85 (1992).
2. Colton, D. - Monk, P.: A modified dual space method for solving the electromagnetic inverse scattering problem for an infinite cylinder, *Inverse Problems* **10**, 87-108 (1994).
3. Devaney, A.J.: A filtered backpropagation algorithm for diffraction tomography, *Ultrasonic Imaging* **4**, 336-350 (1982).
4. Gutman, S. - Klibanov, M.: Regularized Quasi -Newton method for inverse scattering problems, Math. Comput. Modelling **18**, No. 1, pp. 5-31, Pergamon Press Ltd. (1993).
5. Hahn, W.: Stability of motion. Springer 1967.
6. Hartman, P.: Ordinary differential equations, Wiley 1964.
7. Kak, A.C. - Slaney, M.: Principles Computerized Tomographic Imaging, IEEE Press, New York 1987.
8. Kleinman, R.E. - van den Berg, P.M.: A modified gradient method for two-dimensional problems in tomography, *J. Comp. Appl. Math.* **42**, 17-35 (1992).
9. Morse, P.M. - Feshbach, H.: Methods of theoretical physics, McGraw-Hill 1953.
10. Nachman, A.I.: Global uniqueness for a two-dimensional inverse boundary value problem. *Department of Mathematics, Preprint Series*, Number 19, University of Rochester (1993).
11. Natterer, F.: Finite Difference Methods for Inverse Problems, in Ang, D.D. et al. (eds.): Inverse Problems and Applications to Geophysics, Industry, Medicine and Technology. *Publications of the HoChiMinh City Mathematical Society*, **Vol. 2**, 1995.
12. Natterer, F. - Wübbeling, F.: A propagation - backpropagation method for ultrasound tomography. *Inverse Problems* **11**, 1225-1232 (1995).
13. Stenger, F. - O'Reilly, M.: Sinc inversion of the Helmholtz equation without computing the forward solution, Preprint, Department of Computer Science, University of Utah, Salt Lake City, Utah 84112.

Gradient and Newton-Kantorovich Methods for Microwave Tomography

Christian Pichot[1]*, Pierre Lobel*[2]*, Laure Blanc-Féraud*[3]*, Michel Barlaud*[3]*,*
Kamal Belkebir[4]*, Jean-Manuel Elissalt*[5] *and Jean-Michel Geffrin*[6]

[1] Laboratoire d'Electronique, Antennes et Télécommunications, Université de Nice-Sophia Antipolis/CNRS, Bâtiment 4, 250 rue Albert Einstein, 06560 Valbonne, France.

[2] was with the Laboratoire Informatique, Signaux et Systèmes de Sophia Antipolis, Université de Nice-Sophia Antipolis/CNRS, Bâtiment 4, 250 rue Albert Einstein, 06560 Valbonne, France. Now with the Laboratoire d'Electronique, Antennes et Télécommunications.

[3] Laboratoire Informatique, Signaux et Systèmes de Sophia Antipolis.

[4] was with the Laboratoire des Signaux et Systèmes, CNRS/ESE, Plateau de Moulon, 91192 Gif-sur-Yvette, France. Now with the Electromagnetics Division, Faculty of Electrical Engineering, Eindhoven University of Technology, 5600 Eindhoven, The Netherlands.

[5] was with the Laboratoire des Signaux et Systèmes, CNRS/ESE, Plateau de Moulon, 91192 Gif-sur-Yvette, France. Now with Simulog, Les Taissounières HB2, Route des Dolines, 06560 Valbonne, France.

[6] Laboratoire des Signaux et Systèmes, CNRS/ESE, Plateau de Moulon, 91192 Gif-sur-Yvette, France.

1 Introduction

The development of reconstruction algorithms for Active Microwave Imaging, with applications in the medical domain or for non-destructive testing [1], and more generally for electromagnetic and acoustic imaging [2], has gained much interest during the last decade. The first generation of algorithms was based on Diffraction Tomography [2–5], which is a generalization of classical X-ray Computed Tomography, by taking into account diffraction effects. The scattered field data are filtered, mapped onto the Ewald sphere in k-space and inverse transformed. These algorithms provide quasi real-time approximate reconstructions of the polarization current density distribution (qualitative imaging). For a weak scatterer (Born or Rytov approximations), they also yield the complex permittivity distribution (quantitative imaging). They have been used and tested on experimental imaging systems such as a 2.45 GHz planar microwave camera [6], a 2.33 GHz circular microwave scanner [7, 8], and a broad frequency band microwave sensor [1], yielding valuable qualitative images, although artifacts are present for strong and/or inhomogeneous scatterers [6].

The limitations of Diffraction Tomography have stimulated the development of iterative methods for complex permittivity reconstruction of highly contrasted objects [9–17]. The nature of the transmission inverse scattering problem is strongly nonlinear and ill-posed (in the sense of Hadamard) when quantitative imaging is requested.

During the past 15 years, intensive studies have concerned reconstruction algorithms able to give an efficient solution to quantitative imaging. Among them, Newton-Kantorovich [12,16,18] or Levenberg-Marquardt algorithms [19], Gradient [20] and Modified Gradient [17,18,21,22] methods have been applied to this problem. Starting from an exact integral representation of the EM field, the moment method is utilized to generate matrix relations, and then, an optimization procedure for the inverse problem is used. The gradient methods deal with the general nonlinear formulation, while the Newton-type algorithms linearize the system and due to the ill-posedness of the matrices, need also a regularization, generally a Tikhonov regularization with identity operator.

We give in this paper some numerical results, obtained for two-dimensional cylindrical objects under Transverse Magnetic (TM) illumination i.e. with electric field parallel to the cylinder object axis. Three methods have been used : a Conjugate Gradient (CG) method [20], a Newton-Kantorovich (NK) method with identity operator[7] [19] or with gradient-by-zone operator, and a Modified Gradient (MG) method [23]. In order to evaluate and compare their respective performance, the study has been carried out from synthetic data and accomplished by experimental verifications. Investigations on the initial guess of the complex permittivity profile have been made with a backpropagation scheme using the adjoint operator, allowing to provide an estimate of the induced current inside the inhomogeneous object. Different configurations of interest have been studied for applications of microwave imaging in the medical domain and for non-destructive testing.

Last improvements concern an Edge-Preserving (EP) regularization procedure, that we applied successfully, with the CG method, on noisy corrupted synthetic data [24] and also on experimental data [25]. With this regularization procedure, the object to be reconstructed is modeled as a set of homogeneous areas separated by borderlike discontinuities. It involves the use of a non-quadratic regularizing function, which could be seen as a potential function of a *Markov Random Field (MRF)* [26,27]. During the minimization process, this function allows a smoothing in the homogeneous areas of the object, while edges are preserved. The estimation reconstructs alternately the contrast of the object and its edges.

2 Problem Statement

The cylindrical object characterized by a relative complex permittivity $\epsilon(r)$ ($\epsilon(r) = \epsilon'(r) + i\epsilon''(r)$) is contained in a bounded region $\mathcal{D}$ and illuminated successively by different incident TM plane waves e_l^i, $l \in [1, L]$. The receivers are located in the domain $\mathcal{S}$ in the far-field region. For each excitation l, and for $r \in \mathcal{D}$, the forward scattering problem may be formulated as the following

---

[7] This method is a modified Gauss-Newton iterative method, and is equivalent to the distorted Born method [13]

domain integral equation

$$e_l(r) = e_l^I(r) + \int_{\mathcal{D}} k_0^2 c(r') e_l(r') G(r - r') dr', \; r \in \mathcal{D}$$

$$= e_l^I(r) + G^{\mathcal{D}} c e_l(r), \; r \in \mathcal{D} \; , \tag{1}$$

and integral representation for the scattered field

$$e_l^{\mathcal{S}}(s_{lm}) = \int_{\mathcal{D}} k_0^2 c(r') e_l(r') G(s_{lm} - r') dr', \; s_{lm} \in \mathcal{S}$$

$$= G^{\mathcal{S}} c e_l(s_{lm}), \; s_{lm} \in \mathcal{S} \; , \tag{2}$$

with complex contrast function $c(r) = \epsilon(r) - 1$ and k_0 is the wavenumber of background medium and where $G^{\mathcal{D}}$ and $G^{\mathcal{S}}$ are two integral operators mapping respectively $L^2(\mathcal{D})$ (square integrable functions in $\mathcal{D}$) into itself, and $L^2(\mathcal{D})$ into $L^2(\mathcal{S})$, and involving the 2D free space Green's function

$$G(r - r') = \frac{i}{4} H_0^{(1)}(k_0|r - r'|) \; . \tag{3}$$

The direct problem is solved using the moment method (MoM) with pulse basis functions and point matching, which transforms the integral equations (1) and (2), into matrix equations. The rectangular image (or test domain) containing the region $\mathcal{D}$ is discretized into $N = N_{lin} \times N_{col}$ elementary square cells.

Solving the inverse scattering problem leads to reconstruct from the resulting matrix system, the complex contrast of the object, while the incident field, the scattered field, and the Green's matrices are known. We present in the following sections of this paper, three different iterative methods which allow to reconstruct the contrast.

3 Newton-Kantorovich (NK) Method

The matrix system to solve is strongly nonlinear and ill-posed. The Newton-Kantorovich method builds up an iterative solution of the inverse problem, by solving successively the direct problem and a local linear inverse problem [9,12, 16]. At each iteration, an estimate of the complex contrast function c is given by

$$c_{n+1} = \Delta c + c_n \; , \tag{4}$$

where Δc is an update correction obtained by solving in the least squares sense, the linearized forward problem

$$D \Delta c = e^{\mathcal{S}} - F(c_n) = \Delta e^{\mathcal{S}} \; , \tag{5}$$

where the matrix D is a linearized version of the nonlinear operator relating the scattered field to the contrast function c, and $F(c_n)$ represents the measured data vector. The scattered field vector $F(c_n)$ is calculated through the forward problem solver, with a previous estimate of c. Unfortunately, the problem of finding the solution of equation (5) is ill-posed and needs some regularization. For this, we use a Tikhonov regularization and minimize the functional

$$F_{NK}(c) = \left\| \Delta e^S - D\Delta c \right\|_S^2 + \lambda \left\| R\Delta c \right\|_D^2 , \qquad (6)$$

where R is the regularization matrix and λ a regularization parameter, chosen according to an empirical formula [16] or with the General Cross Validation method [28]. Two regularization operators have been used: an identity operator and a gradient-by-zone operator. The gradient-by-zone operator is based first, on the assumption that the object is composed of homogeneous zones of arbitrary geometry, separated by borderlike discontinuities and second, on the notion of neighborhood for each elementary cell of the image.

4 Modified Gradient (MG) Method

With the Modified Gradient method [17, 21, 22], the iterative procedure minimizes two residual errors obtained from equations (1) and (2) at each iteration. We have applied this method directly on experimental data for medical applications with a microwave scanner (§6.2). For perfectly conducting objects concerned with the experimental Ipswich data[8] (§6.3), we have introduced some modifications by adding a priori information about the nature of the object to reconstruct, i.e. high conductivity object ($c = c_{max} \gg 0$). Then, we are interested in finding the location and the shape of the object, using the characteristic binary function ζ (function equal to 1 inside the object and zero outside). But in order to avoid instability and derivability problems, we exhibit an auxiliary function ξ such as $\zeta = \xi^2$, which is relaxed to take any real value. Using the operator notation, the inverse problem yields to find ζ (or ξ^2) for given e_l^S measurements of the scattered field or to solve the equations

$$e_l^S = G^S c_{max} \xi^2 e_l, \, l \in [1, \, L] , \qquad (7)$$

with domain integral equation

$$e_l = e_l^I + G^D c_{max} \xi^2 e_l, \, l \in [1, \, L] . \qquad (8)$$

The iterative procedure minimizes two residual errors at each iteration with the cost functional

$$F_{MG}(\xi, \, e_l) = \frac{\sum_{l=1}^{L} \left\| e_l^I - e_l + G^D c_{max} \xi^2 e_l \right\|_D^2}{\sum_{l=1}^{L} \left\| e_l^i \right\|_D^2} + \frac{\sum_{l=1}^{L} \left\| e_l^S - G^S c_{max} \xi^2 e_l \right\|_S^2}{\sum_{l=1}^{L} \left\| e_l^S \right\|_S^2} , \qquad (9)$$

---

[8] Measured data provided by Rome Laboratory, Electromagnetics & Reliability Directorate, 31 Grenier Street, Hanscom AFB, MA 01731-3010.

where $\| \cdot \|_{\mathcal{D}}^2$ and $\| \cdot \|_{\mathcal{S}}^2$ are the norms associated to the inner product on $L^2(\mathcal{D})$ and $L^2(\mathcal{S})$, respectively. Sequences are constructed with the recurrent relations

$$\begin{cases} e_{l_n} = e_{l_{n-1}} + \alpha_{l_n} v_{l_n} \\ \xi_n = \xi_{n-1} + \beta_n d_n \end{cases} , \qquad (10)$$

where the two functions v_{l_n} and d_n, are the update directions for functions $\{e_{l_n}\}$ and $\{\xi_n\}$, respectively, while the complex numbers α_{l_n} and the real parameter β_n are weights, chosen at each step so as to minimize the cost functional $F_{MG}(\xi_n, e_{l_n})$. Once the v_{l_n} and d_n update directions are found, $F_{MG}(\xi_n, e_{l_n})$ is a nonlinear expression in L complex variables α_{l_n} and one real variable β_n. The minimization of $F_{MG}(\beta_n, \alpha_{l_n})$ is accomplished using a Polak-Ribière conjugate gradient algorithm [29]. This method does not need to compute any matrix inversion as it does for the two other methods.

5 Conjugate Gradient (CG) Method

5.1 General Algorithm

In this method, we choose to minimize a unique functional, resulting from the discretized versions of (1) and (2). This functional is nonlinear and is written as

$$F_{CG}(C) = \sum_{l=1}^{L} \|\rho_l(C)\|_{\mathcal{S}}^2 , \qquad (11)$$

where

$$\rho_l(C) = E_l^S - G^S C\mathcal{L}(C)E_l^I , \qquad (12)$$

and

$$\mathcal{L}(C) = \left(I - G^{\mathcal{D}}C\right)^{-1} . \qquad (13)$$

The matrix C is the $N \times N$ diagonal matrix containing c. We use a conjugate gradient method to minimize (11), with the iterative procedure

$$C^{i+1} = C^i + \alpha^i D^i , \qquad (14)$$

is applied on it. D^i is the update direction ($N \times N$ diagonal matrix formed by the $N \times 1$ vector d^i)[9], and α^i is a complex parameter (weight factor). The value of α^i is found, using a first order approximation and minimizing $F_{CG}(C^{i+1})$ according to α^i :

$$\alpha^i = \frac{\displaystyle\sum_{l=1}^{L} \langle \rho_l(C^i), V_l(C^i) \rangle_{\mathcal{S}}}{\displaystyle\sum_{l=1}^{L} \|V_l(C^i)\|_{\mathcal{S}}^2} , \qquad (15)$$

---

[9] For sake of simplicity, we note d^i the $N \times 1$ update vector as well as the associated $N_{lin} \times N_{col}$ matrix

where

$$V_l(C^i) = G^S \left\{ \mathcal{L}(C^i) \right\}^t D^i \mathcal{L}(C^i) E_l^I \ . \tag{16}$$

Three different update directions d^i have been used. First, *the backpropagation of the error*, using the adjoint (or conjugate transpose) operator G^{S^*} of G^S. Second, *the gradient direction*, and finally *the Polak-Ribière conjugate gradient direction* [29]. The third one gives better results in terms of convergence and stability than the other directions. Using the *Fréchet derivative* [30] of (11), the calculation of the gradient of $F_{CG}(C^i)$ yields to

$$\nabla F_{CG}(C^i) = -2 \sum_{l=1}^{L} \overline{\text{diag}\left(\mathcal{L}(C^i)E_l^I\right)\mathcal{L}(C^i)}G^{S^*} \rho_l(C^i) \ , \tag{17}$$

and d^i is given by

$$d^i = g^i + \frac{\langle g^i, g^i - g^{i-1}\rangle_\mathcal{D}}{\|g^{i-1}\|_\mathcal{D}^2} d^{i-1} \ , \tag{18}$$

with $g^i = -\nabla F_{CG}(C^i)$.

5.2 Edge-Preserving (EP) Regularization

For highly contrasted objects, and/or face with noisy corrupted data, the inverse scattering problem becomes more ill-posed. Some *a priori* informations are needed in order to reconstruct a regular solution. We choose a piecewise constant solution. From general point of view, the additional information takes the form of the following regularization term in the cost functional

$$\lambda \int_\mathcal{D} \varphi(|\nabla c(r)|)dr \ , \tag{19}$$

where λ is the regularization parameter fixing the influence of the regularization term above the data term, and φ is a real function, defined on $[0, +\infty[$, and called regularizing function. Choosing $\varphi(t) = t^2$, yields to the well-known Tikhonov regularization, which produces oversmooth solutions, while choosing $\varphi(t) = t$, yields to the Total Variation criterion [31, 32]. We propose to use a φ function defined in order to perform an isotropic smoothing in the homogeneous areas of the image (corresponding to small gradients), while preserving edges (corresponding to high gradients) [26, 27, 33–35]. Based on a study of the derivative of (19) given by

$$-\nabla \cdot \left(\frac{\varphi'(|\nabla c(r)|)}{|\nabla c(r)|} \nabla c(r) \right) \ , \tag{20}$$

three main conditions for the function $\dfrac{\varphi'(t)}{t}$ must be satisfied [35–37]

1. $\lim\limits_{t \to 0} \dfrac{\varphi'(t)}{t} = M < \infty$: isotropic smoothing in homogeneous areas.

2. $\lim\limits_{t\to\infty} \dfrac{\varphi'(t)}{t} = 0$: preservation of edges.

3. $\dfrac{\varphi'(t)}{t}$ strictly decreasing : to avoid instabilities in the reconstruction algorithm.

A summary of main φ functions is presented in Table 1, and the new discrete cost functional to minimize becomes

$$F_{CG}(C) = \sum_{l=1}^{L} \|\rho_l(C)\|_{\mathcal{S}}^2 + \sum_{p=1}^{N_{lin}} \sum_{q=1}^{N_{col}} \lambda_R^2 \, \varphi \left(\frac{1}{\delta_R} \|\mathrm{Re}(\nabla c)_{p,q}\| \right) +$$

$$\sum_{p=1}^{N_{lin}} \sum_{q=1}^{N_{col}} \lambda_I^2 \, \varphi \left(\frac{1}{\delta_I} \|\mathrm{Im}(\nabla c)_{p,q}\| \right) \ . \tag{21}$$

Table 1. Summary of some φ functions

Name of the φ function	$\varphi(t)$	Convexity	$\dfrac{\varphi'(t)}{t}$	Conditions 1, 2 & 3 satisfied
Total Variation	t	yes	$\dfrac{1}{t}$ (1)	no
Tikhonov	t^2	yes	2	no
Geman & Mc. Clure	$\dfrac{t^2}{1+t^2}$	no	$\dfrac{2}{(1+t^2)^2}$	yes
Hebert & Leahy	$\log(1+t^2)$	no	$\dfrac{2}{1+t^2}$	yes
Green	$\log[\cosh(t)]$	yes	$\dfrac{\tanh(t)}{t}$	yes
Hyper surfaces	$\sqrt{1+t^2}-1$	yes	$\dfrac{1}{\sqrt{1+t^2}}$	yes

(1) $\frac{\varphi'(t)}{t}$ undefined if $t = 0$

When dealing with the reconstruction of a complex matrix, we consider the real part and the imaginary part of the contrast as independent in the regularization scheme. As a matter of fact, there is no link between the real and the imaginary part of the permittivity, and the edge-preserving regularization is applied separately on the real and the imaginary part of the contrast. The weighting parameters λ_R and λ_I fix the influence of the regularization term versus the error matching the scattered field, and the parameters δ_R and δ_I fix the threshold level on the gradient norm above which a discontinuity is preserved, and under which it is smoothed. Based on the work of [27, 35], we can show [24], that if φ satisfies mainly the three conditions 1. 2. and 3., the cost functional (21) can be written as

$$F_{CG}(C) = \operatorname*{Inf}_{b_R, b_I} F^{\dagger}_{CG}(C, b_R, b_I) \ , \qquad (22)$$

where the matrices b_R and b_I (each one belongs to $]0, 1]$) map the discontinuities of the real and imaginary parts of the object respectively[10], and where

$$F^{\dagger}_{CG}(C, b_R, b_I) = \sum_{l=1}^{L} \|\rho_l(C)\|^2_{\mathcal{S}} +$$

$$\left\{ \lambda_R^2 \sum_{p=1}^{N_{lig}} \sum_{q=1}^{N_{col}} (b_R)_{p,q} \left\| \frac{\text{Re}(\nabla c)_{p,q}}{\delta_R} \right\|^2 + \psi((b_R)_{p,q}) + \right.$$

$$\left. \lambda_I^2 \sum_{p=1}^{N_{lig}} \sum_{q=1}^{N_{col}} (b_I)_{p,q} \left\| \frac{\text{Im}(\nabla c)_{p,q}}{\delta_I} \right\|^2 + \psi((b_I)_{p,q}) \right\} \ .(23)$$

The function ψ is convex and analytically defined from the function φ, and the minimization of (21) (which has a non-quadratic regularization term) with respect to c, is replaced by the minimization of (22) (which has a *half-quadratic* regularization term i.e. quadratic in c when (b_R, b_I) is fixed) with respect to (c, b_R, b_I). The following alternate minimization procedure is used :

1. when b_R and b_I are fixed, the regularization term is quadratic in c, and the basic minimization of (11) is not influenced by the regularization term. Of course, new values for the α parameter and for the gradient direction must be calculated [24, 38],
2. when c is fixed, the minima $\hat{b}_R$ and $\hat{b}_I$ are unique and given for each point (p, q) by the analytical expressions

$$(\hat{b}_R)_{p,q} = \frac{\varphi'\left(\frac{1}{\delta_R} \|\text{Re}(\nabla c)_{p,q}\|\right)}{\frac{2}{\delta_R} \|\text{Re}(\nabla c)_{p,q}\|} \qquad (24)$$

$$(\hat{b}_I)_{p,q} = \frac{\varphi'\left(\frac{1}{\delta_I} \|\text{Im}(\nabla c)_{p,q}\|\right)}{\frac{2}{\delta_I} \|\text{Im}(\nabla c)_{p,q}\|} \qquad (25)$$

More details about the minimization procedure can be found in [24, 35, 38].

---

[10] In fact, their value at the point (p, q) tends towards 0 if this point belongs to an edge of the image, and equals 1 if this point belongs to an homogeneous area.

6 Reconstructions from Synthetic and Experimental Data

6.1 Reconstructions from Synthetic Data for a Two Square Cylinders Profile

The test domain $\mathcal{D}$ including the object is a square $3\lambda \times 3\lambda$, where λ is the wavelength in the background medium. The simulated object is discretized into 19×19 subsquares, and the surface S enclosing $\mathcal{D}$ is a circle of radius 9λ. A set of 19 transmitters-receivers is uniformly located on it, and while each transmitter, acting like a line source, illuminates the object, the whole set of receivers collect the scattered field ($L = M = 19$).

The object under investigation, shown in Fig. 1a, is made by two distinct homogeneous square cylinders placed in free space, of diameter $\frac{4}{5}\lambda$, with $\frac{1}{2}\lambda$ separation and relative permittivity $\epsilon' = 1.8$, ($\epsilon'' = 0$). For noiseless data, the reconstruction with the NK method is represented in Fig. 1b, while the reconstruction with the CG method (without regularization) is shown Fig. 1c. A comparison between the convergence of these two methods is presented in Fig. 2. We can see here that with noiseless data, the NK method converges faster than the CG method. The object is perfectly reconstructed with the NK method after 30 iterations, while the CG method needs about 150 iterations (as the computation complexity at each iteration of the NK and CG methods are quite the same, the comparison is reasonable).

We present in Fig. 1d and Fig. 1e, the results obtained from noisy corrupted data. The additive white Gaussian noise is of about 10% of the maximum value of the scattered data. In the Fig. 2, one can see that the NK method diverges at the fourth iteration, while the CG method still converges. But without any additive regularization, the result is still corrupted. The enhancement obtained by the EP regularization is shown for a quite similar object in [24], and also in Fig. 14, where the reconstruction is performed from experimental data.

6.2 Reconstructions from Experimental Data with a Microwave Scanner Prototype

It is now well known that hyperthermia can constitute an efficient adjuvant to radiotherapy and chemotherapy in cancer treatment. A wide variety of hyperthermia systems have been developed on an experimental basis in recent years [39–41]. But successful results are conditioned by the careful control of the heating in order to provide the most efficient treatment protocol. Due to its sensitivity to temperature, microwave imaging could be one possible mean for non invasive hyperthermia monitoring [6]. The complex permittivity varies with temperature, the reconstructed microwave image gives indirect informations on the heating process [6]. As shown in Fig. 3, a microwave imaging system, could be coupled with a deep hyperthermia applicator such as TEM coaxial system. The experimental microwave scanner prototype consists of a water-filled metallic cylinder (inner diameter 59 cm), a 2D mechanical moving system, an emitting antenna, and a receiving antenna which covers the investigation domain. Field

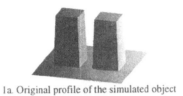

1a. Original profile of the simulated object

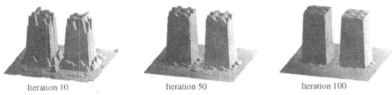

Iteration 5   Iteration 10   Iteration 20

1b. Reconstruction with the NK method (identity operator) from noiseless data

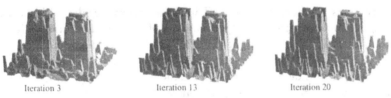

Iteration 10   Iteration 50   Iteration 100

1c. Reconstruction with the CG method from noiseless data

Iteration 3   Iteration 13   Iteration 20

1d. Reconstruction with NK method (identity operator) from noisy corrupted data

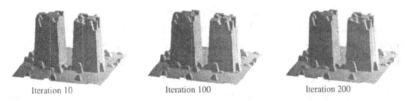

Iteration 10   Iteration 100   Iteration 200

1e. Reconstruction with CG method from noisy corrupted data

Fig. 1. Reconstructions of a two square cylinders profile

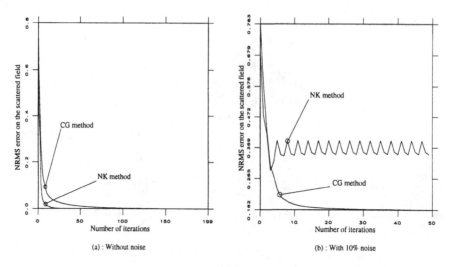

NRMS error on the scattered field

Number of iterations

(a) : Without noise

NRMS error on the scattered field

Number of iterations

(b) : With 10% noise

Fig. 2. Comparison between the convergence of the NK and the CG methods

measurements are carried out by collecting the transmission coefficient S_{12} with a HP 8720 network analyzer working at 434 MHz. The rotating system and network analyzer are both connected to a PC with a GPIB bus (Fig. 3).

For such a geometry, cylindrical coordinates fit better. Then, the domain $\mathcal{D}$ is discretized into N sector cells. For the application considered here, the regularizing operator used with the NK method is the gradient-by-zone operator.

Reconstructions for homogeneous and inhomogeneous circular objects are shown in Fig. 4. The homogeneous object consists of an equivalent muscle ($\epsilon' = 53$, $\epsilon'' = 39$) material with an outer plastic (PET) wall. The background medium is water ($\epsilon' = 76$, $\epsilon'' = 4$). The inhomogeneous object consists of an equivalent muscle material with inside a circular object made of plexiglass ($\epsilon' = 3$, $\epsilon'' = 0$). The reconstruction profiles are more satisfying with the NK method than with the MG method. The values displayed above and under the different images give an indication of the RMS error in the reconstructed profile.

Reconstruction for homogeneous and inhomogeneous elliptic objects having approximatively the same size as a human thorax cross section are shown in Fig. 5. The homogeneous object is filled with an equivalent muscle material with an outer plastic (PVC) wall. The inhomogeneous object consists of two equivalent bone ($\epsilon' = 8$, $\epsilon'' = 2$) circular materials surrounded by an equivalent muscle material with an inner wall of equivalent fat ($\epsilon' = 10$, $\epsilon'' = 4$) material, and an outer plastic (PVC) wall. The thickness of the fat wall is 2 cm. When comparing the reconstruction for the homogeneous object with the NK and MG methods, better results in terms of homogeneity and quantitative values are obtained with the NK method. It gives also satisfactory reconstructions for the inhomogeneous object while no convergence was reached with the MG method.

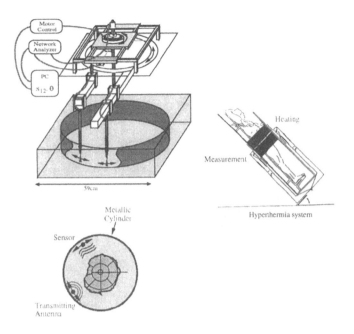

Fig. 3. Experimental setup of a microwave scanner prototype

6.3 Reconstructions from the Experimental Ipswich Data

We present in this section the results obtained from the experimental Ipswich far-field data [20, 23, 25]. The axis of the targets is oriented along the z-axis. The bistatic scattering measurements at 10.0 GHz were made in a plane perpendicular to this axis. The complete Ipswich Test Range system developed at *Rome Laboratory* is described in [42]. The scattered fields of the two metallic objects (cylinder and strip) were collected for eight incident angles of $\{0, 5, 10, 15, 20, 45, 60, 90\}$ degrees, over the observation sector $0 \leq \theta < 360°$, with a sample spacing $\Delta\theta = 0.5°$, while the scattered fields for the dielectric object were collected for six incident angles $\theta_I \in \{0°, 60°, 120°, 180°, 240°, 300°\}$, over an observation sector $\theta_I + 180° \leq \theta_S \leq \theta_I + 375°$, with a sample spacing $\Delta\theta_S = 0.5°$.

Reconstruction of a Metallic Cylinder This target is an alluminium cylinder, of radius 1.59 cm. In order to match the experimental setup with direct problem, a calibration on amplitude and phase has been done on the data, by comparing them with synthetic ones, matching more or less the targets. We present in Fig. 6 a comparison between the calibrated far-field data and the simulated ones. Taking into account the symmetry of the target, we increase the number of illuminations, by symmetrizing the set of illuminations. So, the final scattered field is composed by a set of 28 different illuminations measured on 720 receivers. Reconstructions of the metallic cylinder, using the Newton-Kantorovich (NK) and the Modified Gradient are presented in Fig. 7 and in Fig.

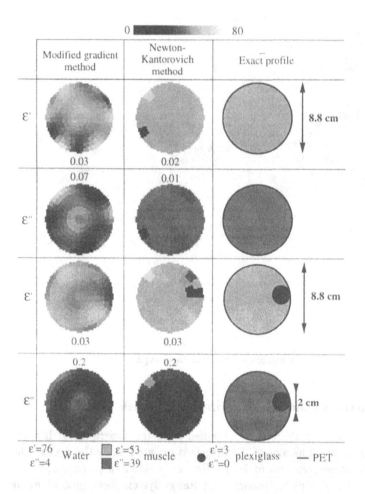

Fig. 4. Results from experimental data for a circular object

8, respectively. The test domain is divided into 11×11 subsquares of $5 \times 5 \, mm^2$. The reconstruction using the Conjugate Gradient (CG) algorithm (without regularization) is shown in Fig. 9. We use in this case a test domain divided into 29×29 subsquares of $1.1 \times 1.1 \, mm^2$, and the representation domain used in Fig. 9, is discretized into 49×49 subsquares.

The three methods succeeded in reconstructing the cylinder. As the inner structure of the metallic cylinder correspond to zero field value, each reconstruction algorithm can find a different solution for the inner profile. We note that the NK method using the identity operator needs more iterations than the other methods. The gradient-by-zone regularization improves greatly the convergence and accuracy of the NK method.

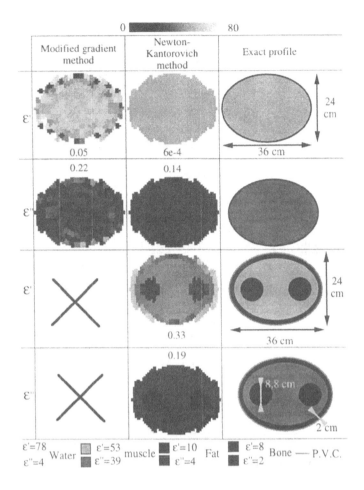

Fig. 5. Results from experimental data for an elliptic object

Reconstruction of a Metallic Strip This target is a metallic strip, circumscribed in a circle of radius 6 cm. The same calibration and symmetrization were applied on this object, than for the metallic cylinder. A comparison between the calibrated far-field data and the simulated ones is also shown in Fig. 6.

Reconstructions of the metallic strip, using the Newton-Kantorovich and the Modified Gradient algorithms, are shown in Fig. 10 and Fig. 11. The test domain is divided into 7×63 subsquares of $2 \times 2\,\mathrm{mm}^2$. Reconstructions of the metallic strip, using the CG algorithm (without regularization) are shown in Fig. 12. We use in this case for the reconstruction a test domain divided into 7×121 subsquares of $1 \times 1\,\mathrm{mm}^2$ and the representation domain used in Fig. 12 is discretized into 27×141 subsquares.

As for the metallic cylinder, the three algorithms succeeded in reconstructing the metallic strip. Using the NK method, only the regularization with the

182

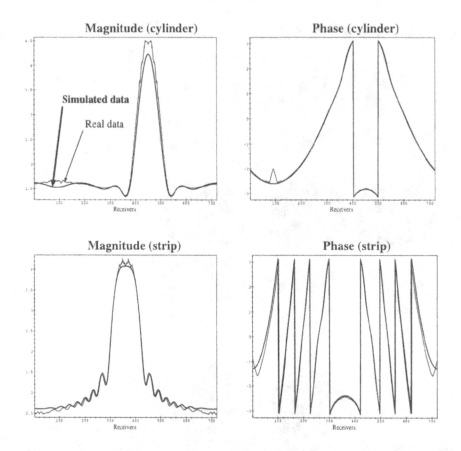

Fig. 6. Comparison for the metallic cylinder and strip, between the calibrated far-field data and the simulated ones

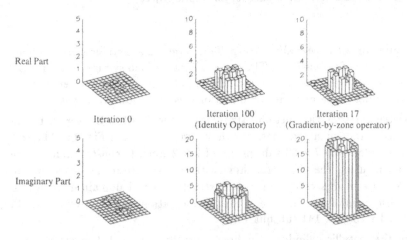

Fig. 7. Reconstruction of the metallic cylinder with NK method

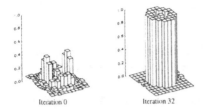

Fig. 8. Reconstruction of the metallic cylinder with MG method

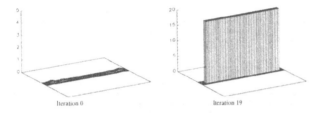

Fig. 9. Reconstruction of the metallic cylinder with CG method

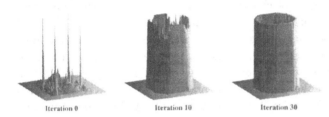

Fig. 10. Reconstruction of the metallic strip with NK method

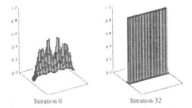

Fig. 11. Reconstruction of the metallic strip with MG method

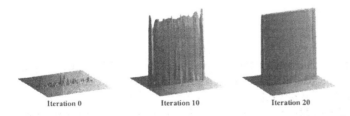

Fig. 12. Reconstruction of the metallic strip with CG method

gradient-by-zone operator gave good results.

Reconstruction of a Polystyrene Square Cylinder The dielectric target is a lossless polystyrene square cylinder with $\epsilon = 1.03$ and side equals to 11.2 cm. We use a domain $\mathcal{D}$ divided into 29×29 subsquares of 5.3×5.3 mm^2. A calibration was made on this object, and we present in Fig. 13, a comparison between the calibrated far-field data and the simulated ones. Using an *a priori* information about the geometry of the target, we symmetrize the object during the iterative reconstruction. A comparative study has been made on results obtained at the same degree of convergence without any regularization, with a Tikhonov regularization and with the edge-preserving regularization scheme (Fig. 14). In the different results, no initial guess were used i.e. the starting value is a zero contrast. The reconstruction without regularization, shows a blurred profile with a coarse shape description. The use of a Tikhonov regularization smoothes the profile and the edges are not preserved. The new regularization scheme improves the performance of the conjugate gradient algorithm : the edges are clearly preserved while the homogeneous areas are smoothed.

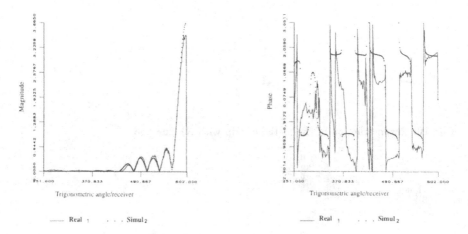

Fig. 13. Comparison for the polystyrene square cylinder, between the calibrated far-field data and the simulated ones

7 Conclusion

Different iterative reconstruction methods have been used or developed, including Newton-Kantorovich, Modified Gradient and Conjugate Gradient algorithm. Each method has their own advantages and drawbacks. The NK methods converges faster than CG and MG but is more instable and needs a good regularization technique even with noiseless data. Several regularization procedures have

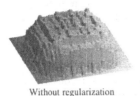 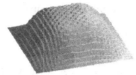 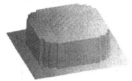

Without regularization   Tikhonov regularization   Edge-preserving regularization

Fig. 14. Reconstruction of the polystyrene square cylinder with CG method and the EP regularization

been studied in order to enhance the quality of the reconstruction, in case of noisy corrupted data or large contrasted objects. Besides the classical Tikhonov regularization with identity operator, a gradient-by-zone operator and an edge-preserving regularization have been investigated. The last regularization associated with the CG algorithm, showed a significant enhancement in case of strongly noisy corrupted experimental data.

References

1. J.Ch. Bolomey and Ch. Pichot. Microwave tomography: from theory to practical imaging systems. *Int. J. Imaging System Technology*, 2:144–156, 1990.
2. W. Tabbara, B. Duchêne, Ch. Pichot, D. Lesselier, L. Chommeloux, and N. Joachimowicz. Diffraction tomography: contribution of the analysis of some applications in microwaves and ultrasonics. *Inverse Problems*, 4:305–331, 1988.
3. A.J. Devaney. Geophysical diffraction tomography. *IEEE Trans. Geosci. Remote Sensing*, GE-22:3–13, 1984.
4. Ch. Pichot, L. Jofre, G. Peronnet, and J. Ch. Bolomey. Active microwave imaging of inhomogeneous bodies. *IEEE Transactions on Antennas and Propagation*, AP-33:416–425, 1985.
5. K.J. Langenberg. Introduction to the special issue on inverse problems. *Wave Motion*, 11:99–112, 1989.
6. J.Ch. Bolomey, Ch. Pichot, and G. Gaboriaud. Planar microwave imaging camera for biomedical applications : Critical and prospective analysis of reconstruction algorithms. *Radio Science*, 26(2):541–549, 1991.
7. L. Jofre, M.S. Hawley, A. Broquetas, E. de los Reyes, M. Ferrando, and R. Elias-Fusté. Medical imaging with a microwave tomographic scanner. *IEEE Transactions on Biomedical Engineering*, BME-37:303–312, 1990.
8. A. Broquetas, J. Romeu, J.M. Rius, A.R. Elias-Fusté, A. Cardama, and L. Jofre. Cylindrical geometry: a further step in active microwave imaging. *IEEE Transactions on Microwave Theory and Techniques*, MTT-39:836–844, 1991.
9. A. Roger. Newton-kantorovitch algorithm applied to an electromagnetic inverse problem. *IEEE Transactions on Antennas and Propagation*, AP-29(2):232–238, March 1981.

10. M.M. Ney, A.M. Smith, and S.S. Stuchly. A solution of electromagnetic imaging using pseudoinverse transformation. *IEEE Transactions on Medical Imaging*, MI-3:155–162, 1984.

11. Y.M. Wang and W.C. Chew. An iterative solution of two-dimensional electromagnetic inverse scattering problem. *Int. J. Imag. Syst.*, 1:100–108, 1989.

12. J. P. Hugonin, N. Joachimowicz, and Ch. Pichot. Quantitative reconstruction of complex permittivity distributions by means of microwave tomography. In P. C. Sabatier, editor, *Inverse Methods in Action*, pages 302–311. Springer-Verlag, Berlin, 1990.

13. W.C. Chew and Y.M. Wang. Reconstruction of two-dimensional permittivity distribution using the distorded Born iterative method. *IEEE Transactions on Medical Imaging*, MI-9(2):218–225, 1990.

14. S. Caorsi, G.L. Gragnagni, and M. Pastorino. Two-dimensional microwave imaging by a numerical inverse scattering solution. *IEEE Transactions on Microwave Theory and Techniques*, MTT-38:981–989, 1990.

15. L. Garnero, A. Franchois, J. P. Hugonin, Ch. Pichot, and N. Joachimowicz. Microwave imaging: complex permittivity reconstruction by simulated annealing. *IEEE Transactions on Microwave Theory and Techniques*, MTT-39:1801–1807, 1991.

16. N. Joachimowicz, Ch. Pichot, and J. P. Hugonin. Inverse scattering : an iterative numerical method for electromagnetic imaging. *IEEE Transactions on Antennas and Propagation*, AP-39:1742–1751, 1991.

17. R.E. Kleinman and P.M. van den Berg. A modified gradient method for two-dimensional problems in tomography. *J. Comput. Appl. Math.*, 42:17–35, 1992.

18. K. Belkebir, R. Kleinman, and Ch. Pichot. Microwave Imaging - Location and Shape Reconstruction from Multifrequency Scattering Data. To appear in *IEEE Transactions on Microwave Theory and Techniques*, MTT-45(4), April 1997.

19. A. Franchois and Ch. Pichot. Microwave Imaging - Complex Permittivity Reconstruction with a Levenberg-Marquardt Method. To appear in *IEEE Trans. on Antennas and Propagation*, AP-45(2), February 1997.

20. P. Lobel, R. Kleinman, Ch. Pichot, L. Blanc-Féraud, and M. Barlaud. Conjugate gradient method for solving inverse scattering with experimental data. *IEEE Antennas & Propagation Magazine*, 38(3):48–51, June 1996.

21. R.E. Kleinman and P.M. van den Berg. An extended range-modified gradient technique for profile inversion. *Radio Science*, 28(5):877–884, October 1993.

22. R.E. Kleinman and P.M. van den Berg. Two-dimensional location and shape reconstruction. *Radio Science*, 29:1157–1169, 1994.

23. K. Belkebir, J.M. Elissalt, J.M. Geffrin, and Ch. Pichot. Newton-Kantorovich and Modified Gradient Inversion Algorithms Applied to Ipswich Data. *IEEE Antennas & Propagation Magazine*, 38(3):41–44, June 1996.

24. P. Lobel, L. Blanc-Féraud, Ch. Pichot, and M. Barlaud. A new regularization scheme for inverse scattering. To appear in *Inverse Problems*, 12, April 1997.

25. P. Lobel, Ch. Pichot, L. Blanc-Féraud, and M. Barlaud. Conjugate Gradient Algorithm With Edge-Preserving Regularization for Image Reconstruction from Experimental Data. In *IEEE AP-S/URSI International Symposium*, volume 1, pages 644–647, Baltimore, Maryland, USA, July 1996.

26. S. Geman and D.E. Mc Clure. Bayesian image analysis : an application to single photon emission tomography. In *Proc. Statist. Comput. Sect.*, pages 12–18, Washington DC, 1985. Amer. Statist. Assoc.

27. S. Geman and G. Reynolds. Constrained restoration and the recovery of discontinuities. *IEEE Transactions on Pattern Analysis and Machine Intelligence*, PAMI-14(3):367–383, March 1992.

28. A. Franchois and Ch. Pichot. Generalized cross validation applied to a Newton-type algorithm for microwave tomography. In M. A. Fiddy Ed., editor, *Proc. Inverse Problems in Scattering and Imaging*, pages 232–240, San Diego, July 1992.

29. E. Polak and G. Ribière. Note sur la convergence de méthodes de directions conjuguées. *Revue Française d'Informatique et de Recherche Opérationnelle*, R1(16):35–43, 1969.

30. M.S. Berger. *Nonlinearity and functional analysis - Lectures on nonlinear problems in mathematical analysis*, chapter 2, pages 84–89. Pure and applied mathematics. Academic Press, 1970.

31. R. Acar and C.R. Vogel. Analysis of bounded variation penalty methods for ill-posed problems. *Inverse Problems*, 10(6):1217–1229, December 1994.

32. P.M. van den Berg and R.E. Kleinman. A total variation enhanced modified gradient algorithm for profile reconstruction. *Inverse Problems*, 11:L5–L10, 1995.

33. T. Hebert and R. Leahy. A generalized EM algorithm for 3-D Bayesian reconstruction from Poisson data using Gibbs priors. *IEEE Transactions on Medical Imaging*, MI-8(2):194–202, June 1989.

34. P. Perona and J. Malik. Scale-space and edge detection using anisotropic diffusion. *IEEE Transactions on Pattern Analysis and Machine Intelligence*, PAMI-12(7):629–639, July 1990.

35. P. Charbonnier, L. Blanc-Féraud, G. Aubert, and M. Barlaud. Deterministic Edge-Preserving Regularization in Computed Imaging. To appear in *IEEE Trans. Image Processing*, IP-6(2), February 1997.

36. L. Blanc-Féraud, P. Charbonnier, G. Aubert, and M. Barlaud. Nonlinear image processing : Modeling and fast algorithm for regularization with edge detection. In *Proc. IEEE-ICIP*, pages 474–477, Washington, USA, October 1995.

37. G. Aubert and L. Lazaroaia. A variational method in image recovery. Research Note 423, Laboratoire Jean-Alexandre Dieudonné, June 1995. To appear in *SIAM Journal of Num. Anal.* (November 1997).

38. P. Lobel, L. Blanc-Féraud, Ch. Pichot, and M. Barlaud. Technical development for an edge-preserving regularization method in inverse scattering. Research Note 95-73, Laboratoire Informatique Signaux et Systèmes de Sophia Antipolis, December 1995.

39. J.W. Strohbehn and E.B. Douple. Hyperthermia and cancer therapy: A review of biomedical engineering contributions and challenges. *IEEE Transactions on Biomedical Engineering*, BME-31:779–787, 1984.

40. G.C. van Rhoon, A.G. Vasser, P.M. van den Berg, and H.S. Reinhold. Evaluation of ring capacitor plates for regional deep heating. *Int. J. Hyperthermia*, 4(2):133–142, 1988.

41. A.A.C. De Leeuw, J. Mooibroek, and J.J.W. Lagendijk. Specific absorption rate steering by patient positioning in the 'Coaxial TEM' system : phantom investigation. *Int. J. Hyperthermia*, 7(4):605–611, 1991.

42. M. G. Coté. Automated Swept-Angle Bistatic Scattering Measurements Using Continuous Wave Radar. *IEEE Transactions on Instrumentation and Measurement*, IM-41(2):185–192, April 1992.

Boundary Modelling in Electrical Impedance Tomography

Michael Pidcock[1] ,Sorin Ciulli[2] and Simona Ispas[2]

[1]   School of Computing and Mathematical Sciences, Oxford Brookes University,
     Oxford, United Kingdom
[2]   Laboratoire de Physique Mathématique et Théorique,Université de Montpellier II,
     Montpellier, France

1 Introduction

Electrical Impedance Tomography (EIT) is a technique which attempts to create images of the electrical conductivity distribution of the material in the interior of an object. In many situations the widely differing electrical properties of the various types of matter within the object mean that the image so created is effectively an image of the distribution of these different type of material. The method proceeds by applying a variety of electric currents to the object using electrodes placed on its surface. A voltage distribution is induced in the object and this is measured on its surface, again via a number of electrodes. These data are used by a reconstruction algorithm to generate the image of the internal conductivity distribution.

It is well known that image reconstruction in EIT is a highly ill-posed, non-linear inverse problem [1] and that the images produced are very sensitive to a wide range of possible errors which can occurr in the technique. These errors are many and varied but it is clear that the interface between the electrodes and the object being imaged is a particularly important aspect of the system which needs to be considered very carefully. It is here that the data is measured and it is important that it is of the highest possible quality.

There are many difficulties associated with the collection of EIT data from these electrodes. For example, in medical applications the electrodes are attached to a patient's skin and it can be quite difficult to know exactly where these electrodes are and to be sure that they remain firmly attached to the patient while the data is being collected. These problems are currently being addressed in a mechanical way by the use of electrode belts but many other ideas involving mechanical, optical or electronic devices are being developed. We will not consider these issues further in this paper.

There is also the problem of the existence of an unknown contact impedance between the electrodes and the body surface which makes the interpretation of the measured data very difficult. This problem is resolved in a variety of ways by different groups working on EIT and it is an analysis of this problem which forms the content of this paper.

2 Mathematical Modelling of EIT

EIT modelling usually assumes that the material within the object is both ohmic and isotropic. Some material are known to be anisotropic e.g. muscle, and in this case the EIT problem becomes much more difficult and, indeed, not uniquely solvable [2]. A limited amount of work has been done on this aspect of the problem [3,4] but here we will follow the usual assumption of isotropy.

Suppose that we are considering an object $\Omega \subset R^n$ $(n = 2,3)$ which has a boundary $\partial\Omega$. If we denote the conductivity distribution within Ω by σ then, as there are no current sources within Ω, the electric potential ϕ satisfies

$$\nabla.(\sigma\nabla\phi) = 0 \qquad\qquad \text{in } \Omega$$

$$B\left(\phi, \sigma\frac{\partial\phi}{\partial n}\right) = 0 \qquad\qquad \text{on } \partial\Omega$$

B is a boundary operator which depends on the particular version of EIT which is being considered. The EIT image reconstruction problem consists of determining σ from a knowledge of B.

In practical implementations of EIT L electrodes $\{\Gamma_l\}$ are placed on the boundary $\partial\Omega$ and an electric current of magnitude I_l is applied to $\Gamma_l, l = 1...L$. No current flows through the region $\Gamma = \partial\Omega - \bigcup_{l=1}^{L}\Gamma_l$. For several years the number of electrodes, L, was restricted to 16 for two dimensional applications. More recently some groups have moved to $L = 32$ or even $L = 64$ in two dimensions and in Oxford we are currently using up to $L = 900$ in laboratory experiments in three dimensions.

The choice of the currents $\{I_l\}$ is a fundamental issue in EIT. For a number of years the only current drive pattern considered was one where current was injected into one electrode (at $\underline{\alpha}$) and drawn from another electrode (at $\underline{\beta}$) while all the remaining electrodes had no current flowing through them. In spite of much discussion about the optimal choice of this pair, most groups using this approach choose them to be adjacent to each other and cycle through the L possibilities. In this approach the electrodes are regarded as either (a) point or (b) of finite size with a uniform current density distribution over the electrode.

More recently, some research groups have adopted a different approach by injecting current into each of the electrodes and choosing the current patterns $\{I_l\}$ in some optimal way. With this approach has come a more sophisticated treatment of the electrodes, firstly (c) by noting that although the potential is constant on each electrode, the current density is not necessarily so and, finally, (d) by including a contribution from the unknown contact impedance, Z. Both of these models use the

Boundary Modelling in Electrical Impedance Tomography

fact that the total current flowing through each electrode is known (I_l).

These four electrode models can be described by the boundary conditions:

(a) $\quad \sigma(\underline{s})\dfrac{\partial\phi}{\partial n}(\underline{s}) = I\Big[\delta(\underline{s}-\underline{\alpha}) - \delta\big(\underline{s}-\underline{\beta}\big)\Big]$ $\qquad\qquad\qquad \underline{s},\underline{\alpha},\underline{\beta}\in\partial\Omega$

(b) $\quad \dfrac{\partial\phi}{\partial n}(\underline{s}) = 0 \qquad \underline{s}\in\Gamma \qquad\qquad \sigma(\underline{s})\dfrac{\partial\phi}{\partial n}(\underline{s}) = \dfrac{I_l}{|\Gamma_l|} \qquad\qquad \underline{s}\in\Gamma_l$

(c) $\quad \dfrac{\partial\phi}{\partial n}(\underline{s}) = 0 \qquad \underline{s}\in\Gamma \qquad\qquad \displaystyle\int_{\Gamma_l}\sigma(\underline{s})\dfrac{\partial\phi}{\partial n}(\underline{s})d\Gamma_l = I_l$

$\qquad\quad\ \phi(\underline{s}) = V_l \qquad \underline{s}\in\Gamma_l \qquad\qquad l = 1,\ldots,L$

(d) $\quad \dfrac{\partial\phi}{\partial n}(\underline{s}) = 0 \qquad \underline{s}\in\Gamma \qquad\qquad \displaystyle\int_{\Gamma_l}\sigma(\underline{s})\dfrac{\partial\phi}{\partial n}(\underline{s})d\Gamma_l = I_l$

$\qquad\quad\ \phi(\underline{s}) + Z_l\big(\underline{s}\big)\sigma(\underline{s})\dfrac{\partial\phi}{\partial n}(\underline{s}) = V_l \qquad \underline{s}\in\Gamma_l \qquad l = 1,\ldots,L$

Models (a) and (b) define Neumann boundary value problems while model (c) defines a mixed Neumann-Dirichlet problem. There is experimental evidence to support the validity of model (d). It represents a mixed Neumann-Robin boundary value problem and it is this model which we will discuss in the rest of this paper.

3 An Integral Equation

Consider the case when $\sigma = 1$ throughout the whole region. Then we can write

$$\phi(\underline{r}) = \int_{\partial\Omega}\dfrac{\partial\phi}{\partial n}(\underline{s})N(\underline{r},\underline{s})d\Omega_s \qquad \underline{r}\in\Omega \qquad\qquad \underline{s}\in\partial\Omega$$

where $N(\underline{r},\underline{s})$ is the Neumann function satisfying

$$\nabla_r^2 N(\underline{r},\underline{r}') = -\delta(\underline{r}-\underline{r}') \qquad\qquad \underline{r},\underline{r}'\in\Omega$$

$$\dfrac{\partial N}{\partial n_s}(\underline{r},\underline{s}) = \dfrac{1}{|\partial\Omega|} \qquad\qquad \underline{r},\underline{s}\in\partial\Omega$$

Using model (d) and continuing the equation to the boundary i.e. let $\underline{r}\in\partial\Omega$, we find that

$$\phi(\underline{r}) = -\sum_{l=1}^{L} V_l \int_{\Gamma_l} \frac{N(\underline{r},\underline{s})}{Z(\underline{s})} d\Omega_s + \sum_{l=1}^{L} \int_{\Gamma_l} \frac{N(\underline{r},\underline{s})}{Z(\underline{s})} \phi(\underline{s}) d\Omega_s \qquad (1)$$

In the rest of this paper we will describe some of the properties of the solution to this Fredholm integral equation of the second kind in the two dimensional case.

4 A Two Dimensional Problem

As a first step in the study of equation (1) we consider the case where Ω is a two dimensional unit disk consisting of material of unit conductivity and containing a concentric anomaly of radius $R < 1$ and conductivity σ. The reasons for considering this problem are:

(i)   By varying R and σ we can vary the conductivity distribution within the region and we are able to see that the distinctive behaviour of the current density distribution which we have found in earlier work, is a consequence of the mixed boundary value problem and not of the internal conductivity distribution

(ii)   We can calculate the Neumann function for this problem [5]

$$N(\underline{r},\underline{s}) = \frac{1}{\pi}\left\{-\log\left|2\sin\left(\frac{\theta-\varphi}{2}\right)\right| + \sum_{m=1}^{\infty}(-\mu)^m \log\left(1 - 2R^{2m}\cos(\theta-\varphi) + R^{4m}\right)\right\} \qquad (2)$$

where $\underline{r} = (1,\theta)$, $\underline{s} = (1,\varphi)$ and $\mu = \dfrac{\sigma-1}{\sigma+1}$.

We see that our integral equation (1) has a weak logarithmic singularity when $\theta = \varphi$.

5 Numerical Solution of the Integral Equation

The numerical solution of equation (1) can be achieved very rapidly by the use of a modified version of the standard Nyström method. The modification is required because of the weak singularity in the Neumann function and the method we have used is to explicitly subtract out the singularity. This approach works very well and requires only a modest number of quadrature points. The speed of this calculation is in rather stark contrast to some earlier work in which we studied a similar problem using a boundary Fourier method [5]. Full details are given in [6].

We have used this method to solve equation (1) for a wide range of functional forms of the contact impedance term $Z_l(\underline{s})$ and current patterns $\{I_l = \cos(N\theta_l), N = 1,2,3...\}$ where θ_l is the polar angular displacement of the centre of Γ_l, $l = 1,...,L$. We have also varied the radius and the conductivity, R and σ, of the anomaly. In all cases we have found that the fundamental result of our earlier work using constant contact impedance remains unchanged. The current density distribution varies smoothly but rapidly over each electrode and shows a sharp peak near the edge of the electrode. This peak diminishes as the magnitude of $Z_l(\underline{s})$ increases near to the edge of the electrode. The detailed nature of this behaviour is unclear from these numerical studies but it has proved extremely expensive in computational terms to devise Finite Element meshes which are sufficiently dense to solve the forward problem of EIT with a satisfactory accuracy. It is typical to find that over 75% of the elements must lie in the region $\{(r,\theta):0.9 < r < 1\}$. Thus a large part of the computational effort is expended on modelling the electrodes which exist merely as a data acquisition device for the main objective of EIT i.e. calculating the conductivity distribution. This is obviously unsatisfactory.

There is, therefore, considerable numerical interest in gaining a detailed understanding of the behaviour of the current density distribution on the electrodes in order that this information can be explicitly built into any numerical scheme for solving the forward problem of EIT. It is known, for example, that in the zero contact impedance case using only two electrodes, the current density distribution has an inverse square root singularity at the edge of an electrode [7]. This behaviour is clearly changed by the inclusion of contact impedance although visually it looks very similar. In the rest of this paper we will outline a method for obtaining similar information about the behaviour of the currents density distribution in the case of non-zero contact impedance.

An Analytic Study of Solutions to the Integral Equation

The method which we have adopted in this two dimensional problem is to reformulate the problem as one in Complex Analysis. We have seen numerically that differing forms for the contact impedance term $Z_l(\underline{s})$ and differing conductivity distributions (represented by varying R and σ) make little difference to the basic results. We have therefore chosen to consider the case where the conductivity distribution is uniform (i.e. take $\mu = 0$ in equation (2)) and here we will also consider only the case where $Z_l(\underline{s}) = Z$ is constant. If we consider the electrodes to be of equal width Δ equation (1) can be written in the form

$$\pi Z \phi(\theta) = \sum_{l=1}^{L} V_l \int_{\theta_l - \frac{\Delta}{2}}^{\theta_l + \frac{\Delta}{2}} \log\left|2 \sin\left(\frac{\theta - \varphi}{2}\right)\right| d\varphi - \sum_{l=1}^{L} \int_{\theta_l - \frac{\Delta}{2}}^{\theta_l + \frac{\Delta}{2}} \log\left|2 \sin\left(\frac{\theta - \varphi}{2}\right)\right| \phi(\varphi) d\varphi \quad (3)$$

The method which we have used to study this equation is developed from techniques introduced in the sixties into Elementary Particle Physics [8] although our problem is considerably more complicated than those considered at that time.

Suppose that the point $(1,\theta)$ lies on one of the electrodes. By a suitable change of variables, both dependent and independent, we are able to rewrite equation (3) as

$$f(x) = g(x) + \lambda \int_0^1 K(x,t)f(t)dt \qquad\qquad 0 \le x \le 1 \qquad (4)$$

where $K(x,t) = \log|x - t|$ and $g(x) = \int_0^1 \log|x - t|w(t)dt +$ regular terms.

$w(t)$ is holomorphic in the neighbourhood of the points $t = 0,1$ which correspond to the edges of the electrodes. We will consider only the behaviour near $x = 0$ as the behaviour near $x = 1$ is similar.

Consider, first, the free term $g(x)$ and define the function

$$F(z) = \int_0^1 \log(t - z)w(t)dt. \qquad (5)$$

We consider z and t to lie in complex $z-$ and $t-$ planes respectively and take the logarithmic function to have a cut along the negative real axis with discontinuity $2\pi i$. Now take $z = x_0 - i\varepsilon$ with $x_0 < 0$ and $\varepsilon > 0$, and allow z to move into the right half complex $z-$ plane and then round the origin in a counterclockwise direction back to its starting value. To avoid the singularity in the integrand of (5) it becomes necessary to deform the contour of integration in the complex $t-$ plane into the form of a hook and when z returns to its starting point, we find that the value of $F(z)$ has changed by an amount $2\pi i \int_0^z w(t)dt$. Hence, the origin is a branch point of F with discontinuity $2\pi i \int_0^z w(t)dt$. Since w is holomorphic near the origin, it has a power series expansion $w(t) = a + bt + ct^2 + \dots$. A function with the required cut along the negative real axis is then given by

$$\left(a + \frac{1}{2}bz + \frac{1}{3}cz^2 + \dots \right) z \log z$$

This expression give the contribution of the free term to the singular behaviour of $F(z)$ near the origin. The consideration of the second term in equation (4) is more complicated but we can use arguments similar to the above if we note that the general solution can be written in the form

$$f(x) = g(x) + \sum_{n=0}^{\infty} \frac{\lambda}{\lambda_n - \lambda} g_n u_n(x)$$

where $u_n(x) = \lambda_n \int_0^1 K(x,t)u_n(t)dt$ are the eigenfunctions of $K(x,t)$ and

$$g_n = \int_0^1 g(x)u_n(x)dx$$

The singular behaviour of f near the origin comes partly from the free term as discussed above and partly form the behaviour of the functions $\{u_n\}$. In considering the behaviour of these functions it is tempting to try to repeat the analysis which was used in connection with the free term on the defining equation for $u_n(x)$. However, considerable care must be taken in the analytic continuation of this relationship as structure unlike the holomorphic function $w(t)$ encountered earlier, the $u_n(x)$ under the integration sign has a cut. The appropriate analytic continuation is

$$U_n^{(1)}(z) = \lambda_n \int_0^1 \log(t-z) \left[\frac{U_n^{(0)}(t) + U_n^{(1)}(t)}{2} \right] dt$$

where $U_n^{(k)}(z)$ is the value of the function $U_n(z)$ on the kth Riemann sheet. Following the earlier analysis we find that

$$U_n^{(1)}(z) - U_n^{(0)}(z) = i\pi\lambda_n \int_0^z \left[U_n^{(0)}(t) + U_n^{(1)}(t) \right] dt.$$

Differentiating this equation with respect to z we find

$$\frac{dU_n^{(1)}(z)}{dz} - \frac{dU_n^{(0)}(z)}{dz} = i\pi\lambda_n \left[U_n^{(0)}(z) + U_n^{(1)}(z) \right]. \tag{6}$$

If we now write

$$U_n^{(0)}(z) = \sum_k a_k z^k + \sum_m \sum_k b_{mk} z^m \log^k(-z) \tag{7}$$

then

$$U_n^{(1)}(z) = \sum_k a_k z^k + \sum_m \sum_k b_{mk} z^m \left[\log(-z) + 2i\pi \right]^k \tag{8}$$

Substituting equations (7) and (8) into equation (6) we find that all the $\{a_k\}$ and $\{b_{mk}\}$ are completely determined except one. Gathering all this together we find, finally, that near to the origin

$$\phi(z) = \sum_k A_k z^k + \sum_m \sum_k B_{mk} z^m \log^k(-z)$$

where the $\{A_k\}$ and $\{B_{mk}\}$ are real constants. Note that this expression does not diverge at the origin, although its derivatives do, a result which is entirely consistent with the numerical results. Full details of this work can be found in [9] for the constant $Z_i(\underline{s})$ and in [10] for the case of non-constant $Z_i(\underline{s})$.

Conclusion

In this paper we have described the electrode models which are normally used in EIT. We have derived an integral equation for the potential in the case of a model which includes the effect of contact impedance. We have described results obtained by solving this equation numerically and used methods of complex analysis to derive an expansion for the potential near the edge of an electrode.

References

1. Breckon W R and Pidcock M K 1987, Mathematical Aspects of Impedance Imaging, *Journal of Clinical and Physiological Measurement*, Vol 8, 77-84.
2. Lee J M and Uhlmann G. 1989, Determining conductivity by boundary measurements II: Interior results, *Comm.Pure Appl.Math*, Vol 42, 1097-1112.
3. Sylvester J 1990, An anisotropic inverse boundary value problem, *Comm.Pure Appl.Math*, Vol 43, 1023-1040.
4. Lionheart W R B 1997, Conformal uniqueness results in anisotropic Electrical Impedance Tomography, *Inverse Problems*, Vol 13, 1-10.
5. Paulson K S, Breckon W R and Pidcock M K 1992, Electrode modelling in Electrical Impedance Tomography, *SIAM Journal on Applied Mathematics*, Vol 52, 1012-1022.
6. Ciulli S, Ispas S and Pidcock M K 1996, Numerical modelling of a mixed Neumann-Robin boundary value problem', submitted for publication.
7. Pidcock M K, Ciulli S and Ispas S 1995, Singularities of mixed boundary problems in Electrical Impedance Tomography, *Physiological Measurement*, Vol 16, 213-218.
8. Eden R J, Landshoff P V, Olive D I and Polkinghorne J C 1966, The Analytic S-Matrix, *Cambridge University Press*.
9. Ciulli S, Ispas S and Pidcock M K 1996, Anomalous thresholds and edge singularities in Electrical Impedance Tomography, J. *Math Phys.*, Vol 37, No 6, 4388-4417.
10. Ciulli S, Ispas S and Pidcock M K 1996, Pinch singularities in Electrical Impedance Tomography, submitted for publication.

Lavrentiev's Method for Linear Volterra Integral Equations of the First Kind, with Applications to the Non-Destructive Testing of Optical-Fibre Preforms

Robert Plato

Fachbereich Mathematik, Technische Universität Berlin,
D - 10623 Berlin, Germany

1 Introduction

1.1 Linear Volterra Integral Equations of the First Kind

In the non-destructive testing of optical-fibre preforms, the problem of determining the axial stress components from measurements of the phase retardation of laser lights sent through the object reduces to a generalized Abel integral equation of the first kind, for more details we refer to Section 4. The methods presented in this paper can be applied to solve those problems efficiently, and we begin more generally with the consideration of a linear Volterra integral equation of the first kind,

$$(Au)(t) := \int_0^t k(t,s)u(s)\, ds \; = \; f_*(t), \qquad t \in [0,a]. \qquad (1.1)$$

Later on we shall present specific equations of type (1.1) like the mentioned generalized Abel integral equations and integral equations with a completely monotone convolution kernel, but for the moment we suppose that $k : [0,a] \times [0,a] \to \mathbb{F}$ in (1.1) denotes an arbitrary kernel, and $f_* : [0,a] \to \mathbb{F}$ is an approximately given function, where either $\mathbb{F} = \mathbb{R}$ or $\mathbb{F} = \mathbb{C}$. We moreover suppose that $A \in \mathcal{L}(\mathcal{H})$ and $f_* \in \mathcal{R}(A)$, where $\mathcal{H}$ is a given Hilbert space, and

$$\mathcal{L}(\mathcal{H}) \; = \; \{\, T : \mathcal{H} \to \mathcal{H} \mid T \text{ is bounded and linear} \,\},$$

and finally,

$$\mathcal{R}(A) \; = \; \{\, Au \mid u \in \mathcal{H} \,\} \subset \mathcal{H}$$

denotes the range of A. If the kernel k in (1.1) is non-degenerated, then $\mathcal{R}(A)$ is non-closed in $\mathcal{H}$, and thus equation (1.1) is ill-posed. This means that if merely an approximation $f \in \mathcal{H}$ for f_* is available,

$$f \in \mathcal{H}, \qquad f_* \in \mathcal{R}(A), \qquad f \approx f_*,$$

then the minimum norm solution of $Au = f$ (if it exists) may have an arbitrarily large distance to the minimum norm solution of (1.1). Thus some careful regularization is needed, and to this end, in this paper we shall consider Lavrentiev's m-times iterated method, see the following subsection for its introduction.

1.2   Lavrentiev's m-Times Iterated Method

In Hilbert spaces, Volterra integral equations of the first kind (1.1) in general may be regularized by methods like Tikhonov regularization, Landweber iteration or the classical conjugate gradient method (the latter applied to the normal equations $A^\star A u = A^\star f_\star$, where $A^\star$ denotes the adjoint operator of A). However, these approaches do not profit from the triangular form of (1.1), or even more worse, the triangular structure is destroyed by any of these methods. Triangularity of the Volterra integral equation (1.1) here means that a discretization of (1.1), e.g. by a projection method, typically leads to a left triangular system or at least to an almost triangular system of equations.

In order to introduce a regularization method that in fact benefits from the triangular structure, we assume that the Volterra operator A in (1.1) is *accretive* with respect to $\mathcal{H}$, i.e.,

$$\mathbf{Re}\,\langle Au, u \rangle \geq 0, \qquad u \in \mathcal{H}.$$

Here, $\mathbf{Re}\,z$ denotes the real part of $z \in \mathbb{C}$, and $\langle \cdot, \cdot \rangle : \mathcal{H} \times \mathcal{H} \to \mathbb{F}$ denotes the inner product in $\mathcal{H}$. Then the mentioned (almost) triangular system of equations associated with the Volterra integral equation (1.1) typically has small positive entries near the diagonal, and thus is seems to be natural and efficient to stabilize this system of equations by adding a small positive constant term on the diagonal. In the infinite-dimensional setting this corresponds to Lavrentiev's classical method, and in this paper we shall consider more generally Lavrentiev's m-times iterated method (with fixed integer m). It generates for a regularization parameter $\gamma > 0$ an $u_\gamma \in \mathcal{H}$ by

$$(A + \gamma I)v_n = \gamma v_{n-1} + f, \qquad n = 1, 2, ..., m,$$

$$u_\gamma := v_m$$

with $v_0 = 0$, and I denotes the identity operator in $\mathcal{H}$. For $m = 1$ one gets Lavrentiev's classical method while for $m > 1$, $m - 1$ stabilized residual corrections are employed. Note, however, that m is fixed so that Lavrentiev's m-times iterated method is a parametric method and not an iterative method. A good choice of the regularization parameter $\gamma > 0$ for Lavrentiev's m-times iterated method is important, and to this end in this paper some discrepancy principles are presented.

1.3   Outline of the Paper

The outline of the paper is as follows: In Section 2 we consider generalized Abel operators as well as integral operators with a completely monotone convolution kernel as examples for Volterra integral operators that are accretive, and in Section 3 some discrepancy principles as specific parameter choices for Lavrentiev's m-times method are considered and the associated convergence results are stated. In Section 4 we present some details about the non-destructive testing of optical-fibre preforms, and numerical illustrations are presented. Finally, in Section 5 we shall consider the case where the underlying space is a Banach space $\mathcal{X}$ and provide some results for Lavrentiev's m-times method for that case; moreover, also a subsection on two stationary iteration methods is included.

2 Specific Linear Accretive Volterra Integral Operators

2.1 Introduction

In this section we present some specific Volterra operators that are accretive in the following sense.

Definition 1. Let $\mathcal{H}$ be a Hilbert space over the field $\mathbb{F} = \mathbb{R}$ or $\mathbb{F} = \mathbb{C}$, and let $\langle \cdot, \cdot \rangle : \mathcal{H} \times \mathcal{H} \to \mathbb{F}$ be the associated inner product. An operator $A \in \mathcal{L}(\mathcal{H})$ is called <u>accretive</u>, if

$$\mathbf{Re}\,\langle Au, u \rangle \geq 0, \qquad u \in \mathcal{H}. \tag{2.1}$$

Accretiveness usually is introduced for unbounded operators, cf. Tanabe [24], but for the applications we have in mind it is sufficient to consider bounded operators. Note that (2.1) is valid if and only if (a) the resolvent set $\rho(-A)$ corresponding to $-A$ contains $(0, \infty)$, and (b) the following estimate is valid,

$$\|(A + \gamma I)^{-1}\| \leq 1/\gamma, \qquad \gamma > 0,$$

where $\| \cdot \|$ denotes the associated operator norm.

2.2 Abel Integral Operators

In the sequel we consider generalized Abel integral operators (cf. Gorenflo & Vessella [9] for an introduction) with respect to specific Hilbert spaces. To this end, throughout this subsection let $\beta > 0$ and $a > 0$ be arbitrary but fixed finite numbers, if not further specified. We then denote by $L^2([0, a], s^{\beta-1}ds)$ the Hilbert space over $\mathbb{F} = \mathbb{R}$ or $\mathbb{F} = \mathbb{C}$ containing all real- or complex-valued, measurable functions u on $[0, a]$, such that $|u|^2$ is integrable with respect to the measure $s^{\beta-1}ds$, and the associated inner product is

$$\langle u, v \rangle \;=\; \int_0^a u(s)\overline{v(s)}\, s^{\beta-1}ds, \qquad u,\, v \in L^2([0, a],\, s^{\beta-1}ds).$$

For the case $\beta = 1$, this space will be simplified denoted by $L^2[0, a]$.

Abel Integral Operators: Part I For $0 < \alpha < 1$, a generalized Abel integral operator $A = A_{\alpha, \beta, a}$ is given by

$$(Au)(t) \;=\; \int_0^t \frac{s^{\beta-1}u(s)}{(t^\beta - s^\beta)^{1-\alpha}}\, ds, \qquad t \in [0, a]. \tag{2.2}$$

The operator A defined by (2.2) is accretive with respect to $\mathcal{H} = L^2([0, a], s^{\beta-1}ds)$; for the details see [17].

Note that the operator A in (2.2) is moderately ill-posed. In fact, if $\beta = 1$ and $a = 1$, then for the singular values $\sigma_n(A)$, $n \geq 1$, of A one has

$$\sigma_n(A) \asymp n^{-\alpha} \qquad \text{as } n \to \infty,$$

cf. Dostanić [7]. Here, $a_n \asymp b_n$ for positive numbers a_n, b_n, $n \geq 1$, means that there are constants $0 < \kappa_1$, κ_2 with $\kappa_1 a_n \leq b_n \leq \kappa_2 a_n$ for $n \geq 1$.

Abel Integral Operators: Part II For $0 < \alpha < 1$, another generalized Abel integral operator $A = A_{\alpha,\beta,a}$ is given by

$$(Au)(t) = \int_t^a \frac{s^{\beta-1}u(s)}{(s^\beta - t^\beta)^{1-\alpha}} \, ds, \qquad t \in [0, a]. \tag{2.3}$$

The lower bound in the integral in (2.3) depends on t, thus A defined by (2.3) has not the form (1.1). This operator A given by (2.3) nevertheless is accretive with respect to $\mathcal{H} = L^2([0, a], s^{\beta-1}ds)$, since A is the adjoint of the operator given by (2.2). We return to this generalized Abel integral operator in Section 4 where the non-destructive testing of optical-fibre preforms is considered.

Other Abel type integral equations with generalized kernels arise in X-ray tomography, see e.g., Cormack [5], Natterer [12].

2.3 Volterra Integral Operators with Convolution Kernels

We next consider the Volterra integral operator

$$(Au)(t) = \int_0^t \kappa(t - s)u(s) \, ds, \qquad t \in [0, a], \tag{2.4}$$

with a Lebesgue-integrable convolution kernel $\kappa : [0, \infty) \to \mathbb{R}$. Here, A as in (2.4) is accretive with respect to $\mathcal{H} = L^2[0, a]$ if κ is completely monotone, i.e.,

$$\mathbf{Re}\,(\mathbf{L}\kappa)(z) \geq 0, \qquad \mathbf{Re}\, z > 0,$$

where $(\mathbf{L}\kappa)(z) := \int_0^\infty e^{-zs}\kappa(s) \, ds$, $\mathbf{Re}\, z > 0$, denotes the Laplace transform of κ. For more details see Nohel & Shea [14] or Gripenberg, Londen & Staffans [10], Theorem 16.2.4.

3 Parameter Choices for Lavrentiev's m-Times Iterated Method

For an arbitrary accretive $A \in \mathcal{L}(\mathcal{H})$, where $\mathcal{H}$ denotes a given Hilbert space, we consider the equation

$$Au = f_*, \tag{3.1}$$

with $\mathcal{R}(A) \neq \overline{\mathcal{R}(A)}$ in general, i.e., equation (3.1) is then ill-posed. Here $\overline{\mathcal{R}(A)}$ denotes the closure of $\mathcal{R}(A)$.

As in the introduction we admit the right-hand side in (3.1) to be disturbed, and in the sequel we additionally suppose that an estimate for the noise level is known, i.e.,

$$f^\delta \in \mathcal{H}, \qquad f_* \in \mathcal{R}(A), \qquad \|f_* - f^\delta\| \leq \delta, \tag{3.2}$$

where $\delta > 0$ is a known error bound, and $\|\cdot\| : \mathcal{H} \to \mathbb{R}$ denotes the underlying norm.

In the sequel we consider (for fixed integer m) Lavrentiev's m-times iterated method which for $\gamma > 0$ generates an $u_\gamma^\delta \in \mathcal{H}$ by

$$\left. \begin{array}{l} (A + \gamma I)v_n = \gamma v_{n-1} + f^\delta, \qquad n = 1, 2, ..., m \\ u_\gamma^\delta := v_m \end{array} \right\} \tag{3.3}$$

where $v_0 = 0$, and for notational convenience we set

$$u_\infty^\delta = 0.$$

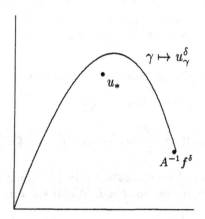

Fig. 1. Semiconvergence of Lavrentiev's m-times iterated method.

For ill-posed equations (3.1), a possible shape of the trajectory $\gamma \mapsto u_\gamma^\delta$ in the space $\mathcal{H}$ is described in Figure 1. Here $\delta > 0$ small is fixed, and for notational convenience it is assumed that $f^\delta \in \mathcal{R}(A)$ and that A has a trivial nullspace, and $u_* \in \mathcal{H}$ denotes the solution of (3.1). In Figure 1, the point $u_\infty^\delta \in \mathcal{H}$ on the trajectory corresponds to the origin, and u_0^δ corresponds to $A^{-1}f^\delta$.

The typical behavior of $\gamma \mapsto u_\gamma^\delta$ as described in Figure 1, also known as semiconvergence, makes it necessary to choose the regularization parameter γ appropriately, and to this end in the following subsections we present certain discrepancy principles.

3.1 Discrepancy Principles

In the sequel we present discrepancy principles as rules for choosing $\gamma_\delta > 0$ in order to get good approximations $u^\delta_{\gamma_\delta} \in \mathcal{H}$ for some solution $u_* \in \mathcal{H}$ of (3.1). To this end, let $\Delta^\delta_\gamma \in \mathcal{H}$ denote the defect, i.e.,

$$\Delta^\delta_\gamma := Au^\delta_\gamma - f^\delta. \tag{3.4}$$

In fact, if $A \in \mathcal{L}(\mathcal{H})$ is accretive, then for fixed $\delta > 0$ the norm of the defect $\|\Delta^\delta_\gamma\|$ is continuous and nondecreasing in γ, and $\lim_{\gamma \to 0} \|\Delta^\delta_\gamma\| \leq \delta$; see Figure 2 for the illustration of a typical situation. Thus the following two versions of the discrepancy principle can be implemented numerically.

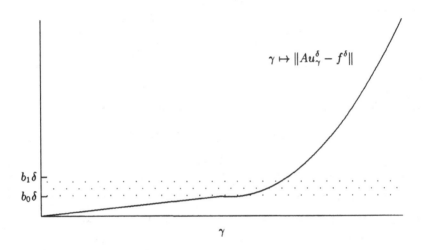

Fig. 2. Illustration for a typical behavior of the functional $\gamma \mapsto \|Au^\delta_\gamma - f^\delta\|$.

Discrepancy Principle 1. Fix positive constants b_0, b_1 with $b_1 \geq b_0 > 1$.
(a) If $\|\Delta^\delta_\infty\| \leq b_1\delta$ then choose $\gamma_\delta = \infty$.
(b) If $\|\Delta^\delta_\infty\| > b_1\delta$ then choose $\gamma_\delta > 0$ such that

$$b_0\delta \leq \|\Delta^\delta_{\gamma_\delta}\| \leq b_1\delta.$$

Discrepancy Principle 2. Fix a real $b > 1$. Moreover, fix $\theta > 0$ and $\tau > 0$, and set $\gamma(k) = \theta/k^\tau$. Terminate computation of $u^\delta_{\gamma(k)} \in \mathcal{H}$, $k = 0, 1, 2, ...$, if for the first time

$$\|\Delta^\delta_{\gamma(k)}\| \leq b\delta,$$

and let $\gamma_\delta := \gamma(k_\delta)$, where k_δ denotes the stopping index.

The following result can be derived from the results in [16]. (3.5) shows that each discrepancy principle for Lavrentiev's m-times iterated method (3.3) with $m \geq 2$ defines a regularization method, and (3.8) provides, under additional smoothness assumptions, order-optimal convergence rates. The asymptotic behavior (3.6) and the estimate (3.9) show that the parameter $\gamma_\delta > 0$ cannot be arbitrarily small, respectively.

Theorem 2. *Let $\mathcal{H}$ be a Hilbert space, let $A \in \mathcal{L}(\mathcal{H})$ be accretive, and suppose that (3.2) is valid. Let $\{u_\gamma^\delta\} \subset \mathcal{H}$ be as in (3.3), with $m \geq 2$. Fix one of the two described Discrepancy Principles 1 or 2, and let the parameter $\gamma_\delta > 0$ be chosen according to it.*
1. If $u_* \in \overline{\mathcal{R}(A)}$ solves (3.1) then

$$\|u_{\gamma_\delta}^\delta - u_*\| \to 0 \qquad \text{as } \delta \to 0, \tag{3.5}$$
$$\delta/\gamma_\delta \to 0 \qquad \text{as } \delta \to 0. \tag{3.6}$$

2. If moreover for some real $0 < \nu \leq m - 1$ and $z \in \mathcal{H}$,

$$u_* = A^\nu z, \qquad \varrho := \|z\|, \tag{3.7}$$

then with some constants $d_\nu, e_\nu > 0$ we have the estimates

$$\|u_{\gamma_\delta}^\delta - u_*\| \leq d_\nu (\varrho \delta^\nu)^{1/(\nu+1)}, \tag{3.8}$$
$$\gamma_\delta \geq e_\nu (\varrho^{-1} \delta)^{1/(\nu+1)}. \tag{3.9}$$

d_ν and e_ν depend also on b_0, b_1 and on b introduced in the Discrepancy Principles 1 and 2, respectively. Moreover, for $0 < \nu < 1$ fractional powers $A^\nu \in \mathcal{L}(\mathcal{H})$ of accretive operators $A \in \mathcal{L}(\mathcal{H})$ can be defined e.g. by formula (6.16) in Chapter 2 of Pazy [15]; for arbitrary $\nu > 0$, fractional powers $A^\nu \in \mathcal{L}(\mathcal{H})$ then are given recursively by $A^\nu := A^{\nu - \lfloor \nu \rfloor} A^{\lfloor \nu \rfloor}$, where $\lfloor \nu \rfloor$ denotes the greatest integer $\leq \nu$.

The proof of Theorem 2 depends basically on the estimate

$$\|u_\gamma^\delta - u_*\| \leq \|[\gamma(A + \gamma I)^{-1}]^m u_*\| + m\delta/\gamma, \tag{3.10}$$

and (3.10) follows immediately from the representation

$$u_* - u_\gamma^\delta = [\gamma(A + \gamma I)^{-1}]^m u_* + \gamma^{-1} \sum_{j=1}^m [\gamma(A + \gamma I)^{-1}]^j (Au_* - f^\delta).$$

For later notational convenience we use for $\gamma = \infty$ the notation $\gamma(A + \gamma I)^{-1} := I$, and then estimate (3.10) is valid also for $\gamma = \infty$.

Remarks. 1. Theorem 2 generalizes similar results for symmetric, positive semi-definite operators $A \in \mathcal{L}(\mathcal{H})$, where $\mathcal{H}$ denotes a Hilbert space, cf. Vainikko [25].

2. For Abel integral operators A as in (2.2) with $0 < \alpha < 1$, $\beta = 1$ and $a > 0$, and for the underlying space $\mathcal{H} = L^2[0, a]$ we shall give an illustration of the smoothness condition (3.7) and the corresponding convergence rates (3.8). To this end for integer $k \geq 1$ we denote by $W^{k,2}[0, a]$ the Sobolev space of all functions $u : [0, a] \to \mathbb{C}$ such that u and its distributional derivates $u^{(j)}$ of order $j \leq k$ all belong to $L^2[0, a]$. If

$$u_* \in W^{k,2}[0, a], \qquad u_*(0) = u_*'(0) = \ldots = u_*^{(k-1)}(0) = 0,$$

for some integer k with $1 \leq k \leq (m-1)\alpha$, then for $\nu = k/\alpha$ one has $u_* \in \mathcal{R}(A^\nu)$, and due to (3.8) we then can expect the following speed of convergence,

$$\|u_{\gamma\delta}^\delta - u_*\| = \mathcal{O}(\delta^{k/(k+\alpha)}) \qquad \text{as } \delta \to 0.$$

The statement (3.5) means by definition that for $m \geq 2$, Lavrentiev's m-times iterated method associated with any of the mentioned discrepancy principles yields a regularization method, respectively. For Lavrentiev's classical method, however, we have the following negative result (the proof is given in [18]):

Proposition 3. *Let $0 \neq A \in \mathcal{L}(\mathcal{H})$ be accretive, and suppose that $0 \in \sigma_{ap}(A)$. Then Discrepancy Principle 1 for Lavrentiev's classical method, this is (3.3) with $m = 1$, yields not a regularization method.*

Here, $\sigma_{ap}(A)$ denotes the approximate point spectrum of A.

Remark. It can be shown similarly that the Discrepancy Principle 2 for Lavrentiev's method also fails. Moreover, Proposition 3 shows that in the case $\{0\} \neq \mathcal{N}(A) \neq \mathcal{H}$, the Discrepancy Principle 1 for Lavrentiev's classical method fails even in the well-posed case $\mathcal{R}(A) = \overline{\mathcal{R}(A)}$.

3.2 Pseudo-Optimal Parameter Choice

It would be desirable to find parameters $\gamma_\delta > 0$ for Lavrentiev's m-times iterated method (3.3) such that an estimate of the following type is fulfilled,

$$\|u_{\gamma\delta}^\delta - u_*\| \leq K \inf_{\gamma > 0} \|u_\gamma^\delta - u_*\|,$$

with some constant K not depending on δ, u_* and f^δ. In the sequel we shall consider a parameter choice that provides a similar estimate at least for the right-hand side in the basic estimate (3.10). To this end we introduce the following notation, which is similar to that used by Leonov, see e.g. [11].

Definition 4. *Let $\mathcal{H}$ be a Hilbert space, and let $A \in \mathcal{L}(\mathcal{H})$ be accretive. A parameter choice strategy for Lavrentiev's m-times iterated method (3.3) is called pseudo-optimal, if it provides, for any $\delta > 0$ and for any u_*, $f^\delta \in \mathcal{H}$ with $\|Au_* - f^\delta\| \leq \delta$, a parameter $\gamma_\delta > 0$ such that*

$$\|[\gamma_\delta(A + \gamma_\delta I)^{-1}]^m u_*\| + \delta/\gamma_\delta \leq K \inf_{\gamma > 0} \left(\|[\gamma(A + \gamma I)^{-1}]^m u_*\| + \delta/\gamma \right), \quad (3.11)$$

with some constant K not depending on δ, u_* and f^δ.

We next introduce a modified discrepancy principle for Lavrentiev's m-times iterated method which is pseudo-optimal, cf. Theorem 5.

Discrepancy Principle 3. Fix real numbers $b_1 \geq b_0 > 1$, and let

$$B_\gamma := \gamma(A + \gamma I)^{-1}, \qquad \gamma > 0.$$

If $\|\Delta_\infty^\delta\| \leq b_1\delta$, then choose $\gamma_\delta = \infty$. Otherwise choose $\gamma_\delta > 0$ such that

$$b_0\delta \leq \|B_{\gamma_\delta}\Delta_{\gamma_\delta}^\delta\| \leq b_1\delta.$$

Here, $\Delta_\gamma^\delta \in \mathcal{H}$ again denotes the defect associated with Lavrentiev's m-times iterated method, cf. (3.4). Note that $B_\gamma\Delta_\gamma^\delta \in \mathcal{H}$ is the defect associated with the $(m+1)$-times iterated method of Lavrentiev, while the approximations $u_\gamma^\delta \in \mathcal{H}$ are generated by Lavrentiev's m-times iterated method.

The following theorem is proved in [19], and it extends analog results for symmetric operators in Hilbert spaces, cf. Raus [20]; similar results for normal equations can be found in Raus [21] and Engl & Gfrerer [8].

Theorem 5. *Let $\mathcal{H}$ be a Hilbert space, and let $A \in \mathcal{L}(\mathcal{H})$ be accretive. Then Discrepancy Principle 3 for Lavrentiev's m-times iterated method (with $m \geq 1$) is pseudo-optimal.*

4 Non-Destructive Testing of Optical-Fibre Preforms and Numerical Tests

4.1 Non-Destructive Testing of Optical-Fibre Preforms

In the sequel we consider the non-destructive testing of optical-fibre preforms, cf. Anderssen & Calligaro [1], or Calligaro, Payne, Anderssen & Ellen [4].

The properties of optical-fibre preforms can be studied in terms of the intrinsic stress components $\sigma_r(r)$, $\sigma_\theta(r)$ and $\sigma_z(r)$, $r \in [0, R]$, in the cylindrical coordinate directions r, θ and z, respectively. Here the independent variable r denotes the distance to the axis, and R denotes the radius of the preform.

In order to determine those intrinsic stress components, laser lights are sent through the optical-fibre preform in the direction normal to the axial direction, and the phase retardation $\psi(x)$, $x \in [0, R]$, of the laser beam then is measured. The required intrinsic stress components then in fact can be recovered from the phase retardation ψ. For example, the retardation ψ and the axial stress component σ_z are related via an Abel integral equation of type (2.3),

$$-\frac{4\pi C}{\lambda} \int_x^R \frac{r\sigma_z(r)}{\sqrt{r^2 - x^2}}\, dr = \psi(x), \qquad x \in [0, R], \tag{4.1}$$

where C denotes the photoelastic constant, and λ denotes the wavelength of the laser light. Moreover, the radial stress σ_r and the retardation ψ are related vice versa,

$$\sigma_r(r) = \frac{\lambda}{2C\pi^2} \cdot \frac{1}{r^2} \int_r^R \frac{x\psi(x)}{\sqrt{x^2 - r^2}} \, dx, \qquad 0 < r \le R.$$

Finally, the tangential stress σ_θ then is easily obtained, $\sigma_\theta = \sigma_z - \sigma_r$.

4.2 Numerical Experiments

In the sequel we solve numerically the classical Abel integral equation

$$(Au)(t) := \frac{1}{\sqrt{\pi}} \int_0^t (t-s)^{-1/2} u(s) \, ds = f_*(t), \qquad t \in [0,1], \qquad (4.2)$$

which (up to a scalar multiple) can be obtained from (4.1) by the substitution $f_*(t) = \psi(R\sqrt{1-t})$, $u(s) = \sigma_z(R\sqrt{1-s})$ for t, $s \in [0,1]$. In our numerical tests we use the right-hand side

$$f_*(t) = \frac{3\sqrt{\pi}}{8} t^2, \qquad t \in [0,1],$$

and then the solution of (4.2) is given by (cf. [9], Chapter 1.1)

$$u_*(s) = s^{3/2}, \qquad s \in [0,1].$$

We choose perturbed right-hand sides $f^\delta = f_* + \delta \cdot v$, where $v \in \mathcal{H} := L^2[0,1]$ has uniformly distributed random values so that $\|v\| \le 1$, and where

$$\delta = \|f_*\| \cdot \%/100,$$

with % noise $\in \{\, 0.11, \ 0.33, \ 1.00, \ 3.00, \ 10.00 \,\}$ in our implementations.

We next present the results of our experiments with Lavrentiev's m-times iterated method for

$$m = 5,$$

and as parameter choice strategy the Discrepancy Principle 2 is applied with $b = 1.5$, $\theta = 1$ and $\tau = 2$. One can show, cf. [17] and Chapter 1.1 in Gorenflo & Vessella [9], that

$$u_* \in \mathcal{R}(A^\nu), \qquad 0 < \nu < 4, \qquad (4.3)$$
$$u_* \notin \mathcal{R}(A^4), \qquad (4.4)$$

and due to (4.4) we cannot derive from Theorem 2 that the entries in the third column stay bounded as % of noise decreases. On the other hand, however, due to (4.3) it is no surprise that these entries in our experiments in fact stay bounded.

Lavrentiev's 5-times iterated method				
% noise	$\|u^\delta_{\gamma_\delta} - u_*\|$	$\|u^\delta_{\gamma_\delta} - u_*\|/\delta^{4/5}$	γ_δ	♯ flops
10.00	0.0839	1.40	1.0	0.3e+06
3.00	0.0918	4.00	0.25	0.5e+06
1.00	0.0292	3.07	0.25	0.5e+06
0.33	0.0084	2.15	0.25	0.5e+06
0.11	0.0029	1.79	0.25	0.5e+06

In Figure 3, the approximations $u^\delta_{\gamma_\delta}$ are shown for two noise levels.

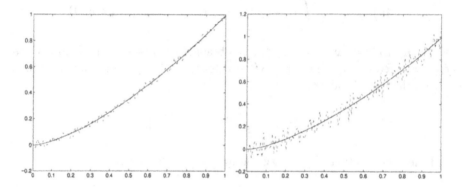

Fig. 3. Reconstruction for 1.0% perturbation (left) and 3.0% perturbation (right) of the right-hand side f_*; solid and dashed lines correspond to u_* and $u^\delta_{\gamma_\delta}$, respectively.

In our implementations, equation (4.2) has been discretized by a Bubnov-Galerkin method with piecewise constant trial functions of length $h = 1/N$, $N = 128$, and Lavrentiev's 5-times iterated method then in fact is applied to the corresponding finite system of equations. All computations are performed in MATLAB on an IBM RISC/6000.

5 Several Extensions

The most important and natural norm is the maximum norm, and therefore it is desirable to provide a theory for the numerical solution of integral equations of the first kind that allows error estimates with respect to this norm. Hence in this subsection we shall drop the assumption that the underlying space is a Hilbert space, and in the sequel $\mathcal{X}$ denotes a general complex Banach space, if not further specified. For ill-posed problems in the Banach space $\mathcal{X}$ we will present briefly some results for Lavrentiev's m-times iterated method. Finally we shall consider two stationary iterative schemes for ill-posed problems in $\mathcal{X}$.

5.1 Lavrentiev's m-Times Iterated Method in Banach Spaces

Introduction In Banach spaces X, the results about Lavrentiev's m-times iterated method presented in this paper can be generalized for those operators $A \in \mathcal{L}(X)$ that are weakly sectorial in the following sense.

Definition 6. Let X be a complex Banach space. An operator $A \in \mathcal{L}(X)$ is weakly sectorial, if $(0, \infty) \subset \rho(-A)$ and if

$$\|(A + \gamma I)^{-1}\| \leq M_0/\gamma, \qquad \gamma > 0, \tag{5.1}$$

for some $M_0 \geq 1$.

This notation is introduced in [17], and the notation is justified by the fact that a weakly sectorial operator A fulfils a resolvent condition over a small sector in the complex plane. Here and in the sequel symbols like $\mathcal{L}(X)$ or the operator norm in (5.1) have the same meaning as in Sections 1 and 2 (for Hilbert spaces).

Example 1. For $0 < \alpha < 1$, $\beta > 0$ and $a > 0$, the Abel integral operators (2.2) and (2.3) are weakly sectorial with respect to the spaces $X = C[0, a]$ and $X = L^p([0, a], s^{\beta-1}ds)$, $1 \leq p \leq \infty$, respectively, with $M_0 = 2$ in each case. For a reasoning we refer to [17].

Here, $C[0, a]$ denotes the complex space of complex-valued continuous functions on the finite interval $[0, a]$, supplied with the maximum norm $\|\cdot\|_\infty$. Moreover, for $1 \leq p < \infty$, $L^p([0, a], s^{\beta-1}ds)$ denotes the complex space of complex-valued, measurable functions u on $[0, a]$, such that $|u|^p$ is integrable with respect to the measure $s^{\beta-1}ds$, and this space is supplied with the norm

$$\|u\| := \left(\int_0^a |u(s)|^p\, s^{\beta-1}ds \right)^{1/p}, \qquad u \in L^p([0, a], s^{\beta-1}ds).$$

Similarly, $L^\infty([0, a], s^{\beta-1}ds)$ denotes the space of complex-valued, measurable functions u on $[0, a]$ which are essentially bounded with respect to the measure $s^{\beta-1}ds$, and then $\|u\|_\infty$ denotes the essential supremum of $|u|$ with respect to the measure $s^{\beta-1}ds$.

Note that the space $L^2([0, a], s^{\beta-1}ds)$ in Example 1 is already considered in Section 2, and there it is already observed that estimate (5.1) for the mentioned Abel integral operators is valid with $M_0 = 1$.

Discrepancy Principle Let X be a Banach space, let $A \in \mathcal{L}(X)$ be weakly sectorial, and let $f^\delta \in X$, $f_* \in \mathcal{R}(A)$ such that $\|f_* - f^\delta\| \leq \delta$ is satisfied. Then the statements in Theorems 2 and 5 remain valid, if in the Discrepancy Principles 1-3, respectively, the conditions "$b_1 > b_0 > 1$" and "$b > 1$" are replaced by "$b_1 > b_0 > M_0^m$", "$b > M_0^m$", and "$b_1 > b_0 > M_0^{m+1}$", respectively. The proofs are given in [16] and in [19], respectively.

Some Related Results It is possible to admit also unbounded operators in Definition 6, and in fact certain a priori parameter choices for Lavrentiev's m-times iterated method for linear weakly sectorial unbounded operators A in Banach spaces are provided in Schock & Phóng [22]. The regularizing properties of Lavrentiev's classical method and other specific regularization methods for Volterra integral equations of the first kind with smooth kernels are e.g. considered in Denisov [6] and in Srazhidinov [23], including error estimates with respect to the maximum norm.

5.2 Iterative Regularization in Banach Spaces

Introduction This subsection is devoted to the iterative solution of ill-posed problems in a Banach space $\mathcal{X}$. More specifically, we consider the discrepancy principle as a stopping rule for the Richardson iteration and an implicit iteration method, respectively, and we present associated order-optimal error estimates for those ill-posed equations $Au = f_*$ where $A \in \mathcal{L}(\mathcal{X})$ is strictly sectorial in the sense of the following Definition 7. To this end we introduce the sector $\Sigma_\theta \subset \mathbb{C}$,

$$\Sigma_\theta := \{ \, \lambda = re^{i\varphi} : r > 0, \; |\varphi| \leq \theta \, \}, \qquad \theta \in [0, \pi].$$

Definition 7. Let $\mathcal{X}$ be a complex Banach space. An operator $A \in \mathcal{L}(\mathcal{X})$ is strictly sectorial, if there is an $0 < \varepsilon \leq \pi/2$ such that $\Sigma_{\pi/2+\varepsilon} \subset \rho(-A)$ and

$$\|(A + \lambda I)^{-1}\| \leq M/|\lambda|, \qquad \lambda \in \Sigma_{\pi/2+\varepsilon},$$

for some $M \geq 1$.

This notation is introduced in [17]. If $A \in \mathcal{L}(\mathcal{X})$ is strictly sectorial, then $-A$ in fact is the infinitesimal generator of a semigroup $T(t) = e^{-tA} \in \mathcal{L}(\mathcal{X})$, $t \geq 0$, that can be extended on a sector Σ_ε (for a small $\varepsilon > 0$) to an analytical, uniformly bounded semigroup (cf. Tanabe [24], Theorem 3.3.1).

Example 2. Let $0 < \alpha < 1$, $\beta > 0$ and $a > 0$. In the spaces $\mathcal{X} = C[0, a]$ and $\mathcal{X} = L^p([0, a], s^{\beta-1}ds)$, $1 \leq p \leq \infty$, the Abel integral operators (2.2) and (2.3) are strictly sectorial, respectively, see again [17] for a reasoning.

In the sequel we suppose that $A \in \mathcal{L}(\mathcal{X})$ is an arbitrary but fixed strictly sectorial operator, where $\mathcal{X}$ denotes some Banach space. Moreover, let again $f^\delta \in \mathcal{X}$, $f_* \in \mathcal{R}(A)$ such that $\|f_* - f^\delta\| \leq \delta$ is fulfilled.

Two Stationary Iteration Methods First we consider the *Richardson iteration* which for initial vector $u_0^\delta = 0$ and $\mu > 0$ small enough generates iteratively the sequence

$$u_{n+1}^\delta = u_n^\delta - \mu(Au_n^\delta - f^\delta), \qquad n = 0, 1, 2, \dots \,.$$

The assumption that $A \in \mathcal{L}(\mathcal{X})$ is strictly sectorial implies that $I - \mu A$ is power bounded for $\mu > 0$ small enough (this follows from Nevanlinna [13], Theorem 4.5.4), and thus the stopping rule discussed below is applicable.

For fixed $\mu > 0$ we next consider the *implicit iteration method*

$$(I + \mu A)u_{n+1}^\delta = u_n^\delta + \mu f^\delta, \qquad n = 0, 1, 2, \dots,$$

for initial vector $u_0^\delta = 0$. Since $A \in \mathcal{L}(\mathcal{X})$ is strictly sectorial, $(I + \mu A)^{-1}$ is power bounded (this can be derived by standard results in semigroup theory, see e.g., Pazy [15], Theorem 1.7.7), and thus the stopping rule discussed below is applicable.

Discrepancy Principle We fix one of the considered iteration methods and denote by

$$\Delta_n^\delta := Au_n^\delta - f^\delta, \qquad n = 0, 1, 2, \dots,$$

the associated defect.

Discrepancy principle 4. For the Richardson iteration let $b > \sup_{n \geq 0} \|(I - \mu A)^n\|$, and for the implicit method let $b > \sup_{n \geq 0} \|(I + \mu A)^{-n}\|$. If $\|\Delta_0^\delta\| \leq b\delta$ then set $n_\delta = 0$. Otherwise stop the iteration after $n_\delta \geq 1$ iteration steps, if

$$\|\Delta_{n_\delta}^\delta\| \leq b\delta < \|\Delta_{n_\delta - 1}^\delta\|.$$

For a strictly sectorial $A \in \mathcal{L}(\mathcal{X})$ and the Discrepancy Principle 4 as a stopping rule for the Richardson iteration and the implicit scheme, respectively, the statements 1. and 2. in Theorem 2 are valid, if the condition "$0 < \nu \leq m - 1$" is replaced by the weaker condition "$0 < \nu < \infty$", and if moreover γ_δ is replaced (a) by n_δ in (3.5), (3.8); and (b) by n_δ^{-1} in (3.6), (3.9). For the proofs see [16].

Pseudo-Optimality For a strictly sectorial $A \in \mathcal{L}(\mathcal{X})$, the Discrepancy Principle 4 as a stopping rule for the Richardson iteration and the implicit scheme, respectively, is even pseudo-optimal in a sense similar to that of Definition 4: for the Richardson iteration we have

$$\|(I - \mu A)^{n_\delta} u_*\| + n_\delta \delta \leq K \inf_{n \geq 0} \left(\|(I - \mu A)^n u_*\| + n\delta \right), \qquad (5.2)$$

with some constant K not depending on $\delta > 0$, $u_* \in \mathcal{X}$, $f^\delta \in \mathcal{X}$ with $\|Au_* - f^\delta\| \leq \delta$. Moreover, an estimate similar to (5.2) also holds for the implicit method; in fact, $I - \mu A$ in (5.2) has to be replaced by $(I + \mu A)^{-1}$ then. The proofs are given in [19].

Concluding Remarks If the strictly sectorial $A \in \mathcal{L}(\mathcal{X})$ is a Volterra integral operator, then Lavrentiev's m-times iterated method is superior to the presented iterative methods due to the reasons mentioned in Section 1. If A is a Fredholm operator and not a Volterra operator, however, then in fact the mentioned iterative methods are more efficient than Lavrentiev's m-times iterated method, since the computation of a parameter $\gamma_\delta > 0$ in the discrepancy principles usually requires a large computational effort then.

210

Some Related Results Early results on the iterative regularization of linear ill-posed problems in Banach spaces can be found in papers by Bakushinskiĭ, see e.g., [2], [3].

Acknowledgements. The author thanks the referee for helpful comments on a first version of this paper.

References

1. **R.S. Anderssen and R.B. Calligaro.** Non-destructive testing of optical-fibre preforms. *Austral. Math. Soc. (Ser. B)*, 23:127–135, **1981**.
2. **A.B. Bakushinskiĭ.** The problem of constructing linear regularizing algorithms in Banach spaces. *U.S.S.R. Comput. Math. Math. Phys.*, 13(1):261–270, **1973**.
3. **A.B. Bakushinskiĭ.** Regularization algorithms in Banach spaces, based on the generalized discrepancy principle (in Russian). In A.C. Alekseev, editor, *Incorrect Problems in Mathematical Physics and Analysis*, pages 18–21, Novosibirsk, **1984**. Nauka.
4. **R.B. Calligaro, D.N. Payne, R.S. Anderssen, and B.A. Ellen.** Determination of stress profiles in optical-fibre preforms. *Electronics Letters*, 18(11):474–475, **1982**.
5. **A.M. Cormack.** Representation of a function by its line integrals, with some radiological applications. *J. Appl. Phys.*, 34(9):2722–2727, **1963**.
6. **A.M. Denisov.** The approximate solution of Volterra equation of the first kind associated with an inverse problem for the heat equation. *Moscow Univ. Comput. Math. Cybern.*, 15(3):57–60, **1980**.
7. **M.R. Dostanić.** Asymptotic behavior of the singular values of fractional integral operators. *J. Math. Anal. Appl.*, 175:380–391, **1993**.
8. **H.W. Engl and H. Gfrerer.** A posteriori parameter choice for general regularization methods for solving linear ill-posed problems. *Appl. Numer. Math.*, 4:395–417, **1988**.
9. **R. Gorenflo and S. Vessella.** *Abel Integral Equations.* Springer, New York, 1st edition, **1991**.
10. **G. Gripenberg, S.-O. Londen, and O. Staffans.** *Volterra and Integral Functional Equations.* Cambridge University Press, Cambridge, 1st edition, **1990**.
11. **A.S. Leonov.** On the accuracy of Tikhonov regularizing algorithms and quasioptimal selection of a regularization parameter. *Soviet Math. Dokl.*, 44(3):711–716, **1991**.
12. **F. Natterer.** Recent developments in X-ray tomography. In E.T. Todd, editor, *Tomography, impedance imaging, and integral geometry*, pages 177–198, Providence, Rhode Island, **1994**. AMS, Lect. Appl. Math. 30.
13. **O. Nevanlinna.** *Convergence of Iterations for Linear Equations.* Birkhäuser, Basel, 1st edition, **1993**.
14. **J.A. Nohel and D.F. Shea.** Frequency domain methods for Volterra equations. *Adv. Math.*, 22:278–304, **1976**.
15. **T. Pazy.** *Semigroups and Applications to Partial Differential Operators.* Springer, New York, 1st, reprint edition, **1983**.
16. **R. Plato.** The discrepancy principle for iterative and parametric methods to solve linear ill-posed equations. *Numer. Math.*, 75(1):99–120, **1996**.

17. **R. Plato**. On resolvent estimates for Abel integral operators and the regularization of associated first kind integral equations. *Submitted for publication.*

18. **R. Plato**. *Iterative and parametric methods for linear ill-posed equations.* Habilitationsschrift, Fachbereich Mathematik, TU Berlin, **1995**.

19. **R. Plato and U. Hämarik**. On the pseudo-optimality of parameter choices and stopping rules for regularization methods in Banach spaces. *Numer. Funct. Anal. Optim.*, 17(2):181–195, **1996**.

20. **T. Raus**. Residue principle for ill-posed problems (in Russian). *Acta et comment. Univers. Tartuensis*, 672:16–26, **1984**.

21. **T. Raus**. Residue principle for ill-posed problems with nonselfadjoint operators (in Russian). *Acta et comment. Univers. Tartuensis*, 715:12–20, **1985**.

22. **E. Schock and Vũ Quôc Phóng**. Regularization of ill-posed problems involving unbounded operators in Banach spaces. *Hokkaido Math. J.*, 20:559–569, **1991**.

23. **A. Srazhidinov**. Regularization of Volterra integral equations of the first kind. *Differential Equations*, 26(3):390–398, **1990**.

24. **H. Tanabe**. *Equations of Evolution.* Pitman, London, 1st edition, **1979**.

25. **G.M. Vainikko**. The discrepancy principle for a class of regularization methods. *U.S.S.R. Comput. Math. Math. Phys.*, 22(3):1–19, **1982**.

Texts and Monographs in Symbolic Computation

Alfonso Miola, Marco Temperini (eds.)

Advances in the Design of Symbolic Computation Systems

1997. 39 figures. X, 259 pages.
Soft cover DM 98,–, öS 682,–. ISBN 3-211-82844-3

Franz Winkler

Polynomial Algorithms in Computer Algebra

1996. 13 figures. VIII, 270 pages.
Soft cover DM 89,–, öS 625,–. ISBN 3-211-82759-5

Jochen Pfalzgraf, Dongming Wang (eds.)

Automated Practical Reasoning
Algebraic Approaches

With a Foreword by Jim Cunningham
1995. 23 figures. XI, 223 pages.
Soft cover DM 108,–, öS 755,–. ISBN 3-211-82600-9

Wen-tsün Wu

Mechanical Theorem Proving in Geometries
Basic Principles

Translated from the Chinese by Xiaofan Jin and Dongming Wang
1994. 120 figures. XIV, 288 pages.
Soft cover DM 98,–, öS 686,–. ISBN 3-211-82506-1

Bernd Sturmfels

Algorithms in Invariant Theory

1993. 5 figures. VII, 197 pages.
Soft cover DM 65,–, öS 455,–. ISBN 3-211-82445-6

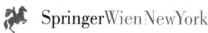 SpringerWienNewYork

Sachsenplatz 4-6, P.O.Box 89, A-1201 Wien, Fax +43-1-330 24 26, e-mail: springer@springer.co.at, Internet: http://www.springer.co.at
New York, NY 10010, 175 Fifth Avenue • Heidelberger Platz 3, D-14197 Berlin • Tokyo 113, 3-13, Hongo 3-chome, Bunkyo-ku

Advances in Computing Science

Springer-Verlag Wien New York starts a new series: "Advances in Computing Science". The title has been chosen to emphasize its scope: "computing science" comprises all aspects of science and mathematics relating to the computing process. The series will include contributions from a wide range of disciplines – numerical analysis, discrete mathematics and system theory, natural sciences, engineering, information science, electronics, and naturally, computer science itself.

Contributions in form of monographs or collections of articles dealing with advances in any aspect of the computing process, or its applications are welcome. They should be written in English, concise and theoretically sound, resulting for example from research projects, advanced workshops and conferences. The books within the series will address not only the specialist in a particular field but also the general scientific audience.

Chris Brink, Wolfram Kahl, Gunther Schmidt (eds.)

Relational Methods in Computer Science

1997. 30 figures. XV, 272 pages.
Soft cover DM 69,–, öS 485,–
ISBN 3-211-82971-7

The calculus of relations turned into an important conceptual and methodological tool in computer science. The methods presented in this book include questions of relational databases, applications to program specification, resource-conscious linear logic, semantic and refinement consideration, nonclassical logics for reasoning about programs, tabular methods in software construction, algorithm development, linguistic problems, followed by a comprehensive bibliography. The reader gets an overview of the wide-ranging applicability of relational methods in computer science.

In preparation:

Franc Solina, Walter G. Kropatsch, Reinhard Klette, Ruzena Bajcsy (eds.)

Advances in Computer Vision 1997

1997. Approx. 260 pages.
ISBN 3-211-83022-7

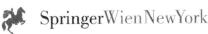
SpringerWienNewYork

Sachsenplatz 4-6, P.O.Box 89, A-1201 Wien, Fax +43-1-330 24 26, e-mail: springer@springer.co.at, Internet: http://www.springer.co.at
New York, NY 10010, 175 Fifth Avenue • Heidelberger Platz 3, D-14197 Berlin • Tokyo 113, 3-13, Hongo 3-chome, Bunkyo-ku

SpringerComputerScience

Walter Kropatsch, Reinhard Klette, Franc Solina (eds.)

in cooperation with Rudolf Albrecht

Theoretical Foundations of Computer Vision

1996. 87 figures. VII, 256 pages.
Soft cover DM 165,–, öS 1155,–
Reduced price for subscribers to "Computing":
Soft cover DM 148,50, öS 1039,50
ISBN 3-211-82730-7
Computing, Supplement 11

Hans Hagen, Gerald Farin, Hartmut Noltemeier (eds.)

in cooperation with Rudolf Albrecht

Geometric Modelling

Dagstuhl 1993

1995. 188 figures. VII, 361 pages.
Soft cover DM 180,–, öS 1260,–
Reduced price for subscribers to "Computing":
Soft cover DM 162,–, öS 1134,–
ISBN 3-211-82666-1
Computing, Supplement 10

David W. Pearson, Nigel C. Steele, Rudolf F. Albrecht (eds.)

Artificial Neural Nets and Genetic Algorithms

Proceedings of the International Conference in Alès, France, 1995

1995. 378 figures. XV, 522 pages.
Soft cover DM 218,–, öS 1525,–
ISBN 3-211-82692-0

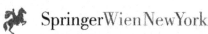

SpringerWienNewYork

Sachsenplatz 4-6, P.O.Box 89, A-1201 Wien, Fax +43-1-330 24 26, e-mail: springer@springer.co.at, Internet: http://www.springer.co.at
New York, NY 10010, 175 Fifth Avenue • Heidelberger Platz 3, D-14197 Berlin • Tokyo 113, 3-13, Hongo 3-chome, Bunkyo-ku

SpringerJournal

Surveys on Mathematics for Industry

Managing Editor: H. Engl, Linz
and an International Editorial Board

"Surveys on Mathematics for Industry" presents mathematical methods relevant for industry and exposing industrial problems which are of interest to mathematicians.

From the Contents:
C. J. Aldridge, A. C. Fowler: Stability and instability in evaporating two-phase flow • F. Bratvedt et al. : Frontline and Frontsim: two full scale, two-phase, black oil reservoir simulators based on front tracking • H. W. Engl: Regularization methods for the stable solution of inverse problems • A. D. Fitt: Mixed systems of conservation laws in industrial mathematical modelling • W. A. Green, E. R. Green, A. K. Mal: Elastic waves in the nondestructive testing of fibre composites • J. Hanson: Visualization techniques for turbulence in computational fluid dynamics • W. Kampowsky, P. Rentrop, W. Schmidt: Classification and numerical simulation of electric circuits • T.-T. Li, Y. Tan: Mathematical problems and methods in resistivity well-loggings • V. I. Mazhukin, A. A. Samarskii: Mathematical modeling in the technology of laser treatments of materials

Subscription Information:
1997. Vol. 7 (4 issues):
for institutional subscribers: DM 298,–, öS 2086,–, plus carriage charges
for individual subscribers: DM 144,–, öS 1008,–, plus carriage charges
Special rates for individual members of societies available: please contact the publisher
ISSN 0938-1953   Title No. 724
For customers in EU countries without VAT identification number
10 % VAT will be added to the subscription price

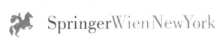
SpringerWienNewYork

Sachsenplatz 4-6, P.O.Box 89, A-1201 Wien, Fax +43-1-330 24 26, e-mail: springer@springer.co.at, Internet: http://www.springer.co.at
New York, NY 10010, 175 Fifth Avenue • Heidelberger Platz 3, D-14197 Berlin • Tokyo 113, 3-13, Hongo 3-chome, Bunkyo-ku

Springer-Verlag
and the Environment

WE AT SPRINGER-VERLAG FIRMLY BELIEVE THAT AN international science publisher has a special obligation to the environment, and our corporate policies consistently reflect this conviction.

WE ALSO EXPECT OUR BUSINESS PARTNERS – PRINTERS, paper mills, packaging manufacturers, etc. – to commit themselves to using environmentally friendly materials and production processes.

THE PAPER IN THIS BOOK IS MADE FROM NO-CHLORINE pulp and is acid free, in conformance with international standards for paper permanency.